NEUROSCIENCE RESEARCH PROGRESS

# CURRENT MANAGEMENT OF CENTRAL NERVOUS SYSTEM MENINGIOMAS

# NEUROSCIENCE RESEARCH PROGRESS

Additional books in this series can be found on Nova's website
under the Series tab.

Additional e-books in this series can be found on Nova's website
under the e-book tab.

NEUROSCIENCE RESEARCH PROGRESS

# CURRENT MANAGEMENT OF CENTRAL NERVOUS SYSTEM MENINGIOMAS

STEVEN D. CHANG
AND
ANAND VEERAVAGU
EDITORS

NOVA BIOMEDICAL

*New York*

**Library of Congress Cataloging-in-Publication Data**

ISBN: 978-1-63483-856-6

Library of Congress Control Number: 2015951297

*Published by Nova Science Publishers, Inc. † New York*

To my wonderful family who have supported me every step of the way

*Dr. Anand Veeravagu*

# Contents

# PREFACE

Meningiomas account for greater than one-third of all primary central nervous system tumors. Though in many cases they are pathologically benign, the presence and growth of such tumors in eloquent central nervous system locations may confer significant risk, potentially resulting in severe morbidity and mortality. Treatment of these tumors varies with tumor location and WHO classification. Rigorous clinical observation, surgical resection and radiation therapy are all appropriate in treating meningiomas. Given the diversity of tumor locations and pathology, it is critical for medical professionals to possess comprehensive knowledge of the diverse management of meningiomas.

This formal reference is critical in understanding the surgical approaches and treatment of meningiomas. Medical practitioners including but not limited to neurosurgeons, radiation oncologists, medical oncologists, neurologists, internal medicine physicians, as well as nurses and physician assistants alike can all benefit from this resource. This text will facilitate the understanding of meningiomas, foster learning of the most current surgical approaches, and comprehensively equip medical providers to deliver comprehensive care to patients with meningiomas.

This text provides a comprehensive and up-to-date resource for the surgical and radiosurgical management of meningiomas. It contains references to the latest peer-reviewed literature in the field and is distinctive in its focus on patient management and outcomes. With extensive clinical experience in the treatment of meningiomas, Dr. Steven Chang and Dr. Anand Veeravagu present a unique perspective and fluency in the treatment of this brain tumor.

Chapter 1 - Meningiomas are tumors that usually arise from the dural coverings of the brain or spinal cord and represent the most common extraaxial brain tumor. Although they may occur in children, their incidence increases steadily with age. Ionizing radiation exposure is a proven risk factor for the development of meningiomas. The WHO has assigned these tumors to Grade I-III of a I-IV grading scale. Most are WHO Grade I although there is great variation in their anatomical and histological appearances. In their most classic forms, meningiomas recapitulate histological features of leptomeningeal arachnoid cap cells, which in turn possess both epithelial and mesenchymal properties. These are manifested in the broad spectrum of microscopic appearances. Aggressive behavior in meningiomas can be predicted by atypical histology or several subtypes with a known propensity for local recurrence and invasive growth.

Chapter 2 - Meningiomas are the most common extra-axial brain tumors seen on radiological imaging, and one of the most common intracranial lesions in general. In this chapter, the authors will explore the role of radiology in the diagnosis and management of central nervous system (CNS) meningiomas. The authors will review the imaging appearance of meningiomas using different modalities, and explore some of the complications associated with meningiomas. Post-operative and treatment-related findings will also be reviewed.

Chapter 3 - Clival and petroclival meningiomas (PCM) are located behind the dorsum sella in the upper 2/3 of the clivus, limited on either side by the trigeminal nerve. The management of these meningiomas is exceptionally complicated because of their central, intradural location in the skull base as it is enclosed by delicate neurovascular structures and the skull base itself. As in other meningiomas, the natural history of a PCM is characterized by slow, relentless growth and invasion of surrounding structures in the majority of cases.

Despite improved resection rates and reduced mortality, debilitating cranial nerve injuries remain a notable source of morbidity and drive surgeons to seek improved treatment strategies that involved combinations of maximally safe resections and adjuvant radiosurgery. Developments in microsurgical anatomy, sparked by microsurgery and skull base surgery, have shown that not all PCM are the same. Small variations at the site of origin resulted in significant deviations in the clinical scenario and the tumor characteristics varied greatly among individual cases. Today, it is commonly accepted that the treatment of PCM must be individualized and centered on the patient's well-being. The absolute standard in PCM has yet to be reached and advances in the understanding of meningioma biology will certainly improve current results.

Chapter 4 - Cavernous sinus Meningiomas (CSM) are defined as lesions that involve the sinus, originating in the cavernous sinus or from neighboring structures. Meningioma growth within the cavernous sinus can encompass vital structures, including cranial nerves and the internal carotid arteries. This results in a tumor that cannot always be treated definitely with surgery. As the understanding of CSM has progressed, successful treatment strategies have been developed. Gross total resection is achieved in a minority of patients as the degree of resection is dictated by the consistency, vascularity and anatomical extent of the tumor. Additionally, radiosurgical methods have been utilized in the treatment of CSM with significant success. Nevertheless, there is currently no consensus treatment paradigm for CSM. Small CSM with minimal mass effects are usually treated with primary radiosurgery. Encouraged by the satisfactory results of radiosurgery in small CSM, newer treatment strategies for larger CSM with significant mass effects combine maximal resection of the extra-cavernous portion with postoperative radiosurgery. Despite these advancements in CSM management, further quality evidence from prospective randomized controlled studies is among several other factors that are needed to help determine and establish optimal treatment strategies.

Chapter 5 - Olfactory groove meningiomas (OGMs) and planum sphenoid meningiomas (PSMs) comprise a significant subset of meningiomas. They encompass the anterior skull base, from the rostral-most portion of the cribriform plate to the posterior aspect of the planum sphenoidale. These lesions present insidiously and are often quite large when discovered. Because of their unique location on the anterior skull base, they can be surgically addressed through multiple access points. From above, smaller or more lateralized lesions may be approached through a unilateral frontal, pterional, or fronto-orbital craniotomy. Larger lesions may be approached through a bifrontal approach, with or without a subcranial component. From below, they can be resected through an expanded endonasal approach. This chapter will discuss OGMs and PSMs with respect to topics such as the removal of these tumors by reviewing their anatomy, some technical and clinical pearls with case presentations, and the associated literature and looking into the future directions of addressing these lesions.

Chapter 6 - Meningiomas arising from the region of the sphenoid wing comprise a significant portion of intracranial and skull base meningiomas and present a diverse array of clinical challenges. These tumors can either be focal (globoid) or diffuse (en plaque) in morphology and present a variety of distinct clinical concerns and surgical challenges depending on the location of the tumor along the sphenoid wing. Clinical presentation is variable but visual symptoms are a prominent concern and a frequent driver of clinical decision-making in the management of these tumors. Surgical resection is the most effective treatment of these lesions and a clear understanding of the relevant surgical anatomy of the sphenoid wing is necessary to minimize surgical morbidity. The frontotemporal craniotomy in combination with an interfascial extracranial dissection technique provides excellent surgical exposure for the resection of most sphenoid wing meningiomas. Lateral sphenoid wing meningiomas are the most readily accessible, but can present challenges related to extracranial tumor invasion or with involvement of the sylvian fissure. Medial or clinoidal tumors are generally more challenging to resect, given their location deep on the sphenoid wing and close association with the optic nerve and the internal carotid artery.

The anterior clinoidectomy, via either extradural or intradural approach, is an essential step in safely resecting many of these tumors. En plaque, or spheno-orbital, meningiomas are a unique entity given their diffuse nature, tendency to induce a marked hyperostostic reaction, and frequent extension into the orbit. Resection of spheno-orbital meningiomas can be difficult due to the extent of bony resection often required as well as the management of reconstruction following resection. Radiosurgery can be an important adjuvant treatment modality for these tumors when complete resection is not possible or would result in excessive morbidity.

Surgical outcomes for resection of sphenoid wing meningiomas are historically poor, but have improved markedly in recent years with improvement in skull base dissection techniques.

Chapter 7 - Meningiomas that originate from the petrous bone are amongst the most challenging lesions that a neurosurgeon may encounter. The surgical decision-making process is difficult and must be approached on a case-by-case basis. Mass effects causing cranial neuropathies, hydrocephalus, or brainstem compression indicate surgical resection due to resulting stigmata such as ataxia, spastic paresis, or somatosensory findings. The tumor's rostral and caudal extension, dural attachment, relation to the internal acoustic canal and size, and the patient's hearing status must all be considered when choosing a surgical approach to achieve maximal safe resection. Stereotactic radiosurgery should be reserved for adjuvant therapy in the cases of residual tumors that demonstrate signs of recurrence or growth as well as for patients who are poor surgical candidates.

Chapter 8 - Cerebellopontine angle (CPA) meningiomas comprise about one percent of all intracranial meningiomas; however, they are the second most common tumor found within the CPA, after vestibular schwannomas. CPA meningiomas commonly present with unilateral hearing loss, tinnitus, ataxia, and diminished facial sensation. Although there is a role for stereotactic radiosurgery, surgery remains the treatment of choice for CPA meningiomas. A detailed understanding of CPA surgical anatomy and operative approaches is critical in preventing severe neurosurgical morbidity.

Chapter 9 - Spinal meningiomas comprise 7.5-15% of all meningiomas and often present between the fifth and seventh decade of life. Presenting symptoms and the neurologic deficits suffered by patients with these tumors are dictated by the anatomic location of the tumor. Surgical resection has been demonstrated to be a safe and effective treatment modality for spinal meningiomas. These lesions are technically challenging to the micro-neurosurgeon, with delicate vasculature and spinal nervous elements in close approximation to tumor tissue. A complete resection has the potential to be curative, with most patients having significant improvement in function. This chapter aims to discuss the epidemiology and histopathology, followed by an in depth discussion of the operative technique.

Chapter 10 - Foramen magnum meningiomas (FMM) are insidious tumors that pose marked challenges to the skull base neurosurgeon. The indolent clinical course of FMM and the gradual onset of symptoms contribute to its delayed diagnosis and relatively large size at presentation. Symptoms are often produced by the compression of surrounding structures (such as the upper cervical spinal cord, lower cranial nerves, and vertebral artery) within a critically confined space. Several surgical approaches have been offered to achieve complete tumor resection. The authors provide an overview of key clinical considerations in the management of patients with FMM and detail important surgical approaches to these lesions.

Chapter 11 - Convexity meningiomas are a benign neoplasm of mesenchymal origin. These tumors account for 15% of all intracranial meningiomas. Most of these tumors are discovered incidentally and patients tend to be asymptomatic at detection. Patients with small, asymptomatic tumors can be monitored with surveillance imaging and strict attention to the onset of new neurological symptoms. Additionally, patients that undergo surgical resection demonstrate favorable outcomes including robust overall survival and low rates of disease recurrence. Surgical intervention for convexity meningioma carries a low morbidity and mortality risk. In this chapter the authors detail the management of patients with convexity meningiomas and discuss the current literature.

Chapter 12 - Tuberculum sellae (TS) and Diaphragma sellae (DS) meningiomas account for 5-10% of all intracranial meningiomas. They usually present with slowly progressive symptoms over several months. Many meningiomas have low proliferative rates and are indolent. However, suprasellar tumors have the risk of causing permanent neurological deficits and are thus often treated surgically. The central skull base location of suprasellar meningiomas and their proximity to critical neurovascular structures pose challenges to treatment. Understanding the bony anatomy of the anterior cranial fossa and the sellar region is critical for treating suprasellar meningiomas. In this chapter the authors will discuss the surgical options, techniques, and indications.

Chapter 13 - Meningiomas are common intracranial tumors in the adult population. The management of intracranial meningiomas depends on specific patient factors and tumor characteristics. When treatment is deemed necessary, surgical resection remains the primary intervention, with gross total resection (GTR) representing the gold standard. When GTR cannot be safely achieved without a significant risk of neurological compromise, residual tumor can be treated with fractionated radiation therapy or stereotactic radiosurgery (SRS) depending on the location and volume of residual disease. The contemporary therapeutic landscape has paved way for SRS as an integral therapeutic modality for patients with meningioma.

SRS was initially confined to the setting of recurrent or residual skull base meningiomas. With broadened experience and progressively successful outcomes for these types of meningiomas, the indications for SRS have gradually expanded to include parasagittal, parafalcine, and convexity meningiomas. SRS can also serve as an upfront treatment for patients presenting with clinical and radiographic features consistent with a benign (WHO grade I) meningioma. SRS has enjoyed particular efficacy as a primary or adjunctive treatment for grade I meningiomas, primarily those tumors located at the skull base, where the operative morbidity is particularly high with aggressive resection.

The majority of contemporary SRS series of patients with WHO grade I meningiomas report tumor control rates in excess of 85%. The role of SRS for WHO grade II and III meningiomas remains less established, with relatively sparse literature describing radiosurgical outcomes for these uncommon, aggressive tumors. Nevertheless, nascent reports suggest that SRS may play an important role in the management of residual or recurrent grade II and III meningiomas. Future studies will hopefully further delineate this role.

As with any modern surgical technique, potential benefits are not devoid of complications. While complications can occur, neurological function is generally preserved. Longitudinal follow-up including neurologic and radiologic assessment is required for an effective radiosurgical therapeutic regimen. Single and multisession stereotactic radiosurgery will likely play an expanding role in the treatment of patients with meningiomas going forward.

Chapter 14 - Meningiomas are often highly vascularized benign tumors that harbor a dural based arterial blood supply. Such vascular characteristics in addition to the pathoanatomical growth of meningiomas have shaped the evolution of various endovascular approaches to meningioma treatment. Skull base locations and involvement of the dural venous sinus, particularly, can present significant surgical challenges. The purpose of this chapter is to review endovascular treatment options, with a particular focus on preoperative embolization, when used as an adjunct to surgical resection in the treatment of meningiomas.

# ACKNOWLEDGMENT

The authors would like to thank Tej Azad, who served as this work's sub-editor, for his tireless efforts in coordinating the publication of this book. Tej edited, organized, and contributed to nearly every chapter. Without his dedication and commitment, this volume would not be possible.

In: Current Management of Central Nervous System … ISBN: 978-1-63483-856-6
Editors: Steven D. Chang and Anand Veeravagu 

*Chapter 1*

# BIOLOGY AND PATHOLOGY OF MENINGIOMAS

***Hannes Vogel, MD***
Department of Pathology, Stanford University
School of Medicine, Stanford, CA, US

## ABSTRACT

Meningiomas are tumors that usually arise from the dural coverings of the brain or spinal cord and represent the most common extraaxial brain tumor. Although they may occur in children, their incidence increases steadily with age. Ionizing radiation exposure is a proven risk factor for the development of meningiomas. The WHO has assigned these tumors to Grade I-III of a I-IV grading scale. Most are WHO Grade I although there is great variation in their anatomical and histological appearances. In their most classic forms, meningiomas recapitulate histological features of leptomeningeal arachnoid cap cells, which in turn possess both epithelial and mesenchymal properties. These are manifested in the broad spectrum of microscopic appearances. Aggressive behavior in meningiomas can be predicted by atypical histology or several subtypes with a known propensity for local recurrence and invasive growth.

## INTRODUCTION

Most meningiomas display easily recognizable diagnostic clinical, radiological, and pathological features. However, the broad diversity of patient demographics and locations and histological subtypes of meningiomas may occasionally present a diagnostic challenge, especially in distinguishing meningiomas from their radiographic and pathological mimics and determining those with either a tendency toward indolent growth versus others that carry the risk of recurrence. The challenge is in recognizing unifying features while distinguishing biological and pathological properties that may provide the basis for a specific therapy and prognosis.

JJ Kepes articulated the dual epithelial and mesenchymal properties of meningeal arachnoid cap cells, the benign counterparts of meningiomas, as a nearly unique feature of these cells, shared only by mesothelial or synovial cells [1]. Another intrinsic attribute of meningeal cells is their avid tendency to form whorls, even in cell culture. Meningeal cells form tight intercellular associations with complex interdigitations and desmosomes, which predict the syncytial appearance of virtually all meningiomas, whereby cell borders are unapparent by light microscopy.

## CLINICAL FEATURES

Meningiomas are defined as meningeal tumors arising from meningothelial arachnoid cap cells, typically arising at the inner surface of the dura mater. Meningiomas account for approximately 30% of all primary brain tumors and are thus the single most common "brain" tumor, excluding glioblastoma as the most common glioma, in persons over the age of 35 [2]. In middle aged adults, meningiomas are distinctly more common in females [3]. Spinal meningiomas are also far more common in women [4], accounting for almost 90% in some series among older patients [5]. Multiple meningiomas are a cardinal feature of neurofibromatosis 2 (NF2) and occur in half of NF2 patients [6].

Meningiomas are also recognized in childhood and represent the most common dural or leptomeningeal-based neoplasm in this age group. Pediatric meningiomas may be characterized by large size at diagnosis, cyst formation, intra-parenchymal location and high-grade histology, and aggressive behavior, particularly in the clear cell and papillary variants [7, 8]. Unlike in adults, there is a male predilection in pediatric meningiomas. Pediatric meningiomas also exist within the spectrum of post-irradiation tumors.

The vast majority of meningiomas arise in obvious association with the dura in intracranial, intraspinal, or orbital locations. Favored locations over the cerebral convexities include parafalcine, the lateral sulcus, and, at the base of the brain, the orbital cortex, sphenoid ridge, posterior clinoid process, and sigmoid sulcus. Common locations in association with the brainstem include the cerebellopontine angle and foramen magnum. Most spinal meningiomas are in the thoracic region. Intraventricular meningiomas may also occur, arising in the tela choroidea at the base of cerebrospinal fluid-producing choroid plexus. Meningiomas have also been a reported in non-neural tissue such as the lung [9-11] and temporal bone [12-14].

## GENETICS

The most common cytogenetic abnormality in meningiomas is loss of chromosome 22, especially of the long arm (22q). The loss includes the region of 22q12 that contains the NF2 gene, which encodes the protein merlin. Predictably, meningiomas are commonly associated with NF2 due to germline mutations [15]. Forty percent of pediatric patients with meningioma have NF2 [7], in which meningiomas may be the presenting manifestation. Among the sporadic meningiomas, 50% to 60% contain NF2 mutations [16, 17], most of which are predicted to result in absence of functional merlin protein.

Atypical higher grade meningiomas and earlier age of onset [6] are more often associated with NF2 mutations, loss of chromosome 22, or other chromosomal abnormalities [18]. Studies suggest that meningiomas associated with NF2 have a higher mitotic index and more aggressive behavior than sporadic meningiomas [19, 20].

NF2 mutations and chromosome 22 losses are less frequent in radiation-induced meningiomas in which 1p and 7p abnormalities are more common by comparison, suggesting different pathways in radiation tumorigenesis [21]. When NF2 mutations are not present, mutations of the SMARCB1 gene have been found in some sporadic meningiomas [22], and in patients with schwannomatosis and multiple meningiomas [23]. TNF-receptor associated factor 7 (*TRAF7)* mutations, either isolated or in association with *AKT1* and *SMO*, were found in 24% of all meningiomas and are apparently exclusive of *NF2* mutations. Mutations in *TRAF7* appear to signify a subset of meningiomas with a lower histologic grade [24].

There is an association between genetic abnormality in meningiomas and both location and tumor subtype. *NF2/chromosome 22 loss*-associated meningiomas are predisposed to locations in the lateral and posterior skull base, whereas the majority of anterior and medial meningiomas are non-NF2 mutant [18]. *SMARCB1*-mutated meningiomas arise predominantly at the falx cerebri [25]. *AKT1-MTOR*, AKT1- and SMO-mutated tumors are located at the skull base [26].

WHO Grade I meningiomas that are NF2-altered are predominantly of the fibroblastic, transitional, or psammomatous histological subtypes [16, 27], whereas NF2 mutations are rarely associated with meningothelial, secretory, and microcystic forms [27, 28].

Combined KLF4, K409Q, and TRAF7 mutations are always associated with the secretory meningioma subtype [29]. SMARCE1 mutations are a cause of clear cell meningiomas, which are WHO Grade II and thus graded atypical, in both spinal and cranial locations [30]. The meningothelial subtype is predominant among meningiomas with mutated *SMO* [26].

## ETIOLOGIES

Meningiomas derive from exposure to ionizing radiation, either therapeutic low, medium or high dosage, or environmental such as in survivors of nuclear bomb explosion. Children are more vulnerable to radiation-induced meningiomas, the best example of which was the development of multiple meningiomas in individuals who underwent low-dose radiation therapy for scalp tinea capitus [31].

The consensus from reports of radiation-induced meningiomas is that they typically present at an earlier age, arise within the prior irradiation field, and are more likely to be multifocal [32]. Average latencies for low-, medium-, and high-dose exposures are 35, 26, and 19.5 years, respectively [33].

A number of dated reports from as early as 1888 make an association between trauma and meningiomas. Cushing and Eisenhardt noted in 1938 that 101 of their 313 patients with meningiomas had a history of head trauma. Association with foreign bodies, prior surgery, and cranioplasty has also been implicated, though a causal relationship has not been formally established in any instance [34].

**Table 1. Molecular genetic abnormalities associated with WHO Grades I-III meningiomas**

| WHO Grade | I | II | III |
|---|---|---|---|
| Chromosomal abnormalities | 22q loss (50%-60%)<br>9p losses (5%) | 1p loss<br>6q loss<br>9p losses (18%)<br>10 loss<br>14q loss<br>18q loss<br>1q, 9q, 12q, 15q, 17q, 20q gains | 1p loss<br>6q loss<br>9p losses (38%)<br>9p21 (p16/p15 *CDKN2A/B, p14 ARF*) loss<br>10 loss<br>14q loss<br>17q23 amplification<br>18q loss |
| Gene expression | NF2 mutations (50%–60%)<br>EGFR activation<br>PDGFRB activation | Telomerase/hTERT activation<br>Notch/Wnt, IGF, VEGF activation<br>Phosphorylated AKT increase<br>SUFU alterations at 10q24 | NDRG2 hypermethylation<br>Phosphorylated AKT increase<br>SUFU alterations at 10q24 |
| Protein expression | PR gain<br>YAP overexpression and nuclear localization<br>Merlin loss (50%)<br>4.1B (DAL-1) loss (50%)<br>TSLC-1 loss (30-85%) | PR loss<br>TSLC1 loss | PR loss<br>TSLC1 loss |

Abbreviations: NF2 - neurofibromatosis type 2; YAP - Yes-associated protein; CDKN2A/B - Cyclin-Dependent Kinase Inhibitor 2A/B; EGFR – epidermal growth factor receptor; PDGFRB - Platelet-derived growth factor receptor beta; hTERT – human telomerase reverse transcriptase; IGF - Insulin-like growth factor; VEGF - vascular endothelial growth factor; AKT - protein kinase B; TSLC1 - Tumor suppressor in lung cancer 1; SUFU - Suppressor Of Fused Homolog (Drosophila); NDRG2 - NMYC downstream-regulated gene 2.

## Prognostic Factors

The key issue in the prognosis of meningiomas is the risk of recurrence, which is closely tied to histological grading, atypical forms, and fatal outcome associated with malignancy. Even benign meningiomas have a 5% recurrence rate by 5 years after gross total resection (GTR), with a marked increase to approximately 30% to 40% over 5 years if only a subtotal resection is achieved. Atypical meningiomas predictably recur even if GTR is achieved [35].

## Gross Pathology

The gross pathology of meningiomas reflects their typically discrete lobulated appearance in association with inner surface of the dura. A well-demarcated surface separating the tumor from underlying brain is often observed.

An *en plaque* variant, usually found over the sphenoid wing, is a flattened mass without formation of the usual globular mass, and is typically associated with hyperostosis of bone.

The external surface of most meningiomas is cobblestoned or bosselated and may be appreciated in cut section as well. Fibrous meningiomas are exceptionally smooth and well demarcated. Psammomatous meningiomas are gritty and may require decalcification for success in producing histological sections. Lipidic or xanthomatous change may be signified by a yellow-orange color. Microcystic meningiomas have a glistening mucoid cut surface. Osseous or cartilaginous metaplasia may display a white cut surface. Necrosis is unusual except in cases of preoperative embolization of the tumor. A necrotic meningioma without a history of embolization may signify an atypical or malignant example.

Gross invasion of leptomeninges and even cranial bone and extracranial soft tissue may occur in low-grade meningiomas. Benign meningiomas may even manifest as a scalp mass as the result of invasion through skull and overlying soft tissue. Frank brain invasion would usually result in adherence between the meningioma and the surface of the brain. Meningiomas may contain macrocysts in 2% to 4% of cases.

Examining neuropathologists should strive to identify any brain tissue in association with the resected tumor. Large specimens are traditionally sampled with one section per centimeter as the largest dimension. Since meningiomas may be histologically heterogeneous, if the initial pathological review discloses borderline atypia or malignancy, the entire specimen should be fully submitted for microscopic examination.

An unusual form of meningothelial cell proliferation is represented by meningioangiomatosis, a lesion of presumed hamartomatous origin that is commonly associated with seizures and a male predominance. It occasionally occurs combined with meningioma [36]. It is radiographically and grossly recognized as a plaque-like firm cerebral mass, most often involving the temporal and frontal lobes.

## Microscopic Pathology

Meningiomas often display heterogeneous histological patterns, both in forms of differentiation described below and in degrees of proliferation. Furthermore, certain combinations are well-recognized, such as angiomatous and microcystic differentiation.

It is generally required that if a histological subtype is to be named, that the tumor be represented by at least 50% of that form of differentiation. This is important, for example, when rhabdoid differentiation occurs; less than 50% rhabdoid histology would not suffice to render a final diagnosis of rhabdoid meningioma, WHO Grade III, and if other atypical or malignant features were lacking, the tumor would remain at WHO Grade I in spite of rhabdoid elements. The same rule applies to other grade-determining histological types such as chordoid, clear cell, and papillary.

The *differential diagnosis* of meningiomas includes the radiologically indistinguishable solitary fibrous tumor/hemangiopericytoma (SFT/HPC), which is usually recognized by the absence of usual meningothelial features and the presence of sheets of epithelioid cells in a variably collagen-rich matrix, with branching “staghorn” vessels. SFT/HPC is now definitively diagnosed by immunohistochemical identification of STAT6-positive tumor nuclei and would be epithelial membrane antigen (EMA)-immunonegative.

**Table 2. WHO 2007 criteria for grading meningiomas**

| Grade | Criteria |
|---|---|
| Grade I | Meningothelial, fibrous (fibroblastic), transitional (mixed), psammomatous, angiomatous, microcystic, secretory, lymphoplasmacyte-rich, metaplastic types |
| Grade II | Chordoid and clear cell types<br>Atypical: mitotic count of 4-19/400X hpf; brain invasion; three of the following: hypercellularity, sheet-like or patternless, spontaneous necrosis, macronucleoli (easily identified at 100X), small cell formation |
| Grade III | Papillary and rhabdoid types<br>Malignant histology resembling carcinoma, melanoma, or high-grade sarcoma; mitotic count $\geq$20/400X hpf |

Abbreviations: hpf - high-powered fields.

Metastatic carcinomas may also mimic meningiomas or on rare occasions be present within a preexisting meningioma. Fibrous meningiomas may bear resemblance to schwannomas, which unlike meningiomas are EMA-immunonegative and diffusely S100-positive. Extranodal marginal cell lymphoma may also present as a meningeal mass.

# WHO Grade I

## Meningothelial

This is the most common and classic variant of meningioma. Cells form lobules or swirling fascicles or nests of cells in a syncytial background, in which cell borders cannot be discerned, but rather the background exists as a delicate interwoven web of cellular processes. Whorls of varying size are usually identifiable, and may be of particular diagnostic utility during intraoperative consultation by performing a cytological touch or imprint preparation (Figure 1); whorls are essentially diagnostic of meningioma in the context of evaluating a mass with typical radiographic and gross features of a meningioma. This histological subtype shows the classic nuclear features of meningiomas, which may be seen in other types as well, namely ovoid nuclei with optically empty nuclear pseudoinclusions (Figure 2). The previous term for this histology was "syncytial meningioma." Nuclear atypia in the form of enlargement, multinucleation, or pleomorphism may be equated with ancient or degenerative change.

## Fibrous (Fibroblastic)

The fibrous meningioma shows broad fascicles of elongated spindle cells with variable amounts of intercellular collagen deposition (Figure 3). Classical whorls may be inconspicuous. Mineralization of the collagen bands may be present. Psammoma bodies are rare. Immunohistochemical staining for EMA may be weak. These tumors may be difficult to distinguish from schwannomas, which unlike meningiomas, would be uniformly S100-immunopositive and not contain psammoma bodies and solitary fibrous tumors that would demonstrate nuclear STAT6 immunopositivity.

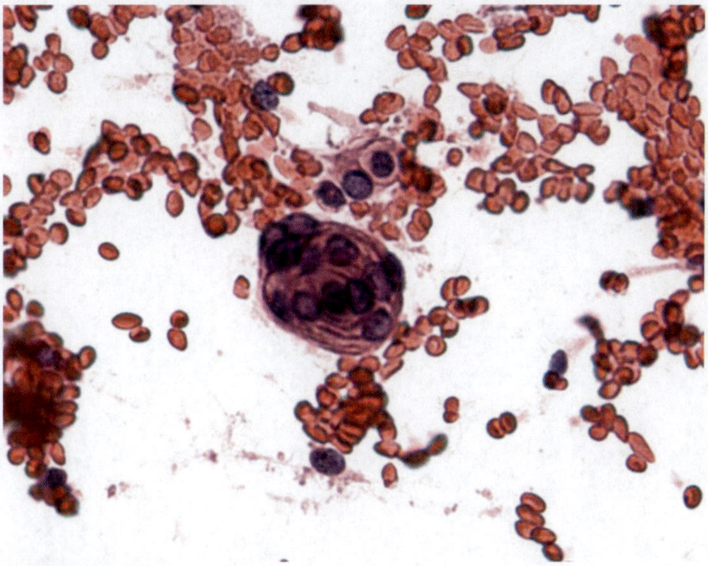

Hematoxylin and eosin – H and E.

Figure 1. Cytological imprint preparation of a meningothelial meningioma demonstrating a tightly cohesive whorl of meningothelial cells. Such a finding during intraoperative consultation is essentially diagnostic of meningioma but may be absent in several subtypes.

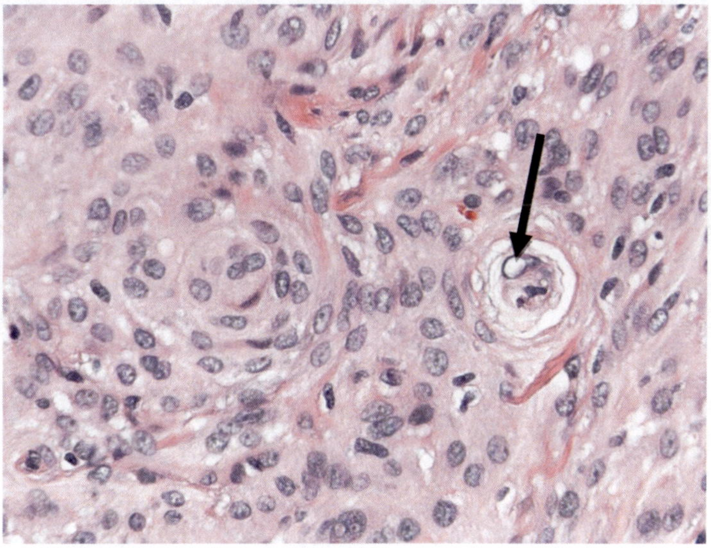

Note the intranuclear clear inclusion (arrow) (H and E).

Figure 2. Classic microscopic appearance of meningothelial meningioma, with whorls of cells in a syncytial background.

## Transitional (Mixed)

The transitional meningioma combines mixed elements of different subtypes, most commonly the meningothelial and fibrous types. Whorls and psammoma bodies may be readily found.

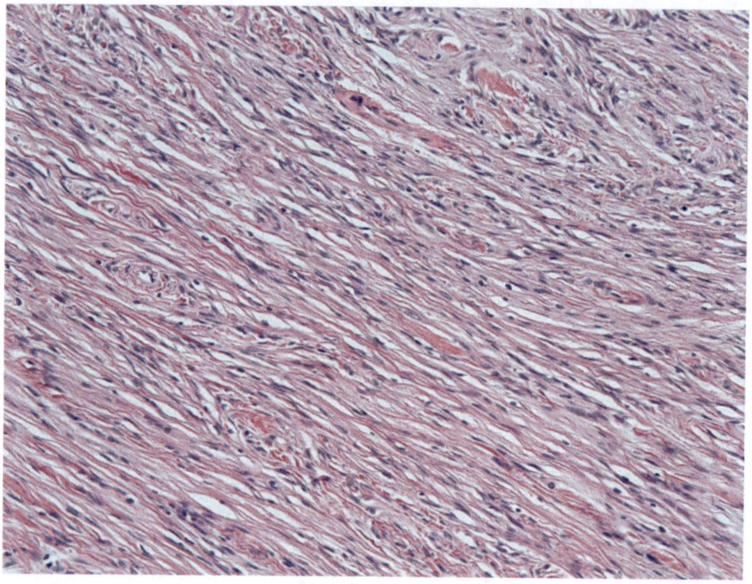

Figure 3. Fibrous meningioma, lacking whorls and resembling other spindle cell tumors such as schwannomas or solitary fibrous tumor.

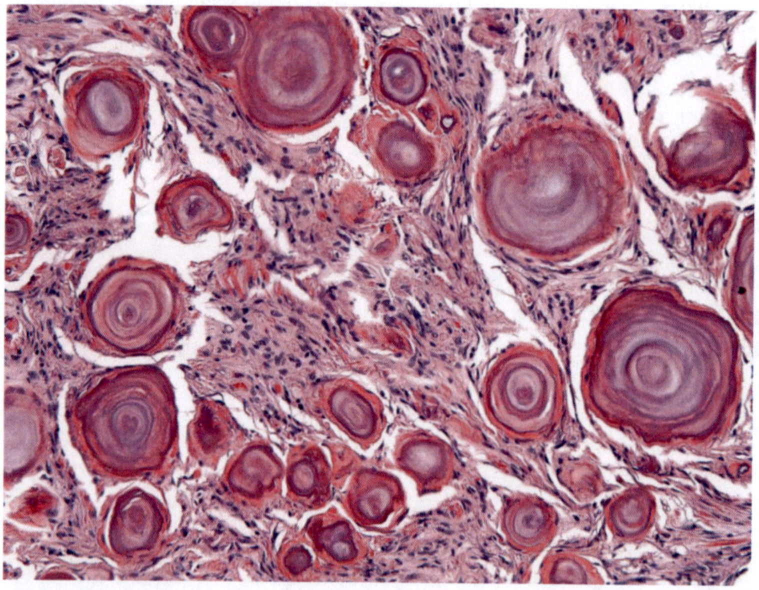

Figure 4. Psammomatous meningioma, with numerous psammoma bodies, which sometimes may completely obscure the intervening tumor cells.

## Psammomatous

The psammomatous meningioma shows innumerable and often back-to-back psammoma bodies (Figure 4), defined as concentric laminated calcified structures, which may allow the identification of calcification in radiographic studies. The density of psammomatous meningiomas for these structures may even obscure recognition of the meningothelial cells.

Widespread calcification may evolve into frank osseous metaplasia. These may be more common among intraspinal meningiomas in older females and in the olfactory grooves.

## Angiomatous

These meningiomas contain conspicuous vascular elements, often dominated by ectatic small- or medium-sized blood vessels and with frequent hyaline change (Figure 5). Significant degenerative nuclear atypia is often present. Features of microcystic meningioma are frequently coexistent in these tumors.

## Microcystic

The microcystic meningioma displays mucin-containing microcysts of varying sizes. There are vacuolated cells and sometimes xanthomatous cells with scattered pleomorphic nuclei and hyalinized blood vessels. Whorls and psammoma bodies are typically scarce although careful microscopic scrutiny of the entire specimen will sometimes reveal small foci of ordinary meningothelial meningioma.

## Secretory

The secretory meningioma more closely resembles the meningothelial or transitional types but contains the distinctive feature of discrete eosinophilic and strongly PAS-positive cytoplasmic inclusions (Figure 6) that are typically strongly immunopositive for epithelial membrane antigen and carcinoembryonic antigen (CEA).

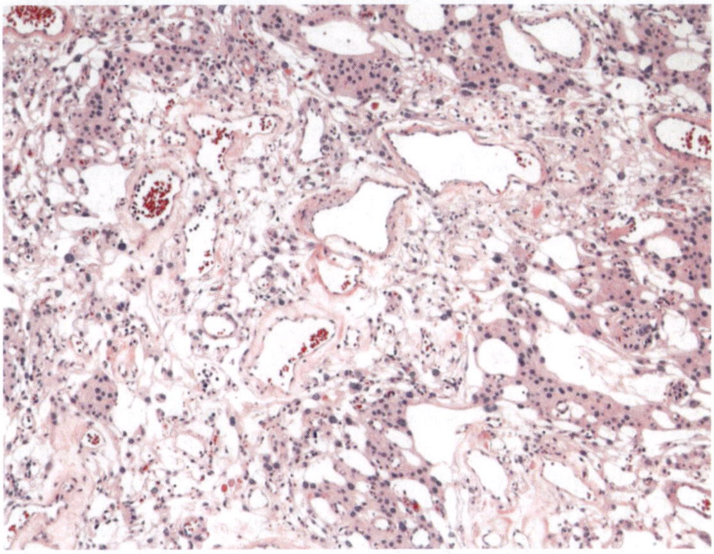

Figure 5. Angiomatous meningioma lacking usual meningothelial differentiation, with prominent and ectatic blood vessels and clear cells as seen in microcystic meningioma.

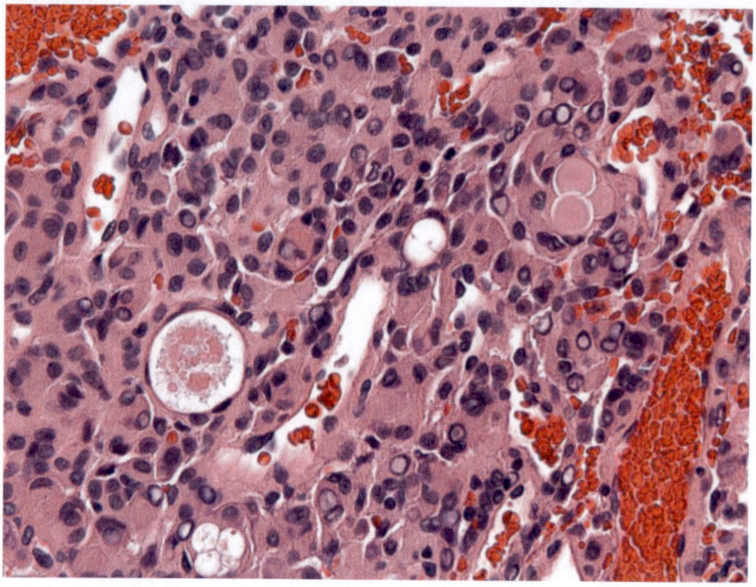

Figure 6. Secretory meningioma with intracytoplasmic round lumina containing eosinophilic material.

At the ultrastructural level these intracytoplasmic inclusions are seen to be microvilli-lined spaces with proteinaceous contents. There may also be an increase in mast cells and histiocytic elements. The secretory meningioma, along with angiomatous and microcystic variants, may be accompanied by significant edema in subjacent brain.

## Lymphoplasmacyte-Rich

These controversial tumors may show massive infiltration by lymphocytes and plasma cells, often with Russell bodies. The lymphocytic infiltrate may be so extensive as to obscure the underlying meningothelial proliferation, but should comprise at least half of the population of cells in the tumor.

Immunohistochemistry for EMA may be of limited usefulness since plasma cells are also EMA-immunopositive. These lesions should always prompt consideration of other primary inflammatory processes such as Rosai-Dorfman disease, plasma cell granuloma, or inflammatory myofibroblastic tumor, involvement by low-grade lymphoma, or a chronic infection.

## Metaplastic

Metaplastic meningiomas are recognized by the WHO as those with widespread mesenchymal components that may include bony, cartilaginous, lipomatous, myxoid, or xanthomatous changes, individually or in combination.

Other types include oncocytic, sclerosing, and mucinous meningioma, which are not formally recognized by the WHO and therefore have not been assigned a grade, however reports do not suggest aggressive behavior in these subtypes.

## MENINGOANGIOMATOSIS

The microscopic pathology includes a wide spectrum of changes, but the essential features are intracortical and leptomeningeal collections of small blood vessels with perivascular spindle cells, and varying degrees of gliosis, hyalinization, and calcification. Entrapped neurons may show unusual changes, including granulovacuolar degeneration and neurofibrillary tangles [36].

## WHO GRADE II

### Atypical Meningiomas

Meningiomas with Grade I morphological features may nonetheless be assigned a WHO Grade of II if certain histologic features are noted either singly or in combination, based on a large case series originating at the Mayo Clinic [37]. Such meningiomas have a 40% 5-year recurrence rate compared with 5% for Grade I meningiomas. The clear cell and chordoid meningiomas are also assigned a WHO Grade of II, as described below. Otherwise, a mitotic count of 4 to 20 mitotic figures per 10 high-powered fields (hpf) is diagnostic of atypical WHO Grade II meningioma. The method in counting the mitotic figures should involve finding the 10 consecutive hpf in regions of the tumor with the highest density of mitotic figures.

Brain invasion is also diagnostic of WHO Grade II meningioma. This determination may be difficult since meningiomas may push into the surface of the brain in the form of knuckles of tumor nodules without true disruption of the pial layer. This determination may be aided by the use of GFAP immunohistochemistry, demonstrating entrapment of GFAP-positive brain tissue between the infiltrating meningioma (Figure 7a and b).

The presence of at least three of the following five histological features will also suffice to diagnose atypical WHO Grade II meningioma: sheeting architecture in which characteristic whorls are not present, hypercellularity defined as 53 nuclei or more spanning an hpf, macronucleoli defined as nucleoli recognizable at 100X magnification, and small cell formation, defined as clusters of small cells resembling lymphocytes, and spontaneous necrosis not attributable to iatrogenic embolization [37].

### Chordoid

These are typically large, supratentorial tumors with an increased rate of recurrence. An infrequent association with Castleman disease has been cited [38]. Chordoid meningiomas show ribbons or trabeculae of cells, often vacuolated, in an abundant mucoid matrix background (Figure 8). Careful inspection of these lesions may focally show more typical meningothelial elements. Mononuclear inflammatory cell infiltrates may be focally prominent. Immunohistochemistry for epithelial membrane antigen may be used to distinguish these from actual chordomas, which are typically EMA-negative and diffusely S100-immunopositive.

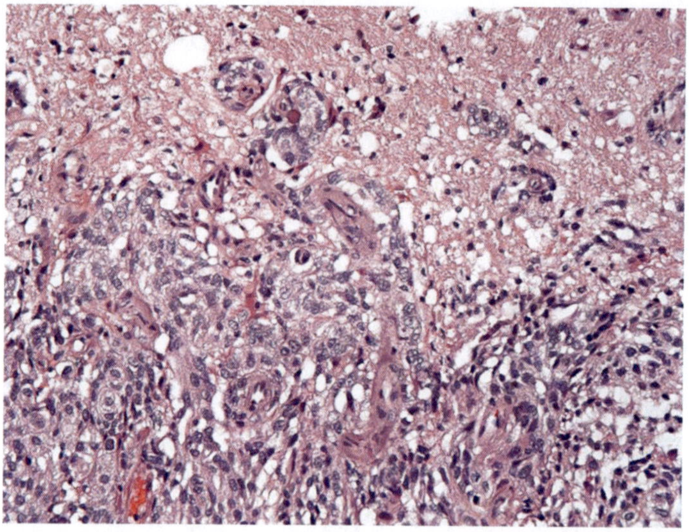

a

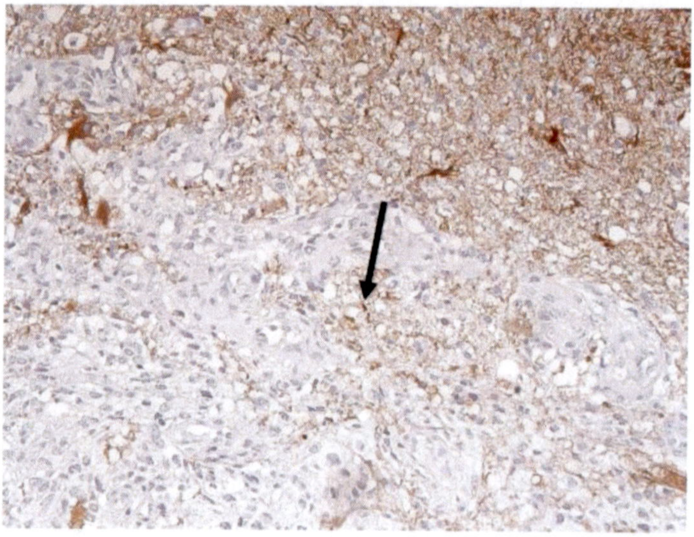

b

Figure 7. a. Brain invasion by meningioma. Brain tissue in the upper field is penetrated by protrusions of meningioma cells. b. Diagnostic value of GFAP immunohistochemistry in documenting invasive meningioma resulting in entrapment of GFAP-positive brain tissue (arrow).

## Clear Cell

The clear cell meningioma is more common at the cerebellopontine angle and cauda equina. It has been reported more frequently in pediatric and young adult patients. Because of a tendency for aggressive behavior and occasional CSF dissemination, this tumor is assigned to WHO Grade II. Histologically, this type of meningioma may be especially difficult to recognize as a meningothelial tumor because of the pattern-less array of clear cells in a collagenous background (Figure 9a) that would nonetheless be immunopositive for EMA (Figure 9b). Cells are typically glycogen rich and thus PAS-positive (Figure 9c). Interspersed among the tumor cells and around blood vessels are bands of hyaline material. Whorl formation and psammoma bodies are essentially nonexistent.

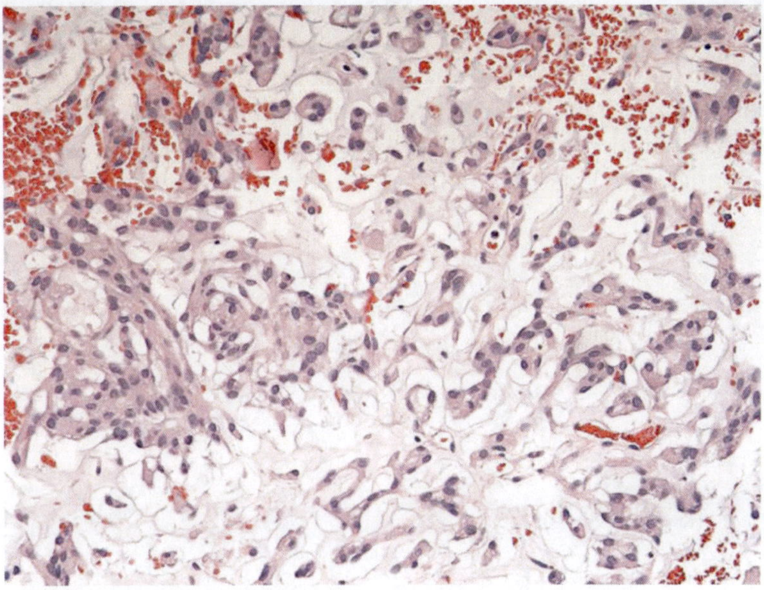

Figure 8. Chordoid menigioma, WHO Grade II, so named because of the ribbons of possibly vacuolated cells in myxoid background, closely resembling chordoma.

## WHO Grade III

### Papillary

This rare type of meningioma tends to occur in the pediatric age group and has a marked tendency for recurrence. Local brain invasion, remote metastases to the lung, and mortality are features of this type of meningioma. The histological pattern consists of a perivascular pseudopapillary arrangement of cells that may not be clearly recognizable as meningothelial in origin (Figure 10). Hyaline thickening of vascular walls may be seen.

Immunohistochemical detection of epithelial membrane antigen, or electron microscopy may be helpful in confirming the diagnosis [39] by demonstrating the characteristic ultrastructural markers of meningioma: interdigitating cell processes, desmosomes, and intermediate filaments.

### Rhabdoid

Rhabdoid meningiomas are also uncommon and are known for frequent recurrence and aggressive clinical course, prompting the WHO Grade of III [40]. Rhabdoid cells are defined as plump cells with eccentric displacement of the nuclei by eosinophilic cytoplasmic masses (Figure 11a) that may be accentuated by anti-vimentin immunohistochemistry (Figure 11b).

The combination of papillary and rhabdoid differentiation may be present. Cellular anaplasia, necrosis, and elevated mitotic activity are typical, and in the absence of these findings, the diagnosis of rhabdoid meningioma on the basis of cells with prominent eosinophilic cytoplasm should be avoided. Some meningiomas may show small foci of truly rhabdoid cells, although in the context of an otherwise WHO Grade I meningioma, the significance of this differentiation is unknown, though retrospective analysis of recurrent rhabdoid meningiomas showed minor or unapparent rhabdoid elements in the primary specimens. The designation of WHO Grade III reflects the very high rate of recurrence, extracranial metastases, and mortality [40].

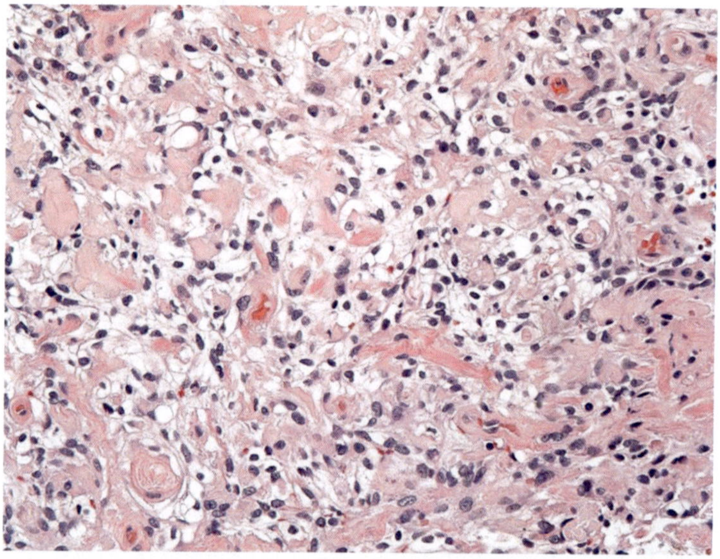

a

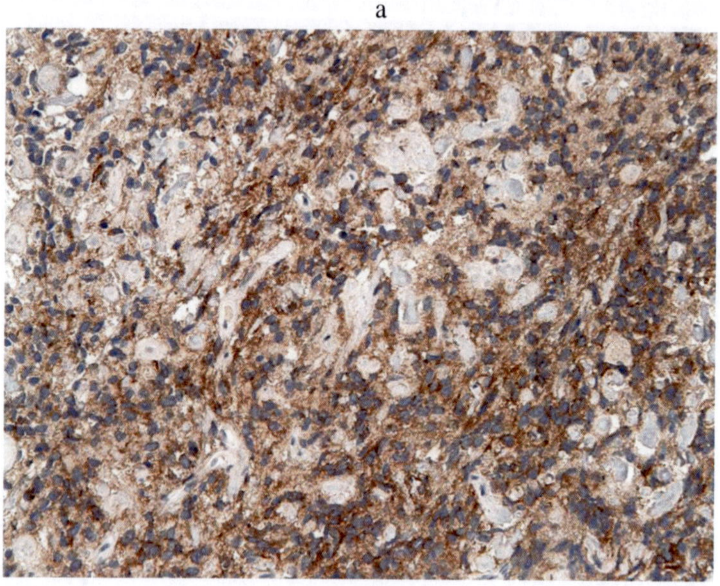

b

Figure 9. (Continued)

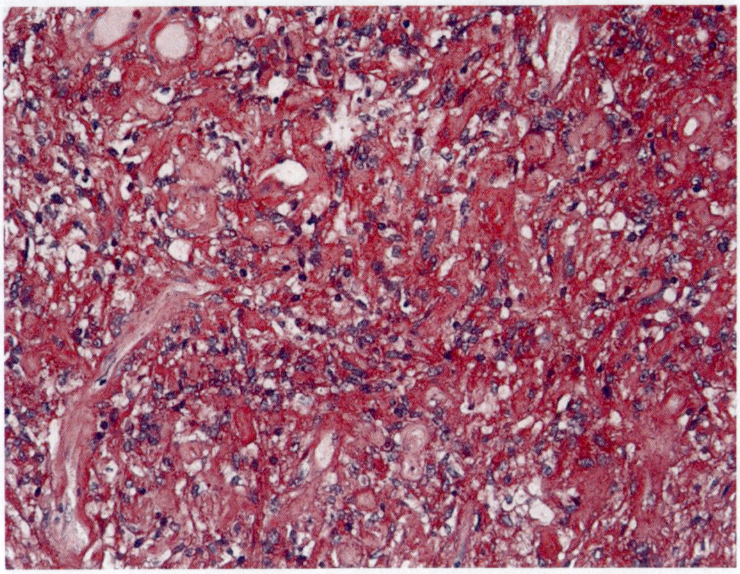

c

Figure 9. a. Clear cell meningioma, WHO Grade II, devoid of typical meningothelial features, with clear cells and interspersed bands of collagen. b. Clear cell meningioma with EMA immunopositivity characteristic of most meningiomas. c. Clear cell meningioma cells are PAS-positive attesting to glycogen content.

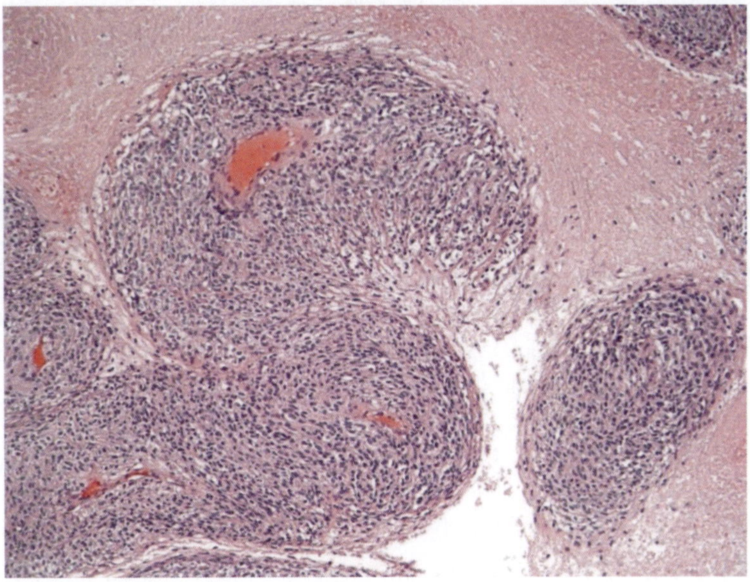

Figure 10. Papillary meningioma, WHO Grade III, with broad papillae in a necrotic background.

## Anaplastic Meningioma

In addition to the papillary and rhabdoid types of WHO Grade III meningiomas, those with greater than 20 mitotic figures per 10 hpf or significant loss of meningothelial differentiation accompanied by frank evidence of carcinomatous, sarcomatous, or malignant melanocytic differentiation are malignant, WHO Grade III lesions [41].

## Immunohistochemistry

The standard immunohistochemical marker in meningioma is EMA, present in the vast majority of meningiomas [42]. However, EMA immunoreactivity is less consistent in atypical and malignant forms. The characteristic intermediate filament of meningiomas is vimentin, which is a reliable if not entirely discriminatory marker in all meningiomas. S100 protein may be present focally and in a cytoplasmic staining pattern without classic nuclear positivity in approximately 40% of meningiomas. As noted above, CEA highlights the cytoplasmic inclusions in secretory meningiomas. Meningiomas are GFAP-negative, but the stain may be especially useful in confirming brain invasion by demonstrating brain enveloped or frankly invaded by meningioma. Progesterone receptor (PR) immunohistochemistry may support the diagnosis of meningioma, but tends to be strongly positive in Grade I examples and of less diagnostic utility in higher grade meningiomas. The pattern varies between strong diffuse or patchy nuclear positivity in Grade I meningiomas to very focal or negative staining in higher grade tumors. The absence of PRs has been linked with poor outcome along with a high mitotic index and malignant grade [43].

## Proliferative Indices in Meningiomas

Just as gliomas show a progression in grade closely linked to their proliferative indices, the mitotic index in meningiomas is related to the risk of recurrence and invasion or even metastatic spread. Mitotic figures are rare, meaning far less than one per 10 hpf in benign examples, 4.8 ± 0.9/hpf in atypical meningiomas, and 19 ± 4.1/hpf in malignant meningiomas [41]. The MIB-1 proliferative index is also useful with average percentages of 3.8%, 7.2%, and 14.7% in benign, atypical, and anaplastic meningiomas, respectively [44]. The challenge for the diagnostic pathologist is in identifying examples of "benign" meningiomas with an increased propensity for recurrence since as a group, there is a recurrence rate of 7% to 25%. A meningioma without diagnostic features of atypicality (WHO Grade II), but with a proliferative index of greater than 4% may be designated as a meningioma with increased proliferative potential and thus signifying a need for close clinical follow-up.

Note that proliferation may vary considerably within a meningioma and the diagnosing pathologist is expected to count mitotic figures in 10 hpf of the most proliferative regions of the tumor.

## Electron Microscopy

Meningiomas have been well-characterized ultrastructurally, and while rarely deployed with low-grade examples, electron microscopy may be of diagnostic utility in poorly differentiated forms.

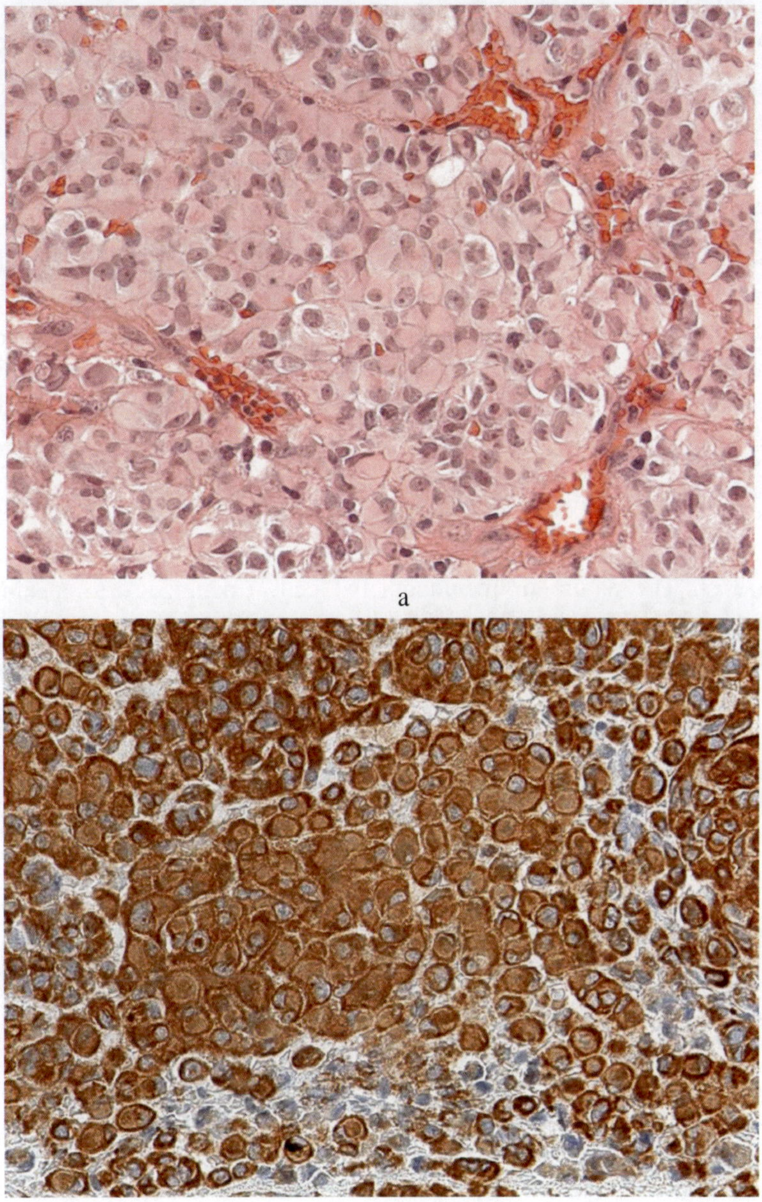

a

b

Figure 11. a. Rhabdoid meningioma, WHO Grade III, a malignant meningioma composed of cells with prominent eosinophilic cytoplasmic aggregates. b. Immunostaining for vimentin, the characteristic intermediate filament of meningiomas, may highlight cytoplasmic aggregates in rhabdoid meningiomas.

Diagnostic features include conspicuous 10-nm intermediate filaments representing vimentin, interdigitating cell processes, and complex intercellular junctions including desmosomes, hemidesmosomes, and gap junctions. The interdigitations account for the light microscopic appearance of a syncytium of nucleated cells in which distinct cell borders are not discernable. Secretory meningiomas display intracytoplasmic lumina lined by microvilli corresponding to intense EMA-immunopositivity.

Interestingly, the clear intranuclear inclusions may be seen ultrastructurally to be an optically empty space with a few glycogen particles and no membrane lining, thus excluding the occasional nuclear inclusion formed by a cytoplasmic invagination.

## CONCLUSION

Meningiomas are most often easily diagnosable dural tumors, however, a wide diversity of gross and microscopic appearances may lead to uncertainty or misdiagnosis because of histological mimicry. Pathological characteristics and biological behavior are closely intertwined and thus the accurate determination of treatment and prognosis of meningiomas as well as possible genetic implications hinge upon precision in the pathological diagnosis.

## REFERENCES

[1] Kepes, J. J. The nature of meningothelial cells (meningocytes, meningoblasts) as reflected in the nomenclature of meningiomas, In: Meningiomas. Biology, Pathology, and Differential Diagnosis. *Masson Monographs in Diagnostic Pathology*, 1982 pp. 3-5.

[2] Claus, E. B., Bondy, M. L., Schildkraut, J. M., Wiemels, J. L., Wrensch, M., Black, P. M. Epidemiology of intracranial meningioma. *Neurosurgery*. 2005;57(6):1088-95.

[3] Longstreth, W. T., Jr., Dennis, L. K., McGuire, V. M., Drangsholt, M. T., Koepsell, T. D. Epidemiology of intracranial meningioma. *Cancer*. 1993;72(3):639-48.

[4] Cohen-Gadol, A. A., Zikel, O. M., Koch, C. A., Scheithauer, B. W., Krauss, W. E. Spinal meningiomas in patients younger than 50 years of age: a 21-year experience. *Journal of neurosurgery*. 2003;98(3 Suppl.): 258-63.

[5] Gezen, F., Kahraman, S., Canakci, Z., Beduk, A. Review of 36 cases of spinal cord meningioma. *Spine*. 2000;25(6):727-31.

[6] Louis, D. N., Ramesh, V., Gusella, J. F. Neuropathology and molecular genetics of neurofibromatosis 2 and related tumors. *Brain pathology* (Zurich, Switzerland). 1995;5 (2):163-72.

[7] Perry, A., Dehner, L. P. Meningeal tumors of childhood and infancy. An update and literature review. *Brain pathology* (Zurich, Switzerland). 2003;13(3):386-408.

[8] Rushing, E. J., Olsen, C., Mena, H., Rueda, M. E., Lee, Y. S., Keating, R. F. et al. Central nervous system meningiomas in the first two decades of life: a clinicopathological analysis of 87 patients. *Journal of neurosurgery*. 2005;103(6 Suppl.):489-95.

[9] Maiorana, A., Ficarra, G., Fano, R. A., Spagna, G. Primary solitary meningioma of the lung. *Pathologica*. 1996;88(5):457-62.

[10] Picquet, J., Valo, I., Jousset, Y., Enon, B. Primary pulmonary meningioma first suspected of being a lung metastasis. *The Annals of thoracic surgery*. 2005;79(4):1407-9.

[11] van der Meij, J. J., Boomars, K. A., van den Bosch, J. M., van Boven, W. J., de Bruin, P. C., Seldenrijk, C. A. Primary pulmonary malignant meningioma. *The Annals of thoracic surgery*. 2005;80(4):1523-5.

[12] Kuzeyli, K., Duru, S., Baykal, S., Usul, H., Ceylan, S., Akturk, F. Primary intraosseous meningioma of the temporal bone in an infant. A case report. *Neurosurgical review*. 1996;19(3):197-9.

[13] Marcelissen, T. A., de Bondt, R. B., Lammens, M., Manni, J. J. Primary temporal bone secretory meningioma presenting as chronic otitis media. *European archives of oto-rhino-laryngology: official journal of the European Federation of Oto-Rhino-Laryngological Societies (EUFOS): affiliated with the German Society for Oto-Rhino-Laryngology - Head and Neck Surgery*. 2008;265(7):843-6.

[14] O'Reilly, R. C., Kapadia, S. B., Kamerer, D. B. Primary extracranial meningioma of the temporal bone. *Otolaryngology-head and neck surgery: official journal of American Academy of Otolaryngology-Head and Neck Surgery*. 1998;118(5):690-4.

[15] Mulvihill, J. J., Parry, D. M., Sherman, J. L., Pikus, A., Kaiser-Kupfer, M. I., Eldridge, R. NIH conference. Neurofibromatosis 1 (Recklinghausen disease) and neurofibromatosis 2 (bilateral acoustic neurofibromatosis). An update. *Annals of internal medicine*. 1990;113(1):39-52.

[16] Wellenreuther, R., Kraus, J. A., Lenartz, D., Menon, A. G., Schramm, J., Louis, D. N. et al. Analysis of the neurofibromatosis 2 gene reveals molecular variants of meningioma. *The American journal of pathology*. 1995;146(4):827-32.

[17] Lekanne Deprez, R. H., Bianchi, A. B., Groen, N. A., Seizinger, B. R., Hagemeijer, A., van Drunen, E. et al. Frequent NF2 gene transcript mutations in sporadic meningiomas and vestibular schwannomas. *American journal of human genetics*. 1994;54(6):1022-9.

[18] Clark, V. E., Erson-Omay, E. Z., Serin, A., Yin, J., Cotney, J., Ozduman, K. et al. Genomic analysis of non-NF2 meningiomas reveals mutations in TRAF7, KLF4, AKT1, and SMO. *Science* (New York, NY). 2013;339(6123):1077-80.

[19] Antinheimo, J., Haapasalo, H., Haltia, M., Tatagiba, M., Thomas, S., Brandis, A. et al. Proliferation potential and histological features in neurofibromatosis 2-associated and sporadic meningiomas. *Journal of neurosurgery*. 1997;87(4):610-4.

[20] Perry, A., Giannini, C., Raghavan, R., Scheithauer, B. W., Banerjee, R., Margraf, L. et al. Aggressive phenotypic and genotypic features in pediatric and NF2-associated meningiomas: a clinicopathologic study of 53 cases. *Journal of neuropathology and experimental neurology*. 2001;60(10):994-1003.

[21] Rajcan-Separovic, E., Maguire, J., Loukianova, T., Nisha, M., Kalousek, D. Loss of 1p and 7p in radiation-induced meningiomas identified by comparative genomic hybridization. *Cancer genetics and cytogenetics*. 2003;144(1):6-11.

[22] Rieske, P., Zakrzewska, M., Piaskowski, S., Jaskolski, D., Sikorska, B., Papierz, W. et al. Molecular heterogeneity of meningioma with INI1 mutation. *Molecular pathology: MP*. 2003;56(5):299-301.

[23] Christiaans, I., Kenter, S. B., Brink, H. C., van Os, T. A., Baas, F., van den Munckhof, P. et al. Germline SMARCB1 mutation and somatic NF2 mutations in familial multiple meningiomas. *Journal of medical genetics*. 2011;48(2):93-7.

[24] Eom, H. S., Kim, M. S., Hur, S. Y., Yoo, N. J., Lee, S. H. Absence of oncogenic AKT1 E17K mutation in prostate, esophageal, laryngeal and urothelial carcinomas,

hepatoblastomas, gastrointestinal stromal tumors and malignant meningiomas. *Acta oncologica* (Stockholm, Sweden). 2009;48(7):1084-5.

[25] van den Munckhof, P., Christiaans, I., Kenter, S. B., Baas, F., Hulsebos, T. J. Germline SMARCB1 mutation predisposes to multiple meningiomas and schwannomas with preferential location of cranial meningiomas at the falx cerebri. *Neurogenetics*. 2012;13 (1):1-7.

[26] Brastianos, P. K., Horowitz, P. M., Santagata, S., Jones, R. T., McKenna, A., Getz, G. et al. Genomic sequencing of meningiomas identifies oncogenic SMO and AKT1 mutations. *Nature genetics*. 2013;45(3):285-9.

[27] Hartmann, C., Sieberns, J., Gehlhaar, C., Simon, M., Paulus, W., von Deimling, A. NF2 mutations in secretory and other rare variants of meningiomas. *Brain pathology* (Zurich, Switzerland). 2006;16(1):15-9.

[28] Kros, J., de Greve, K., van Tilborg, A., Hop, W., Pieterman, H., Avezaat, C. et al. NF2 status of meningiomas is associated with tumour localization and histology. *The Journal of pathology*. 2001;194(3):367-72.

[29] Reuss, D. E., Piro, R. M., Jones, D. T., Simon, M., Ketter, R., Kool, M. et al. Secretory meningiomas are defined by combined KLF4 K409Q and TRAF7 mutations. *Acta neuropathologica*. 2013;125(3):351-8.

[30] Smith, M. J., Wallace, A. J., Bennett, C., Hasselblatt, M., Elert-Dobkowska, E., Evans, L. T. et al. Germline SMARCE1 mutations predispose to both spinal and cranial clear cell meningiomas. *The Journal of pathology*. 2014;234(4):436-40.

[31] Ron, E., Modan, B., Boice, J. D., Jr., Alfandary, E., Stovall, M., Chetrit, A. et al. Tumors of the brain and nervous system after radiotherapy in childhood. *The New England journal of medicine*. 1988;319(16):1033-9.

[32] Perry, A., Gutmann, D. H., Reifenberger, G. Molecular pathogenesis of meningiomas. *Journal of neuro-oncology*. 2004;70(2):183-202.

[33] Perry, A. Chapter 10 "Meningiomas" In: Perry A, Brat DJ, Practical Surgical Neuropathology: A Diagnostic Approach. *J. Churchill* 2010, 185.

[34] Kepes, J. J. Chapter 6. Theories on the etiology of human meningiomas. In: Meningiomas. Biology, Pathology, and Differential Diagnosis. *Masson Monographs in Diagnostic Pathology* 1982, 12-16.

[35] Perry, A. Chapter 10 "Meningiomas," In: Perry A, Brat DJ, Practical Surgical Neuropathology: A Diagnostic Approach. *J. Churchill* 2010, 215-216.

[36] Perry, A., Kurtkaya-Yapicier, O., Scheithauer, B. W., Robinson, S., Prayson, R. A., Kleinschmidt-DeMasters, B. K. et al. Insights into meningioangiomatosis with and without meningioma: a clinicopathologic and genetic series of 24 cases with review of the literature. *Brain pathology* (Zurich, Switzerland). 2005;15(1):55-65.

[37] Perry, A., Scheithauer, B. W., Stafford, S. L., Lohse, C. M., Wollan, P. C. "Malignancy" in meningiomas: a clinicopathologic study of 116 patients, with grading implications. *Cancer*. 1999;85(9):2046-56.

[38] Kepes, J. J., Chen, W. Y., Connors, M. H., Vogel, F. S. "Chordoid" meningeal tumors in young individuals with peritumoral lymphoplasmacellular infiltrates causing systemic manifestations of the Castleman syndrome. A report of seven cases. *Cancer*. 1988;62(2):391-406.

[39] Al-Sarraj, S., King, A., Martin, A. J., Jarosz, J., Lantos, P. L. Ultrastructural examination is essential for diagnosis of papillary meningioma. *Histopathology*. 2001; 38(4):318-24.

[40] Perry, A., Scheithauer, B. W., Stafford, S. L., Abell-Aleff, P. C., Meyer, F. B. "Rhabdoid" meningioma: an aggressive variant. *The American journal of surgical pathology*. 1998;22(12):1482-90.

[41] Perry, A., Louis, D., Scheithauer, B., Budka, H., von Deimling, A. "Meningiomas," In: Louis, D. N., International Agency for Research on Cancer. WHO classification of tumours of the central nervous system. *Lyon: International Agency for Research on Cancer*. 2007:185-72.

[42] Schnitt, S. J., Vogel, H. Meningiomas. Diagnostic value of immunoperoxidase staining for epithelial membrane antigen. *The American journal of surgical pathology*. 1986;10 (9):640-9.

[43] Perry, A., Cai, D. X., Scheithauer, B. W., Swanson, P. E., Lohse, C. M., Newsham, I. F. et al. Merlin, DAL-1, and progesterone receptor expression in clinicopathologic subsets of meningioma: a correlative immunohistochemical study of 175 cases. *Journal of neuropathology and experimental neurology*. 2000;59(10):872-9.

[44] Maier, H., Wanschitz, J., Sedivy, R., Rossler, K., Ofner, D., Budka, H. Proliferation and DNA fragmentation in meningioma subtypes. *Neuropathology and applied neurobiology*. 1997;23(6):496-506.

In: Current Management of Central Nervous System … ISBN: 978-1-63483-856-6
Editors: Steven D. Chang and Anand Veeravagu 

*Chapter 2*

# RADIOLOGY OF MENINGIOMAS

***Wilson B. Chwang, MD, Nancy J. Fischbein, MD and Greg Zaharchuk, MD, PhD***

Department of Radiology, Stanford University School of Medicine, Stanford, CA, US

## ABSTRACT

Meningiomas are the most common extra-axial brain tumors seen on radiological imaging, and one of the most common intracranial lesions in general. In this chapter, we will explore the role of radiology in the diagnosis and management of central nervous system (CNS) meningiomas. We will review the imaging appearance of meningiomas using different modalities, and explore some of the complications associated with meningiomas. Post-operative and treatment-related findings will also be reviewed.

## LIST OF ABBREVIATIONS

Alanine (Ala)
Apparent diffusion coefficient (ADC)
Arterial spin labeling (ASL)
Central nervous system (CNS)
Cerebellopontine angle (CPA)
Cerebral blood flow (CBF)
Cerebral blood volume (CBV)
Cerebrospinal fluid (CSF)
Choline (Cho)
Computed tomography (CT)
CT angiography (CTA)
CT perfusion (CTP)
Diffusion-weighted imaging (DWI)
DOTA-D-Phe1-Tyr3-octreotide (DOTA-TOC)

Fluorine-18 fluorodeoxyglucose (FDG)
Gradient echo (GRE)
Internal auditory canal (IAC)
Magnetic resonance imaging (MRI)
Mean transit time (MTT)
Methoxyisobutylisonitrile (MIBI)
MR angiography (MRA)
MR venography (MRV)
N-acetyl aspartate (NAA)
Neurofibromatosis type 2 (NF2)
Perfusion-weighted imaging (PWI)
Phosphocreatine (Cr)
Positron emission tomography (PET)
Relative cerebral blood volume (rCBV)
Single photon emission computed tomography (SPECT)
Susceptibility-weighted imaging (SWI)
Time to peak (TTP)
Time to maximum residue function (Tmax)

## INTRODUCTION

Meningiomas are commonly identified on CNS imaging studies. Depending on the size and location of the tumor, a patient may present with headache, weakness or sensory deficits, or cranial nerve deficits [1]. Most meningiomas are not symptomatic, however, especially if small, and they are detected as incidental findings on imaging studies that are performed for unrelated reasons. Radiological imaging plays an important role in the diagnosis and management of meningiomas, helping to define the extent of the lesion, to determine what structures are affected, and to assess for complications. Imaging also helps to determine what type of treatment to pursue, if treatment should be pursued at all. We will review imaging characteristics of meningiomas and their potential complications as well as post-treatment findings related to surgical and/or radiation treatment of meningiomas.

## IMAGING CHARACTERISTICS OF EXTRA-AXIAL LESIONS

A meningioma is the prototypical example of an extra-axial lesion, one which arises outside of the brain parenchyma. Extra-axial lesions arise from coverings of the brain, the meninges, which are subdivided into the leptomeninges (pia and arachnoid) and pachymeninges (dura). Extra-axial lesions displace the brain parenchyma, and a layer of cerebrospinal fluid (CSF) can often be seen in between the lesion and the underlying brain, a finding known as the "CSF cleft" sign (Figure 1) [2]. In addition, as there are vessels traversing the subarachnoid space, the presence of vessels between the lesion and underlying brain also indicates that the lesion is likely extra-axial [2]. The dura, a tough fibrous membrane which is the outermost layer of the meninges, may be displaced either away from the brain or towards the brain by an extra-axial lesion, further localizing an extra-axial lesion to the intradural or extradural space. Typically, meningiomas are based on the dura and extend intradurally, though rarely they may extend extradurally if they are found in atypical locations.

By contrast, intra-axial lesions arise from the brain parenchyma itself and will not demonstrate a CSF cleft, expansion of the subarachnoid space, or displacement of the brain. Intra-axial lesions are typically surrounded by brain and cause gyral expansion rather than gyral displacement or compression, and CSF and vessels are seen peripheral to the lesion within the subarachnoid space. The distinction between extra-axial and intra-axial lesions is the first step in identifying and characterizing a potential meningioma.

The differential diagnosis for an extra-axial lesion is broad. Besides meningioma, it includes other neoplasms, such as dural metastases, hemangiopericytoma, and lymphoma, other extra-axial lesions such as arachnoid cysts and epidermoids, and granulomatous diseases such as tuberculosis and sarcoidosis [3]. The differential for meningeal tumors encompasses many different histologic subtypes. Although these may not always be reliably distinguished on imaging, there are features which can indicate either an aggressive or non-aggressive etiology of the lesion. For example, aggressive lesions tend to invade through adjacent spaces and structures, and cause destruction of adjacent bone, whereas non-aggressive lesions often respect spatial and anatomic boundaries and cause smooth bone remodeling rather than destruction.

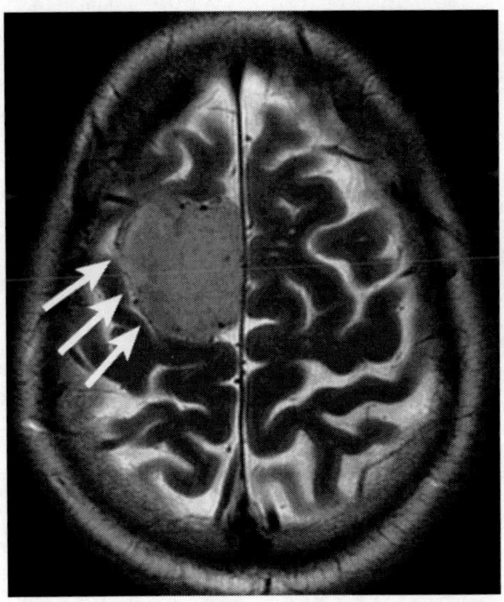

Figure 1. Right frontal meningioma. There is a thin layer of CSF, bright on this T2-weighted image, between the tumor and the underlying brain (arrows). This is known as the "CSF cleft" sign. The dark intensities within the tumor represent flow voids from vessels supplying the tumor.

Adjacent structures may be destroyed by an aggressive lesion, while they are often simply displaced by a non-aggressive lesion. Because most meningiomas are benign, slow-growing tumors, they tend not to demonstrate the aggressive features typically seen with malignant or metastatic tumors. The so-called "malignant" meningiomas represent a rare exception [4].

# Radiology of Meningiomas

## Imaging Features of Meningiomas – General Considerations

In addition to having the general features of an extra-axial lesion, meningiomas have other characteristics that can be helpful for making the diagnosis. They tend to be well-circumscribed, dural-based lesions which displace or buckle adjacent cortex of the brain. Most meningiomas enhance intensely and homogeneously with contrast, although they may have internal areas of calcification or necrosis. They may be associated with adjacent subarachnoid cysts, and variable amounts of peri-lesional edema may be seen in the brain parenchyma. Slow-growing meningiomas tend to have little edema, while rapidly-growing meningiomas often exhibit greater edema. Rarely, meningiomas may have internal hemorrhage.

Two particularly suggestive signs of meningioma are the "dural tail" sign, and hyperostosis of the adjacent bone. The "dural tail" sign refers to a tapering attachment of the lesion to the dura and the formation of obtuse angles between the tumor and the adjacent dura; this is best visualized on contrast-enhanced images [2]. Though this sign is most commonly associated with meningiomas, it is not specific and may be seen with other dural-based lesions. Hyperostosis refers to expansion and sclerosis of bone adjacent to a meningioma, and it can be due to direct tumor infiltration of the marrow space [5] or, more commonly, to reactive changes in the bone. While also not specific, the presence of hyperostosis can help suggest that a lesion in question represents a meningioma. Both the dural tail sign and adjacent hyperostosis are illustrated in a patient with a large left frontoparietal meningioma (Figure 2).

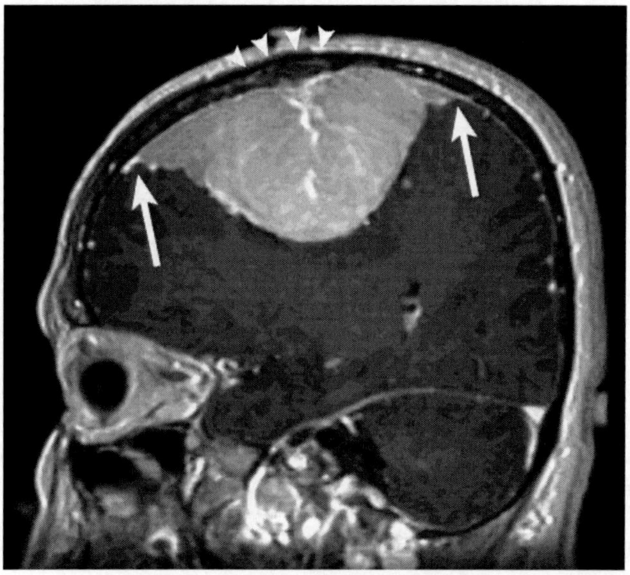

Figure 2. Large right frontoparietal meningioma. T1 post-contrast image shows a broad-based attachment to the dura, or a "dural tail" (arrows), suggestive of meningioma, as well as hyperostosis or expansion of the adjacent bone (arrowheads). Prominent central vessels are also seen in this highly vascular and intensely enhancing tumor.

Another potential finding associated with the presence of an adjacent meningioma is pneumosinus dilatans, a condition of abnormal enlargement or expansion of a paranasal sinus adjacent to a meningioma. Though originally described in the frontal sinus, it may involve any of the paranasal sinuses, [6] and can indicate the presence of a skull base meningioma that might otherwise be difficult to appreciate. The latter point is less of an issue in the era of MR imaging, but on plain films or non-contrast CT scans, this finding can be helpful.

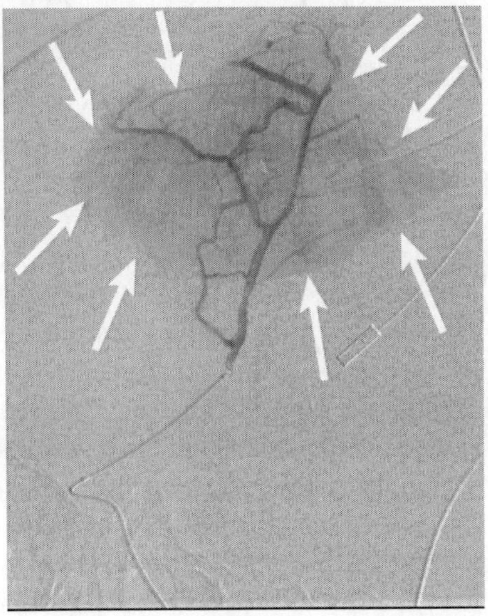

Figure 3. Tumor "blush" of a frontoparietal meningioma (arrows), shown on cerebral angiography. The microcatheter is located within the middle meningeal artery, and multiple branches supplying the tumor are seen.

Meningiomas are typically highly vascular lesions, and the vascular supply to a meningioma results in a characteristic appearance on angiographic imaging. In general, the center of a meningioma is supplied by dural arteries, normally branches of the external carotid artery, and the periphery is supplied by distal pial branches arising from the internal carotid artery. A parenchymal blush or "stain" occurs when the tumor takes up contrast during the initial arterial phase, and then dense venous filling usually remains throughout an extended venous phase. This behavior of a meningioma has been called the "mother-in-law" sign, due to the contrast enhancement's "coming early and staying late" [7]. Figure 3 shows an example of a patient with a large left frontoparietal meningioma, who had a selective injection of the middle meningeal artery that demonstrates the intense vascular stain of the tumor.

These angiographic signs are reflective of the underlying perfusion characteristics of meningiomas. They tend to be high flow lesions with large cerebral blood volume (CBV) and rapid leakage of contrast, accounting for the retained nature of the contrast in the lesion itself. For this reason, imaging modalities that assess cerebral hemodynamics, such as CT perfusion, MR perfusion including arterial spin labeling (ASL), SPECT, and PET have all been used to identify and characterize meningiomas.

CT, MRI, angiography, and other imaging modalities are complementary in providing full characterization of a meningioma. The imaging characteristics of meningioma on different imaging modalities will be further discussed and illustrated below.

## Imaging Features of Meningiomas – CT

For many patients, CT is the first study obtained to evaluate neurologic symptoms due to its rapidity and ease of access. It is the study of choice in the setting of acute trauma, and is usually the best study for evaluating calcification and bony changes. On CT, meningiomas most often appear as extra-axial masses that are isodense to gray matter. About 20% of meningiomas have regions of calcification, and some may be extensively or completely calcified [8]. Small, non-calcified meningiomas are often remarkably difficult to identify on non-contrast CT, given that they are frequently isodense to gray matter, and if small enough, do not create significant mass effect. In larger meningiomas associated with edema, subcortical hypodensity in proximity to a dural-based lesion may be visible. Meningiomas usually avidly enhance following contrast administration, and the dural tail sign due to the broad-based attachment to the dura may be appreciated on contrast-enhanced CT.

As mentioned, CT imaging of meningiomas may demonstrate hyperostosis which can provide an important clue to the diagnosis, especially for meningiomas at the skull base. Hyperostosis itself is a nonspecific sign, and it may be seen in a more generalized fashion in a variety of conditions such as hyperostosis frontalis interna (a benign overgrowth of the inner table of the calvarium), hyperparathyroidism, or Paget's disease, for example. When hyperostosis occurs adjacent to a well-defined extra-axial mass, however, it may represent the meningioma infiltrating the bone and resulting in bony overgrowth and expansion, [5] or may be due to so-called reactive changes of the bone that are not due to actual tumor extension into bone. Different patterns of calcifications have also been described in meningiomas, such as focal or diffuse, or localized versus encompassing the entire meningioma. Calcification and hyperostosis are readily identifiable on CT. In a patient with a right frontoparietal meningioma, bone window images on CT demonstrate hyperostosis of the inner table of the calvarium (Figure 4).

CT angiography (CTA) is used to optimize visualization of the brain vasculature by using thinner slices and a higher contrast dose compared to a routine contrast-enhanced CT, as well as scan acquisition during bolus injection of contrast medium. On CT angiography, the vascular pedicle supplying a meningioma can sometimes be seen, which may be helpful for pre-operative or pre-procedural planning.

A typical "spoke-wheel" vascular pattern reflecting the supply to the center of the lesion from the external carotid artery feeders may be seen. Often, however, the cerebral blood flow (CBF) and leakage are so fast that enhancement appears homogeneous even on CTA.

CT perfusion (CTP) imaging is performed by obtaining multiple images through the same region of brain during the passage of a bolus of contrast. It allows assessment of cerebral hemodynamics such as CBF, CBV, mean transit time (MTT), time to peak (TTP), and/or the time to maximum of the residue function (Tmax) [9]. Given the hypervascularity of most meningiomas, high CBF and CBV are typical findings (Figure 5). True quantitative measurement of CBV is difficult given that the extravasation of contrast during the first pass of the contrast bolus violates many of the assumptions inherent in the CBV measurement;

however, the "light-bulb" bright appearance of meningiomas on perfusion imaging may lend additional support to this diagnosis in the proper clinical context.

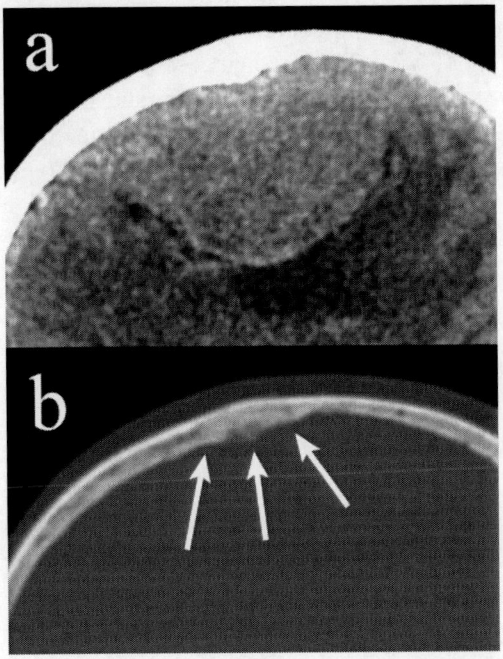


Figure 4. (a) CT soft tissue and (b) bone window images of a frontoparietal meningioma. Hyperostosis, or reactive change of the bone, is demonstrated on the bone window image (arrows).

## Imaging Features of Meningiomas – MRI

MRI has the advantage of superior soft tissue contrast compared to CT, and may be obtained to further evaluate a CT finding or as a primary imaging study for assessment of symptoms that may or may not be related to a meningioma. Meningiomas are not infrequently seen on MRI and are often picked up incidentally. On MRI, like CT, meningiomas demonstrate features of an extra-axial lesion: displacement of brain parenchyma, often with an intervening CSF cleft, as well as the dural tail sign. Central flow voids may be seen on T1- or T2-weighted images, and relatively homogeneous enhancement is seen following contrast administration (Figure 1). Intratumoral cystic regions may be present, but more common are adjacent cysts due to arachnoid adhesions and trapping of CSF to form secondary arachnoid cysts. Associated calcification, which is readily visible on CT, typically appears as a region of signal void on T1 and T2 sequences.

Each of the different sequences on MRI demonstrates a different aspect of the meningioma. On the T1 sequence, meningiomas are typically isointense or hypointense to gray matter, while on T2 they are isointense or hyperintense, depending on the cellularity of the tumor and the presence or absence of calcification. The highly cellular subtypes of tumors tend to be intermediate in signal intensity on T2-weighted images, whereas less cellular subtypes may appear T2 hyperintense. T2 is the best sequence to visualize the CSF cleft sign, since CSF will be hyperintense on T2, and it may also well demonstrate vascular flow voids representing both dural and pial arterial supply or displaced cortical veins (Figure 1). If there is heterogeneous T1 and T2 signal within the tumor, this may reflect other elements such as internal necrosis, hemorrhage, fat, or calcification.

Other sequences that are helpful in characterizing the composition of a meningioma are diffusion-weighted imaging (DWI), T2* gradient echo (GRE), and susceptibility-weighted imaging (SWI). Studies of brain tumors, both primary and metastatic, have shown that the DWI sequence and corresponding apparent diffusion coefficient (ADC) value correlate with cellularity, histologic type, and degree of malignancy [10, 11]. Atypical or malignant variants of meningiomas may differ from ordinary meningiomas in signal characteristics and typically have a lower ADC value [12]. Both T2* gradient echo (GRE) and susceptibility-weighted imaging (SWI) sequences can be used to visualize substances causing magnetic susceptibility differences, such as calcification within a meningioma, if present [13, 14].

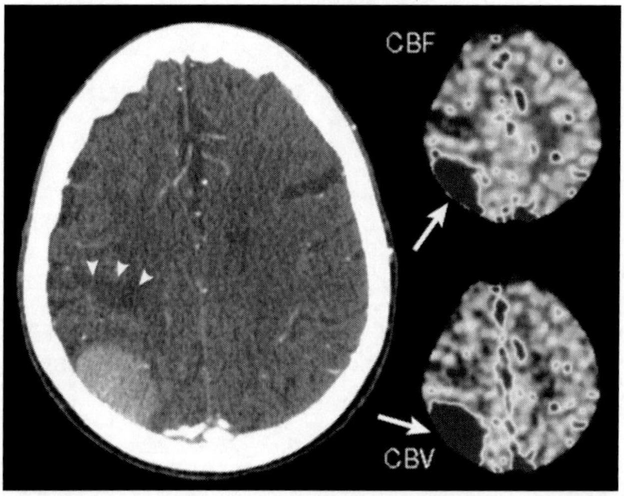


Figure 5. Contrast CT, cerebral blood flow (CBF) and cerebral blood volume (CBV) perfusion maps obtained by CT perfusion imaging of a right parietal meningioma. As seen in this patient, the typical perfusion imaging findings on CTP are very high CBF and CBV (arrows). Note also the edema in the brain parenchyma underlying this meningioma (arrowheads).

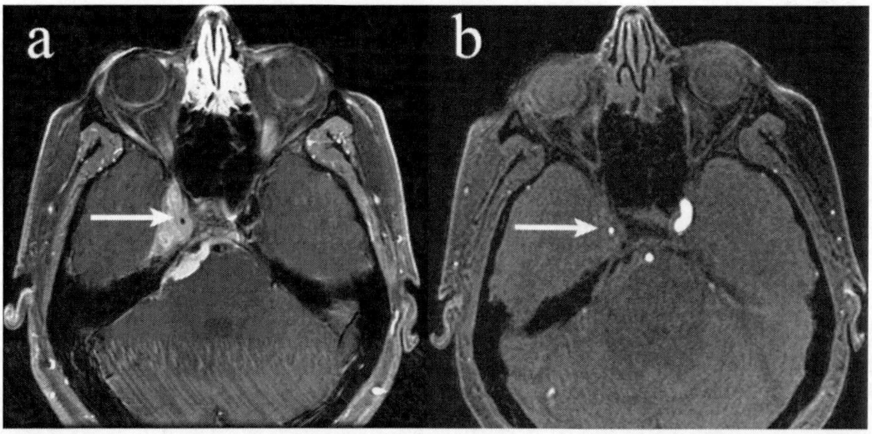


Figure 6. Right cavernous sinus meningioma. (a) T1 post-contrast and (b) MR angiography (MRA) images show encasement and narrowing of the right internal carotid artery by the tumor (arrows).

MR angiography (MRA) and MR venography (MRV) can also be useful in assessing meningiomas. These techniques can help to delineate the vascular supply of a meningioma, but often more importantly they can help to determine whether there is contact, compression, and/or invasion of a major cerebral artery or vein resulting in vascular compromise or an increased likelihood of intraoperative vascular injury. For example, meningiomas of the cavernous sinus will often encase the internal carotid artery and cause luminal narrowing, a finding that can be well depicted on MRA and which helps distinguish meningioma from other mass lesions that occur there, such as lymphoma, which may also encase but generally does not narrow vessels (Figure 6).

Other MRI techniques include MR spectroscopy and MR perfusion. An MR proton spectroscopy pattern that is characteristic of brain tumors and is observed in meningiomas is an elevated choline (Cho) peak, and decreased N-acetyl aspartate (NAA) and phosphocreatine (Cr) peaks [15]. A high ratio of alanine (Ala) to phosphocreatine (Cr) has been found to be relatively specific for meningiomas, due to their high alanine content [16].

MR perfusion-weighted imaging (PWI) provides additional information about a lesion's perfusion characteristics. One PWI method is based on dynamic acquisition following contrast administration and allows calculation of multiple tumor vascular parameters [17]. As mentioned previously, the typical PWI findings in meningiomas are high CBF and CBV. MR perfusion also has the potential to distinguish between external and internal carotid supply to a meningioma following selective intra-arterial contrast injection, both before and after embolization [18]. An alternative MR perfusion method is arterial spin labeling (ASL), a non-invasive method of quantitatively measuring perfusion by magnetically labeling protons in blood which subsequently flow into the imaging plane [19]. It has been applied to meningiomas, which typically show high ASL signal indicative of high CBF (Figure 7). CBF is not always high in meningiomas, however, particularly those that are fibrous or calcified [20]. It can also be used to assess CBF following therapeutic embolization [21].

MRI allows evaluation of many different properties of a meningioma, taking advantage of its ability to discriminate tissue contrast, vascular supply, and tissue susceptibility differences. In general, a meningioma can be readily diagnosed on MRI by taking all of its features into account; however, distinction among different subtypes of meningiomas is not always possible on imaging, and there are times when meningioma can be difficult to distinguish from other dural-based masses, especially in patients with a history of cancer who are at risk of dural metastasis.

## Imaging Features of Meningiomas – Cerebral Angiography

Cerebral angiography, or conventional catheter angiography, provides valuable diagnostic information on dynamic vascular anatomy, with greater spatial and temporal resolution than CT and MRI. Though in the past cerebral angiography was used as an adjunct in the diagnosis of meningioma, diagnostic angiography is now used as a prelude to endovascular embolization to facilitate resection of selected meningiomas. The angiographic appearance of meningiomas is well described and will be presented here, while endovascular treatment of meningiomas will be further described in a later chapter.

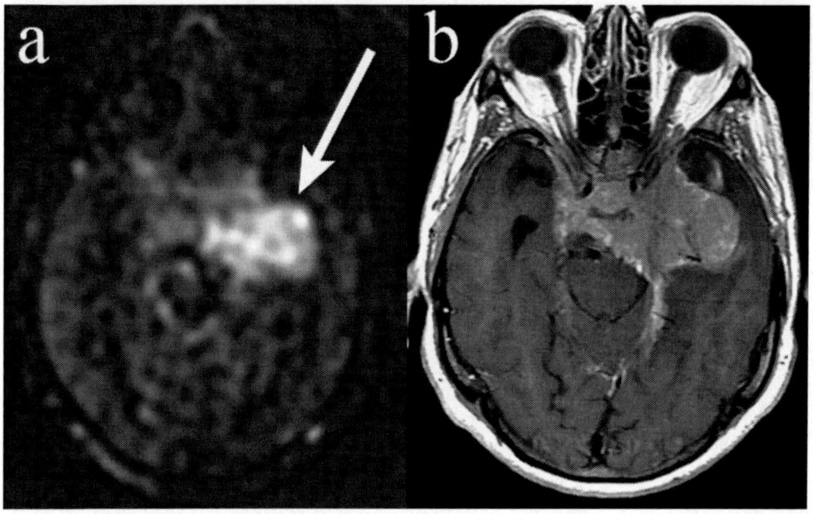


Figure 7. (a) Arterial spin labeling (ASL) and (b) T1 post-contrast images of a large central skull base meningioma. There is high ASL signal (arrow), indicative of high CBF to the tumor.

Because most meningiomas are very vascular tumors, they have a characteristic pattern of vascularity seen on angiography. Dural arteries typically supply the center of the meningioma, and pial arteries typically supply the periphery. This results in a radiating, "spoke-wheel" appearance of the vessels [22]. Most often the dural supply comes from the middle meningeal artery, a branch of the external carotid artery, which becomes enlarged and easy to visualize. It is important to be aware of anatomic variants in the arterial supply, however. A known variant is that the middle meningeal artery originates from the ophthalmic artery, a branch of the internal carotid artery, instead of the external carotid artery [23]. Also, some skull base meningiomas, like sphenoid wing and cavernous sinus meningiomas, may have supply from internal carotid artery branches such as the meningohypophyseal artery or the inferolateral trunk. Therefore, it is vital to fully map the arterial supply to a meningioma prior to a potential interventional procedure, in order to avoid injuring or occluding a blood vessel that supplies the eye or the brain parenchyma.

## Imaging Features of Meningiomas – SPECT and PET

CT and MRI methods have largely supplanted nuclear medicine imaging techniques to evaluate meningiomas. Nuclear medicine studies may, however, provide physiologic information regarding tumor viability, tracer uptake, and other characteristics not assessed by the other imaging modalities. Both single photon emission computed tomography (SPECT) and positron emission tomography (PET) radiotracers have been used for meningiomas.

Tracers used for SPECT imaging emit gamma rays which are measured directly by a gamma camera. SPECT agents which have been used for meningioma detection include thallium-201, various technetium-labeled agents such as methoxyisobutylisonitrile (MIBI) and tetrofosmin, and indium-111 octreotide [24]. Thallium-201 is a potassium analog which is taken up in cells by an active sodium-potassium (Na-K) ATPase pump. There is low uptake of thallium in the normal brain, but there is uptake of thallium within meningiomas, and this may correlate with histologic grade [25]. Technetium-99 is one of the most common radioisotopes used in nuclear imaging, and technetium-labeled MIBI and tetrofosmin may demonstrate uptake within meningiomas as well as other tumors [26, 27]. Indium-labeled octreotide may be used to visualize meningiomas, provided they have a high expression of somatostatin receptors, [28] and may also be used to predict response to somatostatin analog therapy.

PET is an imaging technique based on the emission of positrons, which are annihilated upon their interaction with a nearby electron. A pair of gamma rays moving in opposite directions is produced from this annihilation event, and the coincidence detection of these rays is used to localize their origin. The most common PET tracer is fluorine-18 fluorodeoxyglucose (FDG), which is a radiolabeled glucose analog taken up by metabolically active tumor cells, phosphorylated, and trapped. FDG uptake is nonspecific and may occur in tumors (including meningiomas), infection, or inflammation. In addition, there is high uptake of FDG within the normal gray matter of the brain. Despite its nonspecificity, FDG PET may play a role in the grading of meningiomas by determining tumor-to-gray matter ratio of FDG uptake, as well as predicting tumor recurrence [29].

Gallium-68 DOTA-D-Phe1-Tyr3-octreotide (DOTA-TOC) and DOTA-D-Phe1-Tyr3-octreotate (DOTA-TATE) are somatostatin analogues that show high uptake within meningiomas. They have been shown to be helpful in presurgical planning, demonstrating the extent of the tumor separate from the brain and adjacent bone [24]. In particular, they seem to be useful to detect recurrent meningioma in the post-operative setting, where there is often nonspecific treatment-related contrast enhancement on CT or MRI [30]. Other PET tracers are less common and include radiolabeled amino acids, choline, acetate, and ammonia [24].

Although a detailed comparison between SPECT and PET is beyond the scope of this chapter, suffice it to say that the two techniques differ in sensitivity and spatial resolution in the evaluation of meningiomas.

## Locations and Complications of Meningiomas

Meningiomas may be found anywhere there are arachnoid cap cells. They occur at various locations throughout the supratentorial, infratentorial, extracranial, and spinal compartments. The vast majority of meningiomas are supratentorial, with almost half of those occurring in the parasagittal regions or over the cerebral convexities. The next most common locations are the sphenoid wing and olfactory groove. While many meningiomas are asymptomatic, some can lead to symptoms and complications based on their size, location, and adjacent structures they impinge upon. We will describe some of the important complications that may be seen on imaging, and which must be considered with any treatment plan.

### Convexities and Falx

The most common locations where meningiomas are found are over the cerebral convexities and in the parasagittal region along the falx. These lesions can present with focal neurologic deficits, signs of increased intracranial pressure, or seizures, especially if brain edema is present. For example, a frontal or parietal convexity meningioma may affect primary motor or sensory cortex, resulting in contralateral weakness or sensory deficits. Because of the homunculus representation of somatosensory information, the lower extremities may be affected if the lesion is near midline, while the face and hands may be affected if occurring laterally. Meningiomas which occur overlying Broca's and Wernicke's areas of the dominant hemisphere may result in speech and language deficits, and occipital lesions may result in visual disturbances. In addition, parasagittal meningiomas are adjacent to the superior sagittal sinus. Narrowing or occlusion of the sinus may correlate with symptoms of venous hypertension, and the degree of sinus involvement and the presence or absence of venous collaterals also affects pre-surgical and pre-treatment planning. For example, in a patient with a right parasagittal meningioma, a portion of the tumor could not be safely removed during surgery due to invasion of the superior sagittal sinus (Figure 8).

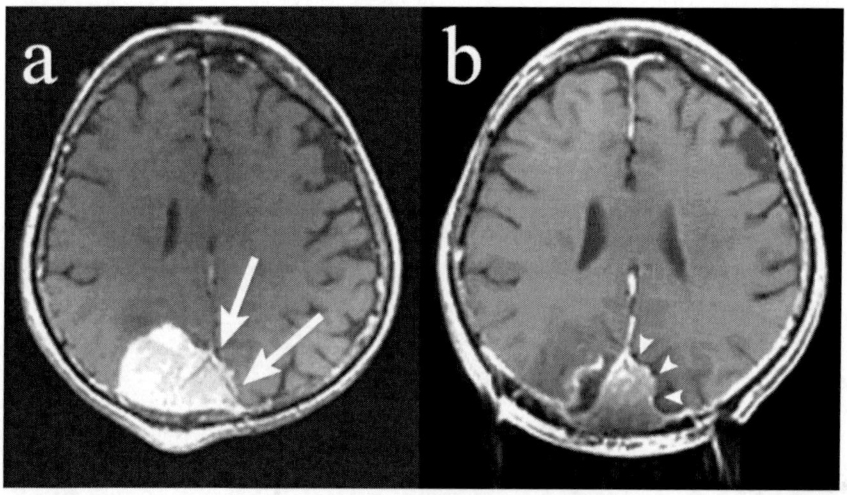


Figure 8. Right parasagittal meningioma. (a) T1 post-contrast image shows the original tumor invading the superior sagittal sinus (arrows) as well as extending to the calvarium and posterior scalp soft tissues. (b) Following surgery, a portion of the tumor was left in place within the superior sagittal sinus (arrowheads).

## ANTERIOR SKULL BASE

Meningiomas of the olfactory groove and planum sphenoidale occur along the cribriform plate and floor of the anterior cranial fossa. These meningiomas may become very large before becoming symptomatic, and may result in cognitive and personality changes, headache, or visual difficulty (if affecting the optic nerves). Olfactory groove lesions may grow into the sinonasal cavity inferiorly. Meningiomas of the tuberculum sellae may impinge upon the optic chiasm, causing visual disturbances, or affect the pituitary gland, causing endocrine dysfunction. Headache and seizure are also possible presenting symptoms. Sphenoid wing meningiomas can cause symptomatic proptosis and visual deficits if they extend into the optic canal or superior orbital fissure, or if they involve bone and extend directly into the orbit through the bony walls of the posterior orbit (Figure 9) [31].

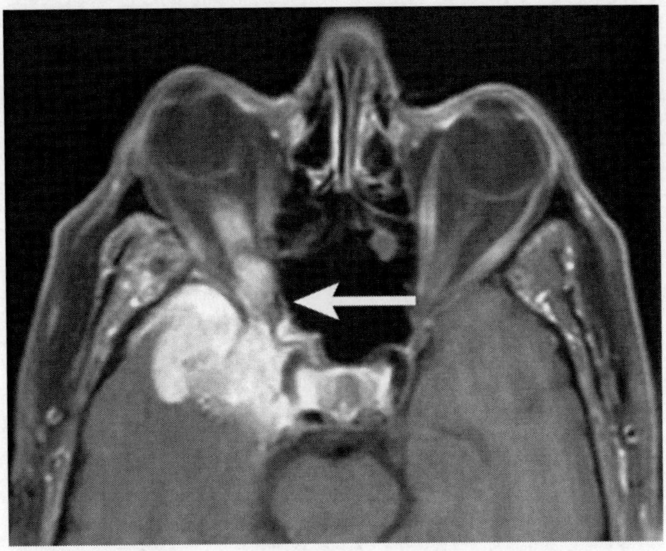

Figure 9. Lobulated right sphenoid wing meningioma. T1 post-contrast image shows extension into the right orbit (arrow) and tumor tracking along the optic nerve sheath complex. There is resultant proptosis of the right globe.

## Central and Posterior Skull Base, Including Cavernous Sinus

Meningiomas of the central and posterior skull base arise along the clivus, petrous apex, tentorium, or foramen magnum. Depending on location, the lesion may exert mass effect upon the middle cranial fossa, posterior fossa, or brainstem. Clival or foramen magnum meningiomas can cause compression of the brainstem and, indirectly, the cerebral aqueduct and fourth ventricle resulting in obstructive hydrocephalus. If a meningioma involves the cavernous sinus, it may cause deficits of cranial nerves III, IV, V1, V2, or VI, and may encase and narrow the internal carotid artery (Figure 6). Also, because of the proximity to the sella and optic chiasm, there may also be pituitary dysfunction and/or visual symptoms if the tumor extends to these adjacent structures.

Cerebellopontine angle (CPA) meningiomas can compress the brainstem and cerebellum, and may also grow into the internal auditory canal (IAC). Imaging of the CPA demonstrates an enhancing dural-based mass centered at this location, which may have a dural tail as well as adjacent hyperostosis. Rarely, these lesions may occur primarily within the IAC, and as such may mimic a vestibular schwannoma [32]. The facial and vestibulocochlear nerves may be compressed and displaced by a meningioma of the cerebellopontine angle, and preservation of these nerves is one of the main goals of surgery in patients who present with hearing loss, tinnitus, or facial weakness [32]. One feature that helps distinguish meningioma from vestibular schwannoma in this region is the lack of IAC widening that is typical of larger vestibular schwannomas, and which should not be present with meningiomas (Figure 10). Additionally, the meningioma will typically demonstrate a broad dural base, while the CPA component of a vestibular schwannoma is typically more round and usually does not demonstrate a dural tail.

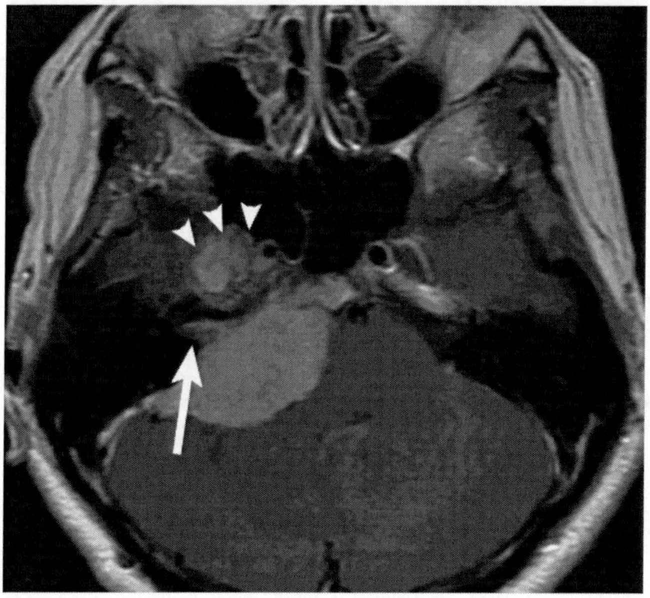

Figure 10. Right cerebellopontine angle (CPA) meningioma. T1 post-contrast image shows growth into the right internal auditory canal, which is not widened (arrow) and appears symmetric compared to the left side. This feature helps distinguish it from another common lesion of the CPA, vestibular schwannoma. Extension to Meckel's cave is also present (arrowheads).

## Optic Nerve

An optic nerve sheath meningioma arises from the arachnoid cap cells surrounding the optic nerve. The appearance of this tumor has been described as "tram-track", due to the enhancing tumor's involving the outer layers of the nerve sheath complex rather than the optic nerve itself [33]. This distinguishes meningioma from other neoplastic lesions that occur here, including optic nerve glioma, which infiltrates and expands the optic nerve. Optic nerve meningiomas may be calcified, and may have associated peri-optic cysts. Typically, visual loss and proptosis are the presenting symptoms of an optic nerve sheath meningioma (Figure 11).

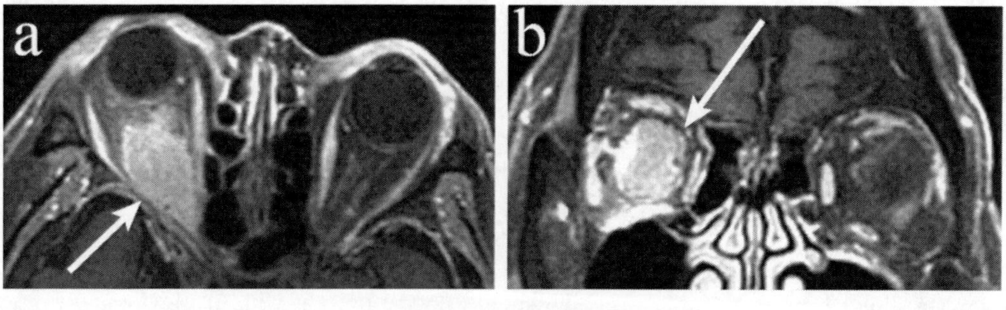


Figure 11. Right optic nerve sheath meningioma. (a) Axial and (b) coronal T1 post-contrast images show the tumor (arrows) eccentric to the right optic nerve, displacing it medially.

## INTRAVENTRICULAR AND INTRAOSSEOUS

Both intraventricular and intraosseous meningiomas are uncommon. Intraventricular meningiomas, usually occurring in the atria of the lateral ventricles, are seen as lobulated enhancing masses expanding the ventricle and potentially causing trapping of the occipital and temporal horns (Figure 12). Intraventricular meningiomas do not typically involve the adjacent brain parenchyma, but malignant lesions may extend into the brain tissue. Intraosseous meningiomas of the calvarium, which truly originate within the bone, are seen as lytic lesions with an associated soft tissue mass (Figure 13). Intraosseous meningiomas may be asymptomatic, unless there is significant scalp swelling, extradural/extracranial extension, or compression of intracranial structures [34]. Rare but described extra-cranial locations of meningiomas include the paranasal sinuses, skin, and parotid gland [35-37].

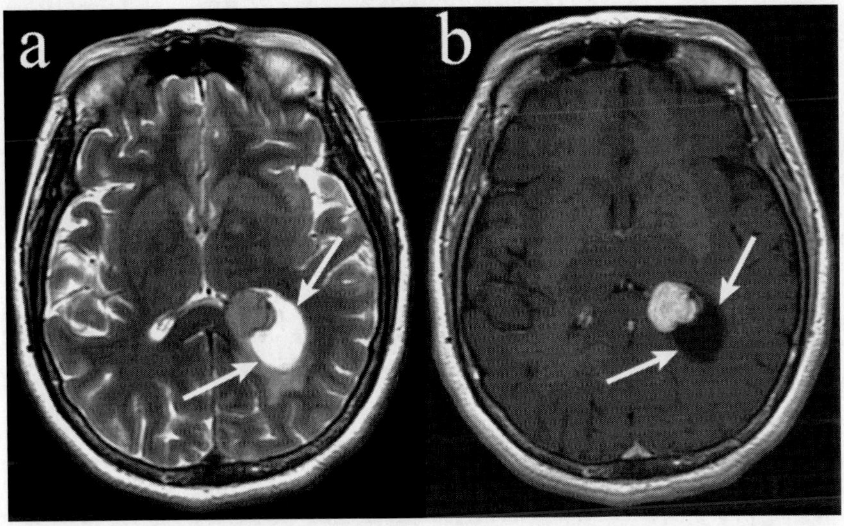


Figure 12. Intraventricular meningioma. (a) T2 and (b) T1 post-contrast images show the tumor expanding the atrium of the left lateral ventricle, with trapping of an enlarged occipital horn (arrows).

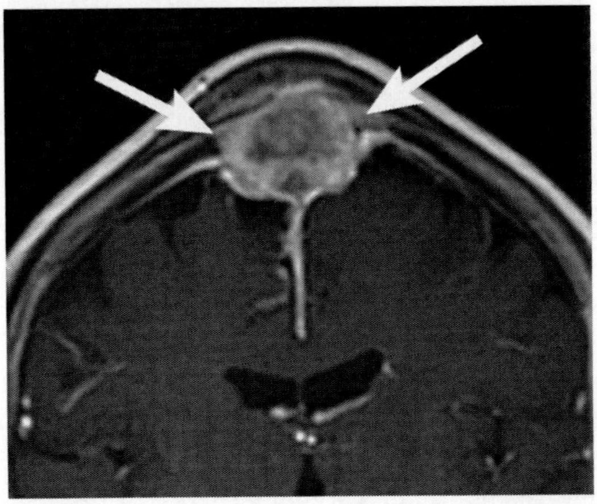

Figure 13. Intraosseous meningioma. T1 post-contrast image shows tumor centered within the diploic space (arrows), growing through the calvarium both intracranially and extracranially.

## SPINE

Spinal meningiomas are typically intradural, extramedullary masses which may occur anywhere along the spine, but most commonly in the thoracic spine of middle aged and older women. They exhibit the usual features of meningiomas elsewhere, such as a broad-based dural attachment, diffuse intense enhancement, and variable calcification [38]. These lesions often present with symptoms related to compression of the spinal cord and associated nerves, and they may extend through variably widened neural foramina into the paraspinous region (Figure 14).

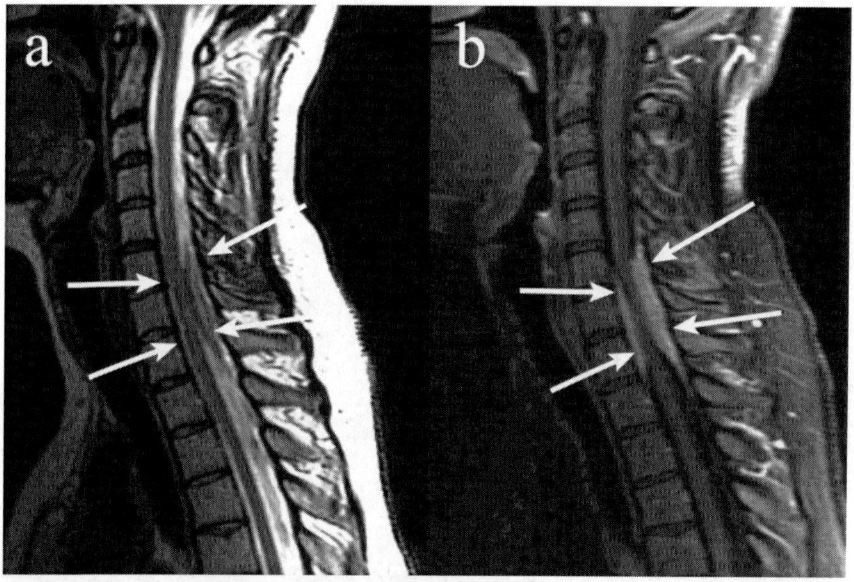


Figure 14. Meningioma of the cervicothoracic spinal canal. (a) Sagittal T2 and (b) T1 post-contrast images show an enhancing extradural tumor compressing the thecal sac and spinal cord (arrows) in this patient with neurofibromatosis type 2 (NF2).

## UNCOMMON MANIFESTATIONS OF MENINGIOMAS

Approximately 15% of meningiomas are atypical, and 2% are malignant [8]. Atypical meningiomas are defined by increased mitotic activity. They often have increased cellularity and intratumoral necrosis, and there can be frank invasion of the brain or adjacent structures (Figure 15). These manifestations of meningiomas can make the diagnosis more challenging, as an atypical meningioma is more likely to mimic a lesion such as a dural metastasis.

Malignant meningiomas are uncommon, but have a propensity to recur intracranially despite treatments with surgery and/or radiation. They have been reported to metastasize to the lung, liver, vertebral bodies, pelvis, and spinal cord [39, 40]. Very rarely, they have been reported to metastasize through the CSF [41]. The many subtypes of meningiomas can have a wide range of pathologic features and varying degrees of aggressive biologic behavior. Because of this, patients may benefit from the addition of adjuvant therapies following surgical resection, a subject of active clinical research [42].

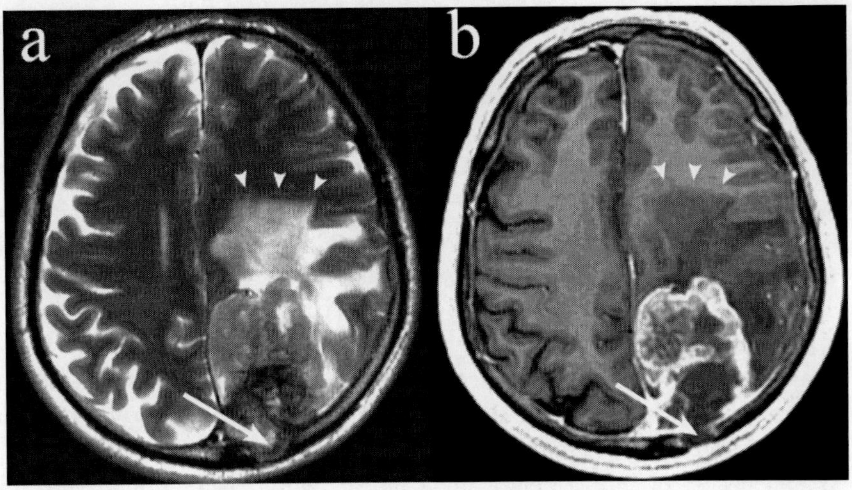


Figure 15. Malignant meningioma. (a) T2 and (b) T1 post-contrast images show a heterogeneously enhancing tumor with an aggressive appearance. There is invasion of the calvarium (arrows) and invasion of the brain parenchyma with extensive edema within the adjacent white matter (arrowheads).

A patient who has had prior radiation exposure may develop radiation-induced meningiomas. It has long been recognized that patients exposed to ionizing radiation at a young age or to large amounts of radiation as adults (e.g., atomic bomb survivors) have a much higher risk of developing meningiomas than the general population [43, 44]. Radiation-induced meningiomas usually look identical to spontaneous meningiomas on imaging, yet there are some important differences: they tend to present at an earlier age, have more aggressive features with respect to histology, and recur more often [45]. They also tend to be multiple within the radiation-exposed field. There is a relationship between initial dose of radiation and tumor grade, age of presentation, and latency period [46]. Obtaining an accurate clinical history is key in linking a meningioma or group of meningiomas to past radiation exposure.

Neurofibromatosis type 2 (NF2) is an autosomal dominant hereditary disease localized to the *NF2* gene on chromosome 22 which results in multiple intracranial schwannomas, meningiomas, and ependymomas. The hallmark of NF2 is bilateral vestibular schwannomas, and the majority of patients present between age 20 and 40 with hearing loss, vertigo, or cranial neuropathies. Meningiomas associated with NF2 have the same imaging appearance as any other meningiomas, but they are more commonly multiple. The presence of multiple meningiomas is sometimes referred to as "meningiomatosis." Rarely, there have been reported cases of meningioangiomatosis, or a condition of meningovascular proliferation and calcification which can occur sporadically or in association with NF2 [47].

## Post-operative and Post-treatment Appearance

Patients with meningiomas are frequently imaged after they have been treated with surgery, radiation, or endovascular embolization. The purpose of such imaging is to assess for complications as well as to visualize any residual or recurrent tumor that may be present. The expected findings on follow up imaging vary widely, depending on the completeness of resection, the occurrence of operative or post-operative complications, and the administration of any adjunctive therapy such as external beam radiation or stereotactic radiosurgery. Radiation can also be used as primary treatment of meningiomas, depending on the size and location of the lesion, among other factors.

With any surgery, there are potential complications such as bleeding, infection, or injury to the adjacent brain. In fact, it is common to see blood products, soft tissue edema, and pneumocephalus on imaging of any post-operative neurosurgical patient. There is often enhancement immediately surrounding a surgical resection cavity which may be due to vascular engorgement or reactive changes. On post-operative imaging studies, the best outcome is complete resection of a meningioma with expected post-operative changes, no evidence of residual tumor, and no evidence of subsequent recurrence. This is ordinarily the case for tumors which are easily accessible to the surgeon, such as over the peripheral convexities, and which do not impinge upon vital structures such as a major artery, venous sinus, or cranial nerve. In this patient with a pineal region meningioma who underwent surgical resection, there was a good post-operative result with no evidence of tumor within the surgical bed even on long-term follow up (Figure 16). Conversely, if there is residual tumor, there may be foci of enhancement which will be thicker and more nodular appearing than expected for ordinary post-operative change (Figure 17), and these may enlarge over time.

Surgical options for the treatment of skull base or optic nerve sheath meningiomas are more limited due to their proximity to or direct involvement of critical structures. In these cases, surgery may be performed in conjunction with other treatment options, or may not be performed at all. In cases where a surgical approach is challenging, stereotactic radiosurgery presents a viable alternative. In a multicenter study of petroclival meningiomas, for example, gamma knife stereotactic radiosurgery resulted in a favorable outcome in 87% of patients as defined by lack of tumor progression and no new or worsening neurologic function [48].

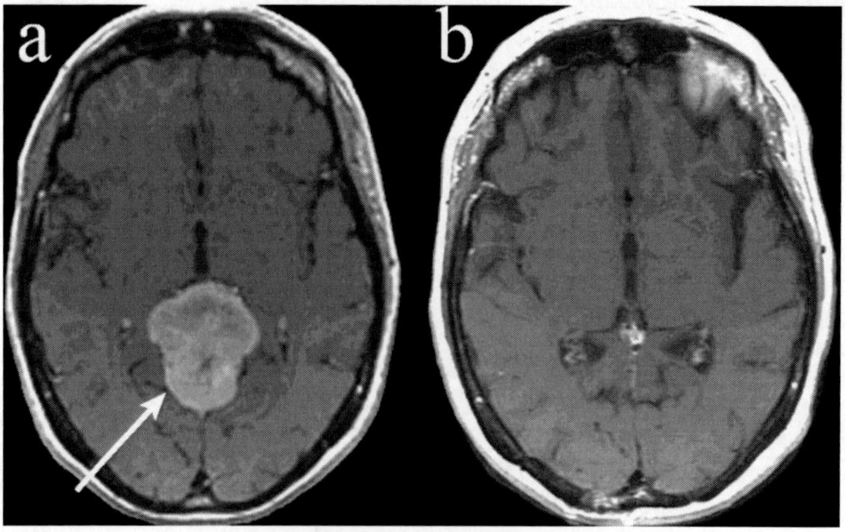


Figure 16. (a) Pre-operative T1 post-contrast image of a pineal region meningioma (arrow), which was surgically excised. (b) Four years later, there is no evidence of residual or recurrent tumor at the resection site.

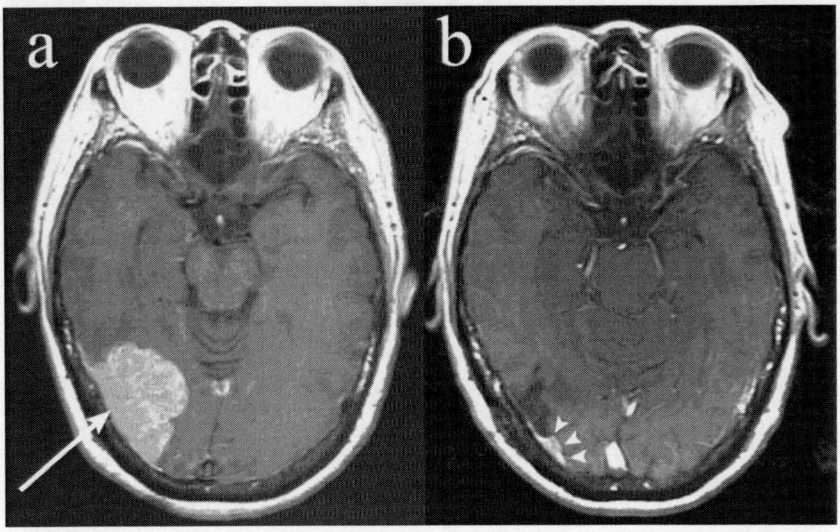


Figure 17. (a) Pre-operative T1 post-contrast image of a right temporal meningioma (arrow), which was surgically excised. (b) On a follow up MRI after surgery, there is focal nodular enhancement along the posteromedial aspect of the resection cavity (arrowheads), suspicious for residual tumor.

The most common imaging finding of a radiation-treated meningioma is stabilization or reduction in tumor size. However, complications of radiation treatment have been reported, including radiation necrosis of the brain, and rarely, late development of an aneurysm [49, 50]. These examples illustrate the importance of long-term follow up imaging in high-risk patients treated with radiosurgery.

Because meningiomas are typically very vascular tumors, preoperative embolization can be performed to reduce the blood supply to the tumor and aid in surgical resection, as previously mentioned [51].

After embolization, the patient may be imaged to evaluate for complications, or to obtain a stereotactic MRI for intraoperative guidance. An embolized or partially embolized tumor will show less vascularity, with decreased contrast enhancement or even no enhancement, and may develop internal necrosis. Embolization materials such as coils may produce artifact on either CT or MRI images. Potential complications following embolization include intra-tumoral or adjacent hemorrhage, scalp necrosis, neurological deficits, and cranial nerve deficits [52]. There can also be re-growth of the tumor, which would be seen on follow up imaging.

## CONCLUSION

Radiology plays a significant role in the diagnosis and treatment planning and follow up of meningiomas. Understanding typical and atypical imaging features of meningiomas, their locations, and potential complications is important for effective management of these patients.

## REFERENCES


[1] Heye S, Maleux G, Van Loon J, Wilms G. Symptomatic stenosis of the cavernous portion of the internal carotid artery due to an irresectable medial sphenoid wing meningioma: treatment by endovascular stent placement. *AJNR Am J Neuroradiol.* 2006 Aug;27(7):1532-4.

[2] Yousem DM, Zimmerman RD, Grossman RI. Neuroradiology: The Requisites, 3rd Edition. Elsevier Health Sciences, Inc., USA 2010.

[3] Demir MK, Yapicier O, Onat E, Toktas ZO, Akakin A, Urqun K, Kilic T. Rare and challenging extra-axial brain lesions: CT and MRI findings with clinic-radiological differential diagnosis and pathological correlation. *Diagn Interv Radiol.* 2014 Sep-Oct;20(5):448-52.

[4] Coke CC, Corn BW, Werner-Wasik M, Xie Y, Curran WJ Jr. Atypical and malignant meningiomas: an outcome report of seventeen cases. *J Neurooncol.* 1998 Aug;39(1):65-70.

[5] Pieper DR, Al-Mefty O, Hanada Y, Buechner D. Hyperostosis associated with meningioma of the cranial base: secondary changes or tumor invasion. *Neurosurgery.* 1999 Apr;44(4):742-6.

[6] Gibbons BA, Miele WR, Florman JE, Heilman CB, Horgan MA. Pneumosinus dilitans and meningioma: a case series and review of the literature. *Neurosurg Focus.* 2011 May;30(5):E13.

[7] O'Brien WT Sr. Top 3 Differentials in Radiology: A Case Review. Thieme Medical Publishers, Inc., USA 2009.

[8] O'Leary S, Adams WM, Parrish RW, Mukonoweshuro W. Atypical imaging appearances of intracranial meningiomas. *Clin Radiol.* 2007 Jan;62(1):10-7.

[9] Wintermark M, Sincic R, Sridhar D, Chien JD. Cerebral perfusion CT: technique and clinical applications. *J Neuroradiol.* 2008 Dec;35(5):253-60.

[10] Hayashida Y, Hirai T, Morishita S, Kitajima M, Murakami R, Korogi Y, Makino K, Nakamura H, Ikushima I, Yamura M, Kochi M, Kuratsu JI, Yamashita Y. Diffusion-weighted imaging of metastatic brain tumors: comparison with histologic type and tumor cellularity. *AJNR Am J Neuroradiol.* 2006 Aug;27(7):1419-25.

[11] Kono K, Inoue Y, Nakayama K, Shakudo M, Morino M, Ohata K, Wakasa K, Yamada R. The role of diffusion-weighted imaging in patients with brain tumors. *AJNR Am J Neuroradiol.* 2001 Jun-Jul;22(6):1081-8.

[12] Nagar VA, Ye JR, Ng WH, Chan YH, Hui F, Lee CK, Lim CC. Diffusion-weighted MR imaging: diagnosing atypical or malignant meningiomas and detecting tumor dedifferentiation. *AJNR Am J Neuroradiol.* 2008 Jun;29(6):1147-52.

[13] Chavhan GB, Babyn PS, Thomas B, Shroff MM, Haacke EM. Principles, techniques, and applications of T2*-based MR imaging and its special applications. *Radiographics.* 2009 Sep-Oct;29(5):1433-49.

[14] Haacke EM, Mittal S, Wu Z, Neelavalli J, Cheng YC. Susceptibility-weighted imaging: technical aspects and clinical applications, part 1. *AJNR Am J Neuroradiol.* 2009 Jan;30(1):19-30.

[15] Majos C, Cucurella G, Aguilera C, Coll S, Pons LC. Intraventricular meningiomas: MR imaging and MR spectroscopic findings in two cases. *AJNR Am J Neuroradiol.* 1999 May;20(5):882-5.

[16] Kinoshita Y, Kajiwara H, Yokota A, Koga Y. Proton magnetic resonance spectroscopy of brain tumors: an in vitro study. *Neurosurgery.* 1994 Oct;35(4):606-13.

[17] Romano A, Rossi Espagnet MC, Calabria LF, Coppola V, Figa Talamanca L, Cipriani V, Minniti G, Pierallini A, Fantozzi LM, Bozzao A. Clinical applications of dynamic susceptibility contrast perfusion-weighted MR imaging in brain tumours. *Radiol Med.* 2012 Apr;117(3):445-60.

[18] Martin AJ, Cha S, Higashida RT, Cullen SP, Halbach V, Dowd CF, McDermott MW, Saloner DA. Assessment of vasculature of meningiomas and the effects of embolization with intra-arterial MR perfusion imaging: a feasibility study. *AJNR Am J Neuroradiol.* 2007 Oct;28(9):1771-7.

[19] Deibler AR, Pollock JM, Kraft RA, Tan H, Burdette JH, Maldjian JA. Arterial spin-labeling in routine clinical practice, part 1: technique and artifacts. *AJNR Am J Neuroradiol.* 2008 Aug;29(7):1228-34.

[20] Kimura H, Takeuchi H, Koshimoto Y, Arishima H, Uematsu H, Kawamura Y, Kubota T, Itoh H. Perfusion imaging of meningioma by using continuous arterial spin-labeling: comparison with dynamic susceptibility-weighted contrast-enhanced MR images and histopathologic features. *AJNR Am J Neuroradiol.* 2006 Jan;27(1):85-93.

[21] Kawaji H, Koizumi S, Sakai N, Yamasaki T, Hiramatsu H, Kanoko Y, Kamiya M, Yamashita S, Takehara Y, Sakahara H, Namba H. Evaluation of tumor blood flow after feeder embolization in meningiomas by arterial spin-labeling perfusion magnetic resonance imaging. *J Neuroradiol.* 2013 Oct;40(4):303-6.

[22] Nelson PK, Setton A, Choi IS, Ransohoff J, Berenstein A. Current status of interventional neuroradiology in the management of meningiomas. *Neurosurg Clin N Am.* 1994 Apr;5(2):235-59.

[23] Osborn AG. Diagnostic Cerebral Angiography. Lippincott Williams & Wilkins, USA 1999.

[24] Valotassiou V, Leondi A, Angelidis G, Psimadas D, Georgoulias P. SPECT and PET imaging of meningiomas. *Scientific World Journal.* 2012;2012:412580.

[25] Jinnouchi S, Hoshi H, Ohnishi T, Futami S, Nagamachi S, Watanabe K, Ueda T, Wakisaka S. Thallium-201 SPECT for predicting histological types of meningiomas. *J Nucl Med.* 1993 Dec;34(12):2091-4.

[26] Ak I, Gulbas Z, Altinel F, Vardareli E. Tc-99m MIBI uptake and its relation to the proliferative potential of brain tumors. *Clin Nucl Med.* 2003 Jan;28(1):29-33.

[27] Choi JY, Kim SE, Shin HJ, Kim BT, Kim JH. Brain tumor imaging with 99mTc-tetrofosmin: comparison with 201Tl, 99mTc-MIBI, and 18F-fluorodeoxyglucose. *J Neurooncol.* 2000;46(1):63-70.

[28] Schulz S, Pauli SU, Schulz S, Handel M, Dietzmann K, Firsching R, Hollt V. Immunohistochemical determination of five somatostatin receptors in meningioma reveals frequent overexpression of somatostatin receptor subtype sst2A. *Clin Cancer Res.* 2000 May;6(5):1865-74.

[29] Lee JW, Kang KW, Park SH, Lee SM, Paeng JC, Chung JK, Lee MC, Lee DS. 18F-FDG PET in the assessment of tumor grade and prediction of tumor recurrence in intracranial meningioma. *Eur J Nucl Med Mol Imaging.* 2009 Oct;36(10):1574-82.

[30] Afshar-Oromieh A, Giesel FL, Linhart HG, Haberkorn U, Haufe S, Combs SE, Podlesek D, Eisenhut M, Kratochwil C. Detection of cranial meningiomas: comparison of 68Ga-DOTATOC PET/CT and contrast-enhanced MRI. *Eur J Nucl Med Mol Imaging*. 2012 Sep;39(9):1409-15.

[31] Mirone G, Chibbaro S, Schiabello L, Tola S, George B. En plaque sphenoid wing meningiomas: recurrence factors and surgical strategy in a series of 71 patients. *Neurosurgery*. 2009 Dec;65(6 Suppl):100-8.

[32] Asaoka K, Barrs DM, Sampson JH, McElveen JT Jr, Tucci DL, Fukushima T. Intracanicular meningioma mimicking vestibular schwannoma. *AJNR Am J Neuroradiol*. 2002 Oct;23(9):1493-6.

[33] Ortiz O, Schochet SS, Kotzan JM, Kostick D. Radiologic-pathologic correlation: meningioma of the optic nerve sheath. *AJNR Am J Neuroradiol.* 1996 May;17(5):901-6.

[34] Tokgoz N, Oner YA, Kaymaz M, Ucar M, Yilmaz G, Tali TE. Primary intraosseous meningioma: CT and MRI appearance. *AJNR Am J Neuroradiol.* 2005 Sep;26(8):2053-6.

[35] Gokduman CA, Iplikcioglu AC, Kuzdere M, Bek S, Cosar M. Primary meningioma of the paranasal sinus. *J Clin Neurosci*. 2005 Sep;12(7):832-4.

[36] Hussein MR, Abdelwahed AR. Primary cutaneous meningioma of the scalp: a case report and review of literature. *J Cutan Pathol*. 2007 Dec;34 Suppl 1:26-8.

[37] Joggerst KH, Langford LA, Williams MD. Aggressive meningiomas involving the parotid gland. *Ann Diagn Pathol*. 2012 Apr;16(2):85-90.

[38] Liu WC, Choi G, Lee SH, Han H, Lee JY, Jeon YH, Park HS, Park JY, Paeng SS. Radiological findings of spinal schwannomas and meningiomas: focus on discrimination of two disease entities. *Eur Radiol*. 2009 Nov;19(11):2707-15.

[39] Kaminski JM, Movsas B, King E, Yang C, Kronz JD, Alli PM, Williams J, Brem H. Metastatic meningioma to the lung with multiple pleural metastases. *Am J Clin Oncol*. 2001 Dec;24(6):579-82.

[40] Enam SA, Abdulrauf S, Mehta B, Malik GM, Mahmood A. Metastasis in meningioma. *Acta Neurochir* (Wien). 1996;138(10):1172-7.

[41] Ramakrishnamurthy TV, Murty AV, Purohit AK, Sundaram C. Benign meningioma metastasizing through CSF pathways: a case report and review of literature. *Neurol India*. 2002 Sep;50(3):326-9.

[42] Kaur G, Sayegh ET, Larson A, Bloch O, Madden M, Sun MZ, Barani IJ, James CD, Parsa AT. Adjuvant radiotherapy for atypical and malignant meningiomas: a systematic review. *Neuro Oncol*. 2014 May;16(5):628-36.

[43] Ron E, Modan B, Boice JD Jr, Alfandary E, Stovall M, Chetrit A, Katz L. Tumors of the brain and nervous system after radiotherapy in childhood. *N Engl J Med*. 1988 Oct 20;319(16):1033-9.

[44] Shintani T, Hayakawa N, Hoshi M, Sumida M, Kurisu K, Oki S, Kodama Y, Kajikawa H, Inai K, Kamada N. High incidence of meningioma among Hiroshima atomic bomb survivors. *J Radiat Res*. 1999 Mar;40(1):49-57.

[45] Mansouri A, Badhiwala J, Mansouri S, Zadeh G. The Evolving Role of Radiosurgery in the Management of Radiation-Induced Meningiomas: A Review of Current Advances and Future Directions. *Biomed Res Int*. 2014;2014:107526. Epub 2014 Jul 17.

[46] Al-Mefty O, Topsakal C, Pravdenkova S, Sawyer JR, Harrison MJ. Radiation-induced meningiomas: clinical, pathological, cytokinetic, and cytogenetic characteristics. *J Neurosurg*. 2004 Jun;100(6):1002-13.

[47] Omeis I, Hillard VH, Braun A, Benzil DL, Murali R, Harter DH. Meningioangiomatosis associated with neurofibromatosis: report of 2 cases in a single family and review of the literature. *Surg Neurol*. 2006 Jun;65(6):595-603.

[48] Starke R, Kano H, Ding D, Nakaji P, Barnett GH, Mathieu D, Chiang V, Yu JB, Hess J, McBride HL, Honea N, Lee JY, Rahmathulla G, Evanoff WA, Alonso-Basanta M, Lunsford LD, Sheehan JP. Stereotactic radiosurgery of petroclival meningiomas: a multicenter study. *J Neurooncol*. 2014 Aug;119(1):169-76.

[49] Lee SR, Yang KA, Kim SK, Kim SH. Radiation-induced intratumoral necrosis and peritumoral edema after gamma knife radiosurgery for intracranial meningiomas. *J Korean Neurosurg Soc*. 2012 Aug;52(2):98-102.

[50] Kellner CP, McDowell MM, Connolly ES Jr, Sisti MB, Lavine SD. Late onset aneurysm development following radiosurgical obliteration of a cerebellopontine angle meningioma. BMJ Case Rep. 2014 May 14;2014.

[51] Dowd CF, Halbach VV, Higashida RT. Meningiomas: the role of preoperative angiography and embolization. *Neurosurg Focus*. 2003 Jul 15;15(1):E10.

[52] Rosen CL, Ammerman JM, Sekhar LN, Bank WO. Outcome analysis of preoperative embolization in cranial base surgery. *Acta Neurochir* (Wien). 2002 Nov;144(11):1157-64.

In: Current Management of Central Nervous System … ISBN: 978-1-63483-856-6
Editors: Steven D. Chang and Anand Veeravagu 

*Chapter 3*

# Clival and Petroclival Meningiomas

***Koray Özduman, MD and M. Necmettin Pamir, MD***
Department of Neurosurgery, Acibadem University,
School of Medicine, Istanbul, Turkey

## Abstract

Clival and petroclival meningiomas (PCM) are located behind the dorsum sella in the upper 2/3 of the clivus, limited on either side by the trigeminal nerve. The management of these meningiomas is exceptionally complicated because of their central, intradural location in the skull base as it is enclosed by delicate neurovascular structures and the skull base itself. As in other meningiomas, the natural history of a PCM is characterized by slow, relentless growth and invasion of surrounding structures in the majority of cases.

Despite improved resection rates and reduced mortality, debilitating cranial nerve injuries remain a notable source of morbidity and drive surgeons to seek improved treatment strategies that involved combinations of maximally safe resections and adjuvant radiosurgery. Developments in microsurgical anatomy, sparked by microsurgery and skull base surgery, have shown that not all PCM are the same. Small variations at the site of origin resulted in significant deviations in the clinical scenario and the tumor characteristics varied greatly among individual cases. Today, it is commonly accepted that the treatment of PCM must be individualized and centered on the patient's well-being. The absolute standard in PCM has yet to be reached and advances in the understanding of meningioma biology will certainly improve current results.

## Introduction

Meningiomas in the region of the clivus and the petrous bones are very rare, reportedly making up only 0.15% of intracranial tumors [21]. Despite their rarity, these lesions require special consideration due to the complexity of their treatment. In fact, among all meningiomas, clival and petroclival meningiomas (PCM) are the most difficult to manage. The difficulty lies in the deep central location of the surgical target, its relation to the brainstem, the vertebrobasillar arterial-system and its perforators, intricate venous drainage of the brainstem and multiple cranial nerves (CNs) and the extensive invasion of the tumor within this very complex anatomy. Despite this complexity, significant advancements in surgical technique, technology and a better understanding of PCM biology have transformed this entity into a routinely treated pathology. This chapter is aimed at summarizing our current understanding of the biology, natural history and surgical and adjuvant treatment of PCM.

## Historical Perspective and Classification

PCM can extend from the dorsum sella to the upper 2/3 of the clivus, from midline to the trigeminal nerve laterally. Growth in the dorsal direction results in displacement of the brainstem and the basilar artery posteriorly with additional displacement to the contralateral side. Cranial nerves (CN) III, IV, V, VI, VII, lower CNs, as well as brainstem perforators and brainstem veins may be involved (impingement, displacement, adherence, encasement, invasion). Extension into surrounding structures (internal acoustic canal, cavernous sinus, Meckel's cave and Dorello's canal) is especially common in large tumors [5]. Invasion of the sphenoid bone can occur in rare cases, especially in sphenopetroclival meningiomas. Further invasion into the retropharyngeal area has not been observed [86]. A small proportion of these lesions can become bilateral [86]. Sphenopetroclival meningiomas by definition involve the petroclival region as well as the cavernous sinus. As mentioned in the chapter on "cavernous sinus meningiomas", a sphenopetroclival meningioma may be the advanced stage of two different entities. It may be caused by posterior fossa invasion of a cavernous sinus meningioma or it may be caused by cavernous and middle fossa invasion from a petroclival meningioma.

As is the case for cavernous sinus meningiomas, the definition and understanding of PCM has undergone considerable evolution. Initial treatment efforts in the 20$^{th}$ century resulted in exceptionally high mortality and morbidity figures and surgical treatment was abandoned. The popularization of microsurgery in the 1960's and 1970's and skull base surgery in the 1990's and 2000's have resulted in renewed interest in the surgery of meningiomas of this region. Routine application of radiosurgical methods has also significantly impacted the management of PCM. Treatment strategies are becoming increasingly refined in the early 21$^{st}$ century. Therefore, the evolving understanding of PCM and its definition shall be considered in detail.

Despite the rarity of these lesions, their complex nature attracted early attention. In the initial description by Cushing and Eisenhardt a "gasseropetrosal group" was defined [18]. This was followed by the classification of posterior fossa meningiomas by Castellano and Ruggiero [11]. They used autopsy studies as the basis for their classification system and divided posterior fossa meningiomas into 6 groups consisting of 1, cerebellar convexity meningiomas; 2, tentorium meningiomas; 3, posterior surface of the petrous bone meningiomas; 4, clivus meningiomas; 5, foramen magnum meningiomas; and 6, Meckel's cave-meningiomas. Due to exceptionally high mortality and morbidity figures, however, petroclival meningiomas were considered inoperable at the time [11]. This concept was challenged for the first time by Hakuba et al. [30], who showed complete surgical removal in the pre-computed tomography, pre-microsurgery era. Development of microsurgery and subsequent skull base surgery had a significant impact on our understanding of PCM. In 1980 Yaşargil et al. [85] published a seminal study on basal meningiomas of the posterior fossa, based on their experience using microsurgery. This study differentiated between 5 groups: 1, clival; 2, petroclival; 3, sphenopetroclival; 4, foramen magnum; and 5, cerebellopontine angle (CPA) meningiomas [85]. Yaşargil et al. noted three important characteristics for meningiomas of this region: 1, meningiomas at this location lacked a large area of insertion; 2, they had a "wide area of firm adherence" to the dura; and 3, they did not have any hyperostosis (enostosis) of the underlying clival bone (except for CPA meningiomas). In this report the mortality was down to 10% [85].

Another significant step forward came from skull base surgery. The initial belief that petroclival meningiomas were "unresectable" was challenged after microsurgery. The surgical results dramatically improved after the introduction of skull base surgery [23, 31, 65] Application of skull base technologies has also undergone a considerable evolution. Extensive approaches fell out of favor due to their unacceptably high surgical mortality and morbidity. This gave way to simpler, more optimized and standardized basic skull base approaches [7, 26, 64, 78]. With advancements in surgical technique and technology, intraoperative monitoring, and development of adjuvant treatment strategies, mortality and morbidity have significantly lessened and PCM have largely, but not uniformly, become routinely treated (Table 1). Newer classification schemes were also introduced. Ichimura and Kawase classified petroclival meningiomas into 4 groups (upper clival, cavernous sinus, tentorium and petrous apex) [32]. Al-Mefty classified meningiomas at the petroclival junction into 5 groups (petroclival, sphenopetroclival, clival, petrous apex and Meckel's cave meningiomas) [2].

Development of skull base techniques also necessitated a better understanding of microsurgical anatomy. Anatomical studies and experience from surgical explorations made it clear that the relation to the trigeminal nerve and the sphenooccipital synchondrosis are of clinical importance. Surgical mortality and morbidity, as well as surgical techniques, differ significantly when the meningioma is based ventral or dorsal to the trigeminal nerve. The treatment and outcome are different for cerebellopontine angle meningiomas and petroclival meningiomas. Similarly, the surgical approach is significantly different when the meningioma is located in the lower half of the clivus, where it is considered a foramen magnum meningioma. Today, we differentiate between clival meningiomas, petroclival meningiomas, and sphenopetroclival meningiomas. The term petroclival meningioma refers to a meningioma that arises at the petroclival borderline in the upper half of the clivus, medial to the trigeminal nerve. A new era of PCM management began after radiosurgery achieved broad adoption in skull base pathologies. Even with the most recent advances in technology and surgical technique, there is still no standard universal treatment for all PCM as treatment strategies continue to mature.

## Pathogenesis

It has been noted since the earliest reports that petroclival meningiomas are localized around the sphenooccipital synchondrosis.

**Table 1. Major surgical series of petroclival meningiomas: Different eras are marked in different shades of gray**

| Study | n | Mortality (%) | Permanent morbidity (%) | Permanent Cranial Nerve morbidity (%) | Gross-total resection rate (%) |
|---|---|---|---|---|---|
| Hallopeau [31] | 1 | | | | |
| Hakuba et al. [30] | 6 | | | | 16.7 |
| Yaşargil et al. 1980 [85] | 20 | 10 | 26 | 50 | 35 |
| Mayberg and Symon 1986 [46] | 35 | 9 | 34 | 54 | 26 |
| Hakuba et al. 1988 [29] | 6 | 16.6 | 60 | | 100 |
| Al-Mefty et al. 1988 [4] | 13 | 0 | 8 | 31 | 85 |
| Samii et al. 1989 [62] | 24 | 0 | 21 | 70 | 71 |
| Nishimura et al. 1989 [51] | 24 | 8 | 33 | 20 | 71 |
| Kawase et al. 1991 [35] | 10 | 0 | | 8 | 70 |
| Spetzler et al. 1992 [70] | 18 | 0 | 11 | 39 | 78 |
| Bricolo et al. 1992 [9] | 33 | 9 | 39 | 76 | 79 |
| Samii and Tatagiba 1992 [63] | 36 | 0 | N/A | N/A | 75 |
| Kawase et al. 1994 [36] | 42 | 0 | 0 | N/A | 76 |
| Sekhar et al. 1994 [68] | 48 | N/A | | | N/A |
| Couldwell et al. 1996 [17] | 109 | 4 | 15 | 33 | 69 |
| Zentner et al. 1997 [87] | 19 | 3.4 | | 5 | 68 |
| Goel 1999 [25] | 24 | 0 | 58 | N/A | 67 |
| Samii et al. 1999 [64] | 70 | 0 | 4 | N/A | N/A |
| Abdel Aziz et al. 2000 [1] | 35 | 0 | | 11 | 37 |
| Carvalho et al. 2000 [10] | 70 | | | | N/A |
| Jung et al. 2000 [33] | 64 | N/A | 3 | N/A | 41 |
| Roberti et al. 2001 [58] | 110 | 1 | 45 | 47 | 45 |
| Cho and Al-Mefty 2002 [15] | 7 | 0 | | | 71 |
| Seifert et al. 2003 [66] | 19 | 0 | 0 | 26 | 63 |
| Goel and Muzumdar 2004 [26] | 28 | 7 | 8 | N/A | 75 |

| Study | n | Mortality (%) | Permanent morbidity (%) | Permanent Cranial Nerve morbidity (%) | Gross-total resection rate (%) |
|---|---|---|---|---|---|
| Erkmen et al. 2005 [22] | 97 | 0 | | 7 | N/A |
| Little et al. 2005 [44] | 137 | 0.8 | 24 | 22.6 | 40 |
| Zhu et al. 2006 [88] | 25 | | | | 56 |
| Park et al. 2006 [54] | 49 | 2 | 29 | 29 | 20 |
| Bambakidis et al. 2007 [7] | 46 | 0 | 24 | 30 | 43 |
| Natarajan et al. 2007 [49] | 150 | 0 | 13 | 20 | 32 |
| Mathiesen et al. 2007 [45] | 29 | 0 | | N/A | 41 |
| Tahara et al. 2009 [75] | 15 | | | | 50 |
| Li et al. 2010 [43] | 57 | | | | 58 |
| Seifert 2010 [65] | 93 | 0 | 32 | 31 | 37 |
| Watanabe et al. 2011 [80] | 37 | | | | N/A |
| Yamakami et al. 2011 [82] | 32 | | | | 59 |
| Nanda et al. 2011 [48] | 50 | 0 | | 32 | 28 |
| Chen et al. 2011 [13] | 82 | | | | 56 |
| Yang et al. 2011 [84] | 41 | | | | 61 |
| Yang et al. 2011 [83] | 39 | | | | 64 |
| Kusumi et al. 2012 [39] | 23 | | | | N/A |
| Xiao et al. 2013 [81] | 21 | 0 | | | 57.1 |
| Li et al. 2013 [42] | 259 | 1 | 54 | | 53 |
| Al-Mefty 2014 [5] | 64 | 0 | | 32.8 | 76.4 |
| TOTAL | 2217 | | | | |

Synchondroses are cartilaginous ossification centers and play important roles in the growth of the skull base. Along the middle cranial base there are 3 synchondroses: the sphenoethmoidal, intersphenoid and sphenooccipital synchondrosis. It has also been noted that upper clival meningiomas arise in close proximity of the sphenooccipital synchondrosis [14]. The calcification of this cartilage occurs late in puberty [40]. Although the sphenooccipital synchondrosis is frequently given as an anatomical reference for PCM, and although an association between meningiomas and the synchondrosis has been suggested, no experimental study so far has reported any pathophysiological link.

Although the exact origin and the oncogenic mechanisms for meningioma development are still unknown, important molecular clues and oncogenic programs have recently been reported. Several studies in 2013 identified at least 4 different genetic programs with distinct genetic alterations in meningiomas [8, 16, 56, 61]. The site of origin of meningiomas follows a distinct anatomical pattern and the genetic changes associated with these locations are not random. Clark et al. have shown that meningiomas with NF2/chr22 loss originate in the lateral and posterior regions of the skull base, while most of the anterior and medial meningiomas were non-NF2 mutant [16]. When supplementary data from this study were analyzed with a focus on PCM, none of the 12 PCM cases were mutant for NF2; 7/12 (58.3%) cases carried TRAF7 mutations, 4/12(33.3%) cases carried KLF4 mutations, 3/12 (25%) cases were mutant for AKT1 and 2/12 (16.7%) cases had allelic loss of chromosome 22. No SMO1 mutations were observed among petroclival meningiomas [16].

The incidence of TRAF7 mutations in petroclival meningiomas was higher than the generally reported rate of 24% in all meningiomas [16]. Co-mutations of KLF4 and TRAF7 were observed in 4/12 (33.3%) cases. It has been shown by independent groups that co-mutation of KLF4/TRAF7 is observed in 100% of secretory meningiomas. In the cohort reported by Clark et al., secretory meningiomas were observed in 2/12 cases. In our institutional cohort, 3/10 (30%) meningiomas cases were of secretory morphology, which is the highest incidence of secretory meningiomas among all anatomical locations. When all secretory meningiomas operated on at our institution were analyzed 3/13 (23.1%) cases were located in the petroclival region. In summary, these findings indicate that TRAF7, KLF4 mutations and the secretory morphology are enriched for the PCM and that no PCM is associated with NF2 [16].

## Clinical Presentation

PCM are most commonly encountered in middle-aged or elderly women, as is the case in other meningiomas. Pediatric cases are exceptionally rare. Most cases stay undetected for extended periods of time without becoming symptomatic. Headaches, gait disturbances or CN palsies are the most common presenting symptoms. Tumor size varies greatly in clinical series but patients most commonly present with tumors of 2-4 cm in diameter.

## Therapeutic Decision-Making

There is limited scientific evidence to support a definitive treatment algorithm for PCM [21]. All existing literature on the topic is based on the individual experience of very skilled and proficient surgeons. Also, management strategies have varied over time according to technical abilities and technological advancements. The therapeutic approach to petroclival meningiomas can be studied in 4 consecutive periods. The first period is the "pre-microsurgery era", when there were only a few case reports of heroic treatment efforts. Initial attempts by pioneers such as Hallopeau, Cushing, Olivecrona, Dechaume & Wertheimer, Dandy-Delcour-Laine, Cherrington & Schneck and Hakuba were done with conventional subtemporal and retrosigmoid approaches [11, 14, 18-20, 27, 30, 31, 41, 52]. During this period, there was only one reported case of gross-total resection, which was reported by Hakuba et al. [30], but the operative mortality was in excess of 50% [11, 14, 18-20, 27, 30, 31, 41, 52]. Therefore, PCM were still considered inoperable and patients succumbed to progressive disease. The second, "microsurgical era" starts with the popularization of microsurgery when selected cases were operated on with acceptable mortality rates, but when most meningiomas at the petroclival area were still considered inoperable. However, microsurgical techniques gave us a better understanding of the pathoanatomy [85] and reports by Yasargil and Mayberg & Symon reported operative mortalities below 10% [46, 85]. The third period, which started in the 1990's and continued into the 2000's, is the "early skull base surgery era" when development of novel skull-base approaches enabled extensive tumor resections. Pioneers such as Hakuba, Al-Mefty, Sekhar, Kawase, Spetzler and Fukushima devised novel approaches to the region and challenged the dogma that extensive resections comparable to other anatomical sites are not possible in PCM [4, 24, 28, 29, 35, 62, 67, 70]. The motto "remove the bone and leave the brain alone", emphasized the importance of comprehending the anatomy, getting close to the pathology and chasing the tumor to all its extensions. This period sparked renewed general interest in petroclival meningiomas, redefined the operability criteria for PCM, provided a better understanding of unique pathologies (such as different subtypes), and also sparked general interest in its microsurgical anatomy. However, despite impressive tumor resection rates, operative morbidity was still very significant for benign skull base pathologies. Such skull base approaches were not routine "everyday procedures" but performed by specialized skull base surgeons. The fourth and most recent phase is the "maturation phase of skull base surgery" when results and patient outcomes were re-evaluated. A report by Sekhar et al. on the long-term follow-up of 150 PCM patients emphasized that gross-total resections are a rarity rather than the rule even in the hands of master surgeons, and that debilitating CN morbidities as well as other complications are very common. The gross-total resection rate, as determined by early postoperative magnetic resonance imaging (MRI) ranges from 28% to 54% in surgical series published from 2009 to 2014 and the permanent CN morbidity ranges from 31% to 32.8%. These findings forced the neurosurgical community to re-evaluate results, to improve and refine surgical techniques with a strong emphasis improving patient outcomes and minimizing adverse events.

After standardization and optimization, skull base approaches were adopted by the general neurosurgical community and became a part of the standard armamentarium of the neurosurgeon. The popularization of teaching skull base surgery by neurosurgical societies and federations has also played an important role in the worldwide acceptance of standard skull base approaches. Standardization also made complication avoidance a reality. Skull base approaches to the petroclival region are not harmless; permanent morbidity in the form of CN VI and VII paralysis, hearing loss and lower CN palsies can devastate the life of the patient. Other major morbidities such as hemiparesis, cerebrospinal fluid (CSF) fistula, venous infarctions (in the brainstem, temporal lobe or the cerebellum), hematoma in the tumor bed, or hydrocephalus are also not negligible. With the patient's quality of life prioritized above everything, new strategies were sought to reduce the complication rate and complement the management strategy in cases of subtotal resection. Another major improvement in the fourth phase was the popularization of Gamma Knife radiosurgery (GKRS), which gained widespread acceptance as a primary and adjuvant tool in the hand of the neurosurgeon. Simultaneously, the experience of the previous decades made clear that not all PCM are the same and that treatment should be individualized. In this latest period it was universally accepted that the quality of life comes first before all other considerations. Petroclival meningiomas are rare lesions and for each case there are several variables, such as patient age, comorbidities, symptomatology, exact anatomical localization, and size of the tumor, all of which influence treatment results. Patient expectations and preferences also play important roles. Therefore the management strategy for PCM should be individualized. There is no doubt that with a better understanding of the tumor and its disease biology, more effective treatment paradigms will be possible.

The intention to treat should be based on the predicted course of the disease; therefore the natural history of petroclival meningiomas is of crucial importance. PCM are rare pathologies, therefore specific information on its natural history is not easy to come by. The most widely cited study by van Havenbergh et al. reported conservative follow-up of 21 patients with PCM for periods longer than 4 years. During this follow-up period 76% of the lesions demonstrated continued growth and 63% of the patients experienced neurological worsening [79]. This is consistent with other studies reporting volumetric growth in 70.4% of meningiomas, independent of the anatomical site [53]. Park et al. reported a follow-up of 9 cases for a mean of 63 months and reported that 22.2% eventually required surgical treatment [54]. Studies of the natural history of meningiomas have also shown that growth is more likely in meningioma patients younger than 60 years of age, in meningiomas that are hyperintense on T2-weighted MRI, in meningiomas with peritumoral edema, in meningiomas that did not harbor calcifications, and those that have a diameter greater than 25 mm [12, 53, 60, 79].

Asymptomatic and small tumors may be followed in elderly patients and treated only if they continue to grow. In young patients, however, such asymptomatic and small tumors require treatment either in the form of radiosurgery or surgical resection. All studies agree on the superiority of gross-total resection when it can be safely achieved. Fibrous tumors with hard consistency, adherence to the brainstem, CNs and perforating arteries, encasement of major vessels and cavernous sinus invasion are the most common causes of failure in total resection. The most common morbidity in petroclival meningioma surgery results from iatrogenic CN palsies, which are reported in 22% to 76% of surgeries. CN palsies result in a significant decrease in functionality and thus quality of life of patients.

Therefore most authors favor preservation of function to a more "impressive" postoperative MRI. With current surgical techniques, petroclival meningiomas can be resected with minimal mortality and morbidity, in the range of 30% with radical surgery and less with more conservative approaches [23, 31, 65]. Tumor progression has been reported in 42% of petroclival meningiomas with a mean time to progression of 36 months, and in such cases radiosurgery or radiotherapy provides adequate tumor growth control [65]. Fractionated radiation therapy may be used in tumors of all sizes, however, this modality does not alleviate the mass effect on the brainstem and therefore should be reserved only for selected cases. Use of fractionated radiotherapy is widely accepted for anaplastic meningiomas. Poor patient health and low performance levels may also be an indication for this treatment.

## Surgical Approach

Approaches to the temporal bone and the petroclival region can be grouped into 3 basic strategies: anterolateral, lateral and posterior approaches.

## Retrosigmoid

A commonly utilized surgical corridor to the petroclival region is the classic retrosigmoid (lateral suboccipital) approach. This approach, along with the subtemporal approach was the standard approach to PCM in the pre-microsurgical and microsurgical eras. The retrosigmoid approach was first used by Sir Charles Balance in 1894 for a "fibrosarcoma of the meninges" on the posterior surface of the petrous bone, and the patient survived with trigeminal and facial injuries [73]. The procedure remained largely unaltered since its first use. Refinements in anesthesia, patient positioning, surgical technique, instrumentation and intraoperative monitoring have made it one of the most reliable modern surgical approaches. Several pioneers of skull base approaches later came to the conclusion that extensive skull base approaches are not required for most PCM. It was evaluated that most cases could be resected with the standard retrosigmoid approach with excellent results and a comparatively far smaller complication rate [6, 50, 76]. This is especially true for large PCM that naturally retract the brainstem and create a surgical corridor. Tumors that invade the cavernous sinus can be safely managed with a second staged anterolateral approach to the cavernous sinus or managed by radiosurgery if the tumor is small. Today the retrosigmoid approach remains the workhorse in PCM surgery.

## Anterolateral and Middle Fossa Approaches

Presigmoid approaches use drilling of the petrous bone to varying extents and mobilization of the transverse-sigmoid junction posteriorly to gain a more lateral view in front of the brainstem. For small lesions anterior to the brainstem or those that have an extension into the cavernous sinus (sphenopetroclival meningiomas), anterolateral approaches provide access to the anterior aspect of the brainstem. Anterior approaches include the cranioorbitozygomatic (COZ) approach and cavernous sinus explorations. These two basic anterolateral approaches are the workhorses of skull base surgery if the tumor extends into the cavernous sinus. Staged combinations of COZ and the retrosigmoid approach are classic, safe and effective [7]. Another anterolateral approach is the "middle fossa approach", which was described and popularized by Kawase et al. in 1985 [37]. This approach was initially described for treatment of proximal basilar artery aneurysms, but results of petroclival meningioma surgery using this approach were later reported again by Kawase et al. [35]. Similar to the anterolateral approaches, the middle fossa approach uses a small window to expose the area around the petrous apex. This is a small and limited approach with limited use, but is attractive because hearing and facial nerve functions are safely preserved. Combinations of these approaches are possible but seldom used as increased complexity of the approaches results in increased morbidity and mortality. Instead there is a trend to stage surgeries or combine maximally safe resections with adjuvant radiosurgery.

## Presigmoid Approach

Before the popularization of skull base surgery, subtemporal and suboccipital paramedian approaches were commonly utilized for petroclival meningiomas. The first systematic lateral approach to the petroclival region was provided by King [38]. Morrison and King cited that the approach was initially pioneered by Henderson [47]. This translabyrnthine/transtentorial approach was later modified by Hakuba et al. with the addition of the suboccipital paramedian approach [30]. The presigmoid approach was reported by Hakuba et al. in 1985, for the treatment of 8 retrochiasmatic craniopharyngiomas [28]. In 1989 Al-Mefty et al. and Samii et al. simultaneously and independently reported the results of the transpetrous approach [3, 62]. In the report by Al-Mefty et al., the results of 13 petroclival meningiomas were reported [3]. Later on this approach was popularized in the neurosurgical community by Al-Mefty as the "petrosal" approach. Other skull base surgeons have devised technical improvements in presigmoid approaches [67]. Combinations with other skull base approaches (e.g., with the anterior petrosal approach to result in the "combined petrosal approach") have been defined [15]. Throughout the history of skull base surgery, the presigmoid approach has also evolved and has been standardized. Nevertheless, even less invasive modifications have been devised [78]. The advantages of the presigmoid approach include the minimal retraction on the temporal lobe or the cerebellum, the close distance to the tumor, exposure of the lateral and anterior surface of the brainstem even with small tumor, preservation of the sigmoid sinuses and the vein of Labbé and the devascularization of the tumor at the initial stage of the operation [4].

Presigmoid approaches consist of the combination of temporo-occipital craniectomies, a simple mastoidectomy and varying degrees of petrosectomy. The extent of the petrosectomy is tailored to the need of the particular operation and depends on the anatomical target and preoperative symptomatology. It can range from petrosal apicectomy to partial labyrinthectomy, total labyrinthectomy (trans-labyrinthine) and to total petrosectomy (transcochlear approach). The hearing function can be preserved with resections up to partial labyrinthectomy. More extensive approaches result in loss of hearing and involve drilling of the facial canal at the risk of a facial palsy, however these approaches may be indicated for widely invasive tumors.

Temporal bone anatomy, once a foreign territory to neurosurgeons, has become a familiar structure with the introduction of skull base techniques to everyday neurosurgery. Several landmarks are indispensable for proper guidance of surgical approaches. On the lateral surface of the mastoid bone are the external auditory meatus (EAM), the Henle's spine (located at the posterosuperior margin of the EAM), the temporal line (which is a virtual continuation of the zygomatic arcus posteriorly towards the asterion), and the mastoid tip, which are the main landmarks [57, 77]. These landmarks will help to identify the mastoid during temporal bone dissection, which will in turn guide the surgeon to the compact bone surrounding the labyrinth and the facial nerve. The triangle formed between the superior temporal line and the Henle's spine is known as the suprameatal triangle and roughly corresponds to the mastoid antrum [4, 57, 77]. Before drilling of the mastoid bone begins, a linear cut is placed along the superior temporal line, which is connected with another perpendicular cut extending through the EAM and the Henle's spine. Drilling of the temporal bone ensues under constant irrigation to expose the sigmoid sinus and the posterior fossa dura. The middle fossa dura is then exposed. The mastoid antrum is located roughly at a depth of 1.5 cm [4, 57, 77]. The fallopian canal housing the facial nerve and inner ear structures, including the semicircular canals, are located anterior and deep to the mastoid antrum [57, 77]. The labyrinth lies inferoposterior to the mastoid antrum and is identified by the surrounding compact bone [57]. This is the limit for the petrous approach, but according to the need, partial labyrinthectomy, total labyrinthectomy (trans-labyrinthine approach) or total petrosectomy with facial nerve skeletonization (transcochlear approach) may be added to temporal bone dissection [57]. Preoperative detailed analysis of tumor extension is crucial to judge the optimal approach. Additionally, the venous anatomy of the region should be studied in detail to avoid complications during surgery (whether the transverse sinuses meet at the torcula, which sinus is dominant, the size and dominance of the vein of Labbé, the location and size of other basal veins) [4].

## Extension of the Presigmoid Approach

For the standard presigmoid approach, the patient is placed in the lateral or park-bench position and the head is positioned with the petrous bone in the most apical position. Skin incision can vary from a hockey-stick incision centered on the ear to a small "c" shaped incision [4, 78]. The temporalis muscle fascia is preserved and prepared for closure and the temporalis muscle is dissected subperiosteally and retracted anteriorly. The craniotomy for the presigmoid approach consists of the combination of a temporo-occipital craniotomy and mastoidectomy centered on the junction of transverse and sigmoid sinuses. Burr holes are placed on the transverse sinus. The first burr hole is located inferomedially to the asterion, the second placed at the junction of the superior temporal line with the line connecting the squamal and petrous parts of the temporal bone. These two burr holes expose the infratentorial and supratentorial compartments, respectively. At the transverse-sigmoid junction the sinus may be tightly adherent to the bone, so care should be given not to injure the sinus. In the classic presigmoid approach the mastoid bone and the petrous corner are drilled to expose the Meckel's cavity [4, 28]. During the dissection of the petrous bone, the mastoid antrum constitutes the most important landmark. A posterior extension exposes the sigmoid sinus and the fallopian canal, both of which are spared. The dura is opened along the middle fossa base and this cut is combined with another in front of the sigmoid sinus. The superior petrosal sinus is clipped and divided at this stage. The division of the tentorium, to the tentorial hiatus, creates a wide exposure to the front of the brainstem. However, the tentorial incision should be posterior to where CN IV enters the tentorial hiatus. The temporal lobe is retracted superiorly and the sigmoid sinus-cerebellum posteroinferiorly. CSF drainage from the CPA cistern aids in relaxation of the brain. Care should be taken not to harm the anterior and posterior inferior cerebellar arteries, which may be engulfed by the tumor.

Variations in venous anatomy may limit the presigmoid approach. The approach may present higher risk for the patients who have a single or dominant ipsilateral sigmoid sinus or one that does not connect with the confluens. Venous drainage through the layers of the tentorium is also of concern. A large or high-lying sigmoid bulb may block access to the petroclival area. In these patients, the combined petrosal approach may be considered if the hearing is intact. If the hearing is already affected the translabyrinthine or complete petrosectomy approaches may be considered [15].

## Petrosal "Keyhole" Approach

The presigmoid approach is based on two main components: posterior mobilization of the transverse-sigmoid sinus junction and drilling of the mastoid bone to gain lateral exposure. To achieve this exposure, the standard presigmoid approach starts with a combined subtemporal and posterior fossa craniotomy. In our experience, however, we have noted over the years that the main limiting factors for superior mobilization of the temporal lobe are the temporal draining veins and the main limiting factor for posterior mobilization of the transvers-sigmoid sinus junction is the sigmoid sinus. Even large craniotomies do not provide extra room for retraction, as the main limits (the temporal draining veins and the sigmoid sinus) cannot be sacrificed. Therefore, in our view, most of the advantages of the presigmoid approach depend on mastoid and petrous bone drilling rather than on subtemporal or posterior fossa craniotomies. It is the petrosectomy that provides the necessary anterior view to the brainstem, and decreases the working distance to the tumor (Figure 1). Because we noted that apertures comparable to that of the presigmoid approach could be achieved with simple petrosectomy, we devised the small petrosal approach in 2004 [78].

In the small petrous approach, the petrous bone removal is limited and is not accompanied by a posterior fossa craniotomy or subtemporal craniotomy to retract the sinus (Figure 1). The two factors that are the basic components of the presigmoid/petrous approach are challenged, and rather than retracting the sinus, the craniotomy is shifted to in front of the sinus with a more anterior point of view.

The small aperture provides the necessary access to the front of the brainstem for removal of PCM. The petrosectomy for this approach starts, as in the standard procedure, with a mastoidectomy.

The sigmoid sinus is skeletonized under operating microscope using a high-speed drill under constant irrigation. Sufficient exposure of the presigmoid dura from the superior petrosal sinus to the level of the jugular bulb, is gained while the inner and middle ear structures are preserved. This also exposes the sigmoid and transverse sinuses, After completion of the extradural bone removal, the temporal dura is incised parallel to the floor of the temporal fossa in the anterior portion of the vein of Labbé. The presigmoid dura covering the posterior fossa is then incised up to the superior petrosal sinus, which is coagulated or closed with hemoclips and transected. CSF is released from the CPA cistern. The temporal lobe is slightly elevated and the tentorium is completely transected, parallel to the petrous bone, in the direction of the trochlear nerve. Preservation of the vein of Labbé during elevation of the temporal lobe and during cutting of the tentorium is very important. After the tentorium has been completely cut, the transverse and sigmoid sinuses and the remaining part of the tentorium can be retracted using self-retaining retractors. The ambient cistern and crus cerebri are then exposed as well as the PCM. After tumor removal, the dura is closed with a fascial graft.

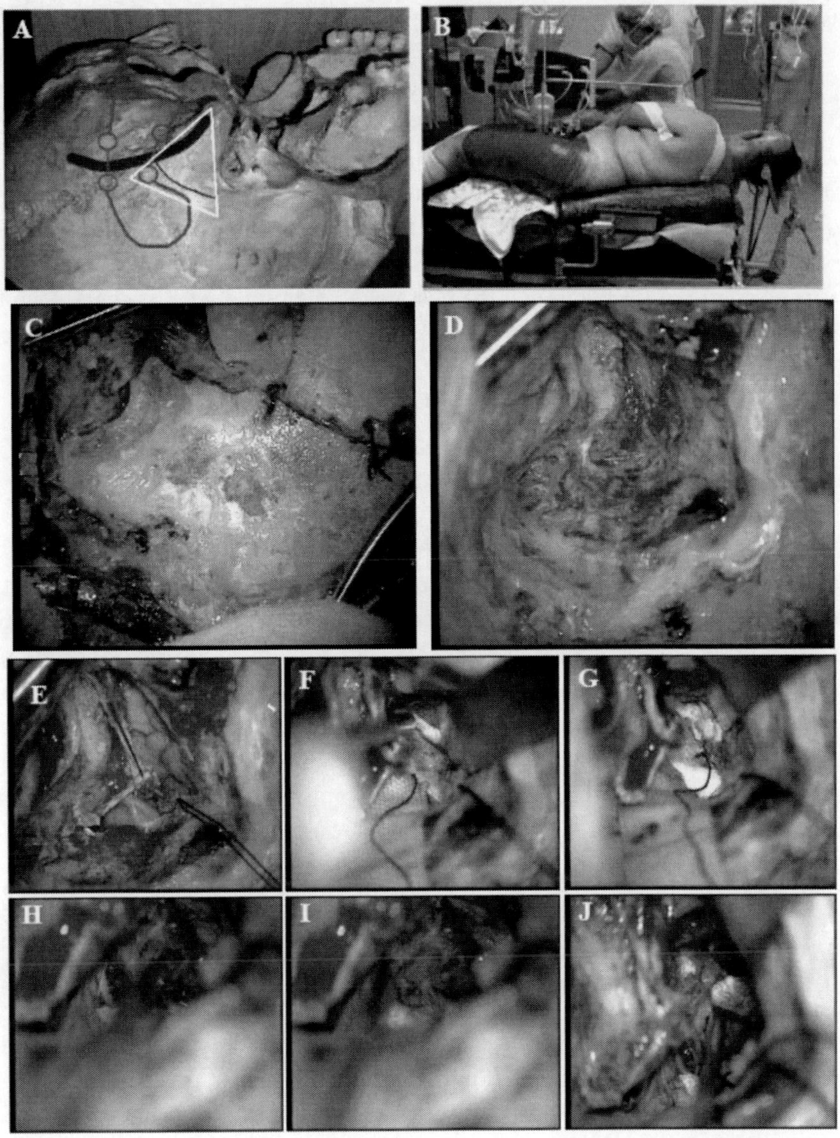


Figure 1. The small petrosal approach is a modification of the original presigmoid/petrosal approach. We have noted over the years that the main limiting factors for superior mobilization of the temporal lobe are the temporal draining veins, and the main limiting factor for posterior mobilization of the transverse-sigmoid sinus junction is the sigmoid sinus; therefore temporal and posterior fossa craniotomies in a petrosal approach (marked in red in A) do not add to the surgical exposure as the temporal draining veins and the sigmoid sinus cannot be sacrificed. Therefore, the small petrosal approach is only limited to the temporal bone dissection. The patient position is lateral, identical to the one used in the retrosigmoid approach (B). Transverse and sigmoid sinuses are skeletonized and a triangular area anterior to sigmoid sinus is exposed (C and D). After finishing the work with the bone, the temporal dura is opened parallel to the floor of the temporal fossa (E). The temporal lobe is gently elevated with retractors (arrow) and the tentorium is divided parallel to the petrous bone towards the trochlear nerve (F and G). Attention should be given to not damaging the trochlear nerve and vein of Labbé in this stage of the operation (H). This approach provides a more anterior view to the brainstem compared with the retrosigmoid approach (I and J).

The mastoid bony defect is then packed with fat graft, Gelfoam and thrombin/fibrinogen sealant to prevent CSF leakage. Muscle layer, subcutaneous tissue and skin are closed primarily. Most of the complications during the standard presigmoid approach occur during the retraction of the mobilized sigmoid sinus or while cutting the tentorium. Therefore, mobilization is limited in the small petrosal approach, which avoids some of the possible complications. Using this keyhole approach, functional structures within the petrous bone are spared and protected. The operative time is shorter than the standard presigmoid approach and due to the more limited exposure, complications related to the closure like CSF leaks are less common. The cosmetic result is fair and the postoperative bony defect is small. A comparably conservative strategy was also utilized by Fukushima and the "parapetrous approach" was devised [24].

## Surgical Outcomes

There is compelling evidence that an extensive resection is the optimal treatment for intracranial meningiomas. Simpson grade-I resections have been associated with significantly longer progression-free survival [5, 69]. However, it should be noted that a skull base approach is required for aggressive removal, which comes at the cost of increased complication rates. An acceptable compromise is gross-total resection of the tumor and coagulation of its dural-base, but even this goal is a considerable challenge for the surgeon (Figure 2). The most common causes of surgical failure in PCM surgery are: 1, hard consistency; 2, adherence to the brainstem; 3, adherence to the CNs; 4, encasement of perforating arteries; 5, cavernous sinus invasion; and 6, individual variations in the trigeminocardiac reflex that result in severe bradycardia. Brainstem infarctions, secondary to perforator or venous injury, and temporal or cerebellar infarctions, secondary to Labbé's vein or basilar occipital vein injury, are the most dreaded complications. Hematoma in the surgical bed may also be devastating, oftentimes related to hemorrhage from small veins that are collapsed during surgery (which can be avoided by performing maneuvers that increase the venous pressure at the end of the operation after completing meticulous hemostasis). Injury to lower CNs is another dreaded complication. CSF fistulas are common complications in surgeries that involve temporal bone drilling. Defects from the mastoid antrum may communicate through the Eustachian tube to result in fistula. A limited approach, meticulous waxing of the air cells, obliteration by fat and muscle, and use of vascularized fascial flaps, will significantly decrease the risk. Prophylactic lumbar drainage is not indicated.

PCM frequently invade surrounding anatomical structures including the middle cranial fossa, cavernous sinus, and Meckel's cave. This is marked for sphenopetroclival meningiomas in particular. Even bilateral cavernous sinus and sphenoid sinus invasion can be observed (Figure 3). Resection of the portion extending into the cavernous sinus is not possible in most cases and requires a second stage with an anterolateral exposure.

As indicated above, PCM are distinct from most meningiomas of other nearby locations such as the retromastoid meningiomas in the CPA. Although hyperostosis is frequently seen in a cerebellopontine angle, meningioma it is not observed in PCM. Similarly, a dural origin cannot be demonstrated, but rather the tumor presents with a wide firm attachment to the dura. It is also noted that meningiomas in the midline caudal basal skull base are enriched for the secretory variant that is associated with significantly higher pial invasion and peritumoral edema.

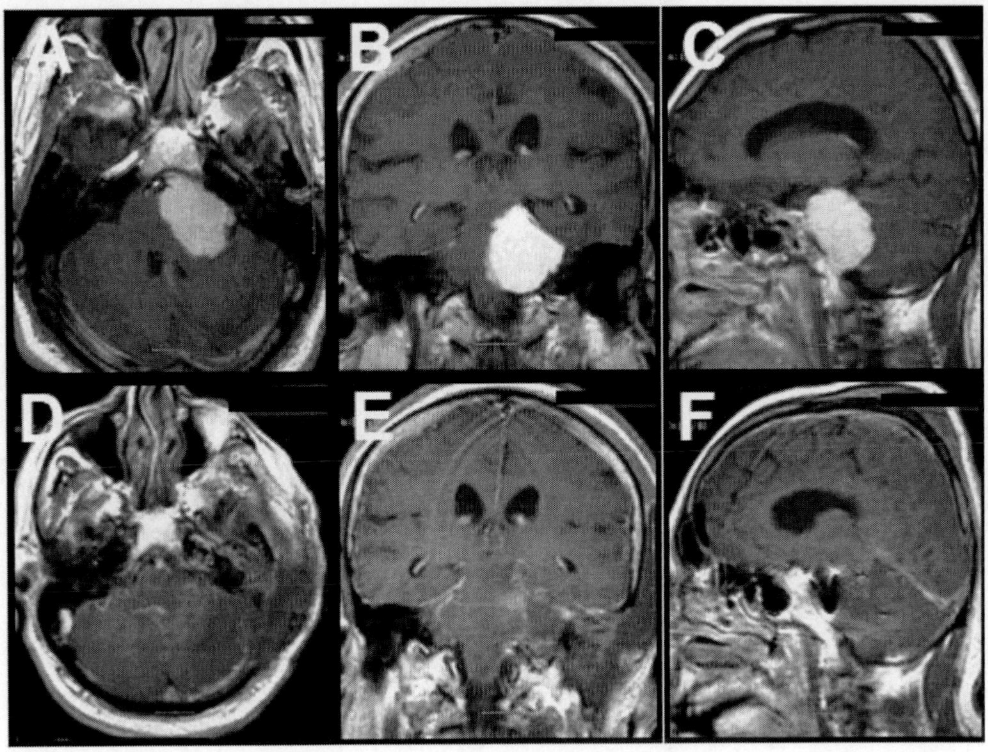


Figure 2. Preoperative contrast enhanced T1-weighted images of a left-sided petroclival meningioma reveal brainstem compression (A, B, C). The tumor was removed using a retrosigmoid approach (D, E, F).

The relation of the tumor to surrounding neurovascular structures including the brainstem and CNs is also variable and can take the form of impingement, displacement, adherence, encasement, and pial or intimal invasion. This invasion pattern of the meningioma is determined by its anatomical origin and intrinsic biology. The anatomical origin, above all, is of paramount importance, as demonstrated by Al-Mefty [2]. An arachnoidal plane between the tumor front and the confronted compartment (e.g., brainstem) will be to the advantage of the surgeon and facilitate safe resection. As expected, such a plane is not entirely present in a large tumor, which is one of the factors complicating the resection of large PCM.

The tumor impinging on the brainstem is encountered in the last stage of the operation and the temptation to remove this last piece of the tumor may risk injuring the brainstem, its perforators, or the small draining veins [65]. Preoperative evaluation of the interface between the tumor and the brainstem is therefore critical.

Brainstem edema on MRI is a good indicator of pial invasion, but is not exclusive. With current diagnostics, neither the consistency of the tumor nor its relation to surrounding neurovascular structures (impingement, displacement, adherence, encasement, and invasion) can be predicted preoperatively with enough confidence. Current neuromonitoring techniques also fall short of preemptive determination of any possible brainstem damage. Some authors advocate intentionally leaving a sheath of residual tumor on the brainstem to avoid brainstem injury, which is subsequently managed with radiosurgery [65].

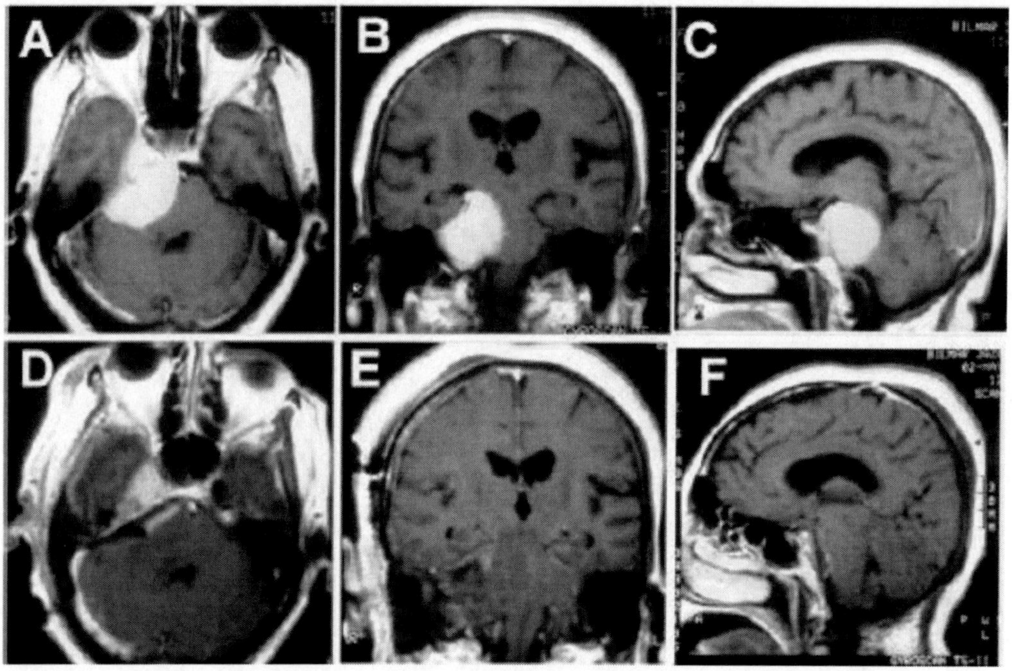


Figure 3. Preoperative contrast enhanced T1-weighted images of a right-sided sphenopetroclival meningioma reveal brainstem compression (A, B, C). The tumor was removed using a retrosigmoid approach (D, E, F) and the cavernous sinus portion was subsequently treated with Gamma-Knife radiosurgery.

## Radiosurgery

A complete surgical resection provides the patient with long-lasting well-being, and in many cases, practically a cure. However, this is not always possible. As observed in Table 1, total resection rates are still significantly low, even in the hands of most masterful surgeons. Some biological factors such as the origin of the tumor or problems from increasing size cannot be overcome with purely surgical strategies.

To avoid complications that can cripple patients for the rest of their lives, subtotal resections are commonly accepted. GKRS has emerged as an important adjunct in such cases. Tumor growth control rates well above 90% at 5 years has made Gamma-Knife an appealing candidate for pre-planned combinations of maximally safe resections and radiosurgery [6, 23, 34, 50, 59, 71, 72, 74]. For small and asymptomatic petroclival meningiomas GKRS is an attractive alternative to microsurgical excision. With larger tumors, the efficacy of radiosurgery decreases; volumetric size is the primary limiting factor for the efficiency of radiosurgery. In these patients, maximally safe resections both alleviate brainstem compression and decrease the volume of the tumor.

Results of radiosurgery for skull base tumors are widely reported, but studies reporting specific results on PCM are few. Nevertheless, the long-term results of radiosurgery on PCM are encouraging. One of the earliest studies on the subject was that of Roche et al. [59] in 2003 that reported the results on 32 patients with a mean follow-up of 56 months. In this study, tumor growth control was achieved in all patients, but neurological worsening due to brainstem vascular infarcts occurred in 6.3%.

Flannery et al. [23] published the long-term results of the Pittsburgh series of 168 PCM and reported 5- and 10-year tumor growth control rates of 91% and 86% respectively with a marginal dose of 13 Gy and median tumor volume of 6.1 mL. The most recent study on the radiosurgical management of petroclival meningiomas evaluated the results of 140 patients treated with upfront GKRS and 114 patients treated with GKRS as an adjuvant treatment after microsurgical excision [71]. The median follow-up in this report was 71 months, with 5-year and 10-year tumor growth control rates of 93% and 84% respectively using a mean marginal dose of 13.4 Gy for tumors with a median volume of 7.8 $cm^3$. This study used a multivariate analysis and concluded that smaller tumors, female patients, and those with no previous history of radiotherapy favored better.

## Conclusion

PCM, once considered inoperable, are treated routinely due to the advancements in microsurgery and skull base surgery. Modern management strategies also incorporate radiosurgery to minimize possible complications. Patient well-being is at the center of all current management strategies. Treatment strategies should be individualized, tailored to each patient and to the capabilities of the managing institution and surgeon.

## References

[1] Abdel Aziz KM, Sanan A, van Loveren HR, Tew JMJ, Keller JT and Pensak ML: Petroclival meningiomas: predictive parameters for transpetrosal approaches. *Neurosurgery* 47: 139, 2000.

[2] Al-Mefty O (2010) Overview of petroclival meningiomas. In *Meningiomas: Expert Consult - Online and Print, 1e* (eds Pamir MN, PMcL B and Fahlbush R), pp. 800. Saunders.

[3] Al-Mefty O, Ayoubi S and Smith RR: The petrosal approach: indications, technique, and results. *Acta Neurochir Suppl* (Wien) 53: 166, 1991.

[4] Al-Mefty O, Fox JL and Smith RR: Petrosal approach for petroclival meningiomas. *Neurosurgery* 22: 510, 1988.

[5] Almefty R, Dunn IF, Pravdenkova S, Abolfotoh M and Al-Mefty O: True petroclival meningiomas: results of surgical management. *J Neurosurg* 120: 40, 2014.

[6] Bambakidis NC et al. Evolution of surgical approaches in the treatment of petroclival meningiomas: a retrospective review. *Neurosurgery* 61: 202, 2007.

[7] Bambakidis NC et al. Evolution of surgical approaches in the treatment of petroclival meningiomas: a retrospective review. *Neurosurgery* 62: 1182, 2008.

[8] Brastianos PK et al. Genomic sequencing of meningiomas identifies oncogenic SMO and AKT1 mutations. *Nat Genet* 45: 285, 2013.

[9] Bricolo AP, Turazzi S, Talacchi A and Cristofori L: Microsurgical removal of petroclival meningiomas: a report of 33 patients. *Neurosurgery* 31: 813, 1992.

[10] Carvalho GA, Matthies C, Tatagiba M, Eghbal R and Samii M: Impact of computed tomographic and magnetic resonance im aging findings on surgical outcome in petroclival meningiomas. *Neurosurgery* 47: 1287, 2000.

[11] Castellano F and Ruggiero G: Meningiomas of the posterior fossa. *Acta Radiol suppl* 104: 1, 1953.

[12] Chamoun R, Krisht KM and Couldwell WT: Incidental meningiomas. *Neurosurg Focus* 31: E19, 2011.

[13] Chen LF, Yu XG, Bu B, Xu BN and Zhou DB: The retrosigmoid approach to petroclival meningioma surgery. *J Clin Neurosci* 18: 1656, 2011.

[14] Cherington M and Schneck SA: Clivus meningiomas. *Neurology* 16: 86, 1966.

[15] Cho CW and Al-Mefty O: Combined petrosal approach to petroclival meningiomas. *Neurosurgery* 51: 708, 2002.

[16] Clark VE et al. Genomic analysis of non-NF2 meningiomas reveals mutations in TRAF7, KLF4, AKT1, and SMO. *Science* 339: 1077, 2013.

[17] Couldwell WT, Fukushima T, Giannotta SL and Weiss MH: Petroclival meningiomas: surgical experience in 109 cases. *J Neurosurg* 84: 20, 1996.

[18] Cushing H and Eisenhardt L: Meningiomas: Their Classification, Regional Behavior, Life History, and Surgical End Results. 785, 1962.

[19] Dandy A, Delcour J and Laine E: Les meningiomas du clivus. *Neurochirurgie* 9: 249, 1963.

[20] Dechaume J and Wertheimer P: Les meningiomes retrosellaires. *Sud. Med. Chir.* 68: 1072, 1936.

[21] Diluna ML and Bulsara KR: Surgery for petroclival meningiomas: a comprehensive review of outcomes in the skull base surgery era. *Skull Base* 20: 337, 2010.

[22] Erkmen K, Pravdenkova S and Al-Mefty O: Surgical management of petroclival meningiomas: factors determining the choice of approach. *Neurosurg Focus* 19: E7, 2005.

[23] Flannery TJ et al. Long-term control of petroclival meningiomas through radiosurgery. *J Neurosurg* 112: 957, 2010.

[24] Fukushima T (1993) Comibined supra- infrapetrosal approach for petroclival lesions. In Surgery of cranial base tumors (eds Sekhar LN and Janecka IP), pp. 661-669. Lippincott raven, Philadelphia.

[25] Goel A: Extended lateral subtemporal approach for petroclival meningiomas: report of experience with 24 cases. *Br J Neurosurg* 13: 270, 1999.

[26] Goel A and Muzumdar D: Conventional posterior fossa approach for surgery on petroclival meningiomas: a report on an experience with 28 cases. *Surg Neurol* 62: 332, 2004.

[27] DW G: Surgical management of petrous apex meningioma. *Laryngoscope* 89: 204–213, 1979.

[28] Hakuba A, Nishimura S and Inoue Y: Transpetrosal-transtentorial approach and its application in the therapy of retrochiasmatic craniopharyngiomas. *Surg Neurol* 24: 405, 1985.

[29] Hakuba A, Nishimura S and Jang BJ: A combined retroauricular and preauricular transpetrosal-transtentorial approach to clivus meningiomas. *Surg Neurol* 30: 108, 1988.

[30] Hakuba A, Nishimura S, Tanaka K, Kishi H and Nakamura T: Clivus meningioma: six cases of total removal. *Neurol Med Chir* (Tokyo) 17: 63, 1977.

[31] Hallopeau H: Note sur deux faits de tumeur de mesocephale. Gaz Med (Paris) 3: 2, 1874.

[32] Ichimura S, Kawase T, Onozuka S, Yoshida K and Ohira T: Four subtypes of petroclival meningiomas: differences in symptoms and operative findings using the anterior transpetrosal approach. *Acta Neurochir* (Wien) 150: 637, 2008.

[33] Jung HW, Yoo H, Paek SH and Choi KS: Long-term outcome and growth rate of subtotally resected petroclival meningiomas: experience with 38 cases. *Neurosurgery* 46: 567, 2000.

[34] Kano H et al. Stereotactic radiosurgery for patients with trigeminal neuralgia associated with petroclival meningiomas. *Stereotact Funct Neurosurg* 89: 17, 2011.

[35] Kawase T, Shiobara R and Toya S: Anterior transpetrosal-transtentorial approach for sphenopetroclival meningiomas: surgical method and results in 10 patients. *Neurosurgery* 28: 869, 1991.

[36] Kawase T, Shiobara R and Toya S: Middle fossa transpetrosal-transtentorial approaches for petroclival meningiomas. Selective pyramid resection and radicality. *Acta Neurochir* (Wien) 129: 113, 1994.

[37] Kawase T, Toya S, Shiobara R and Mine T: Transpetrosal approach for aneurysms of the lower basilar artery. *J Neurosurg* 63: 857, 1985.

[38] King TT: Combined translabyrinthine-transtentorial approach to acoustic nerve tumours. *Proc R Soc Med* 63: 780, 1970.

[39] Kusumi M et al. Tentorial detachment technique in the combined petrosal approach for petroclival meningiomas. *J Neurosurg* 116: 566, 2012.

[40] Lang J: Skull Base and Related Structures: *Atlas of Clinical Anatomy*. 326, 1995.

[41] Ledinski G: Proceedings: experience with meningiomas in the posterior fossa. *Acta Neurochir* (Wien) 31: 284–285, 1975.

[42] Li D et al. Surgical management and outcomes of petroclival meningiomas: a single-center case series of 259 patients. *Acta Neurochir* (Wien) 155: 1367, 2013.

[43] Li PL, Mao Y, Zhu W, Zhao NQ, Zhao Y and Chen L: Surgical strategies for petroclival meningioma in 57 patients. *Chin Med J* (Engl) 123: 2865, 2010.

[44] Little KM, Friedman AH, Sampson JH, Wanibuchi M and Fukushima T: Surgical management of petroclival meningiomas: defining resection goals based on risk of neurological morbidity and tumor recurrence rates in 137 patients. *Neurosurgery* 56: 546, 2005.

[45] Mathiesen T, Gerlich A, Kihlstrom L, Svensson M and Bagger-Sjoback D: Effects of using combined transpetrosal surgical approaches to treat petroclival meningiomas. *Neurosurgery* 60: 982, 2007.

[46] Mayberg MR and Symon L: Meningiomas of the clivus and apical petrous bone. Report of 35 cases. *J Neurosurg* 65: 160, 1986.

[47] Morrison AW and King TT: Experiences with a translabyrinthine-transtentorial approach to the cerebellopontine angle. Technical note. *J Neurosurg* 38: 382, 1973.

[48] Nanda A, Javalkar V and Banerjee AD: Petroclival meningiomas: study on outcomes, complications and recurrence rates. *J Neurosurg* 114: 1268, 2011.
[49] Natarajan SK, Sekhar LN, Schessel D and Morita A: Petroclival meningiomas: multimodality treatment and outcomes at long-term follow-up. *Neurosurgery* 60: 965, 2007.
[50] Nicolato A et al. Gamma knife radiosurgery in meningiomas of the posterior fossa. Experience with 62 treated lesions. *Minim Invasive Neurosurg* 44: 211, 2001.
[51] Nishimura S, Hakuba A, Jang BJ and Inoue Y: Clivus and apicopetroclivus meningiomas--report of 24 cases. *Neurol Med Chir* (Tokyo) 29: 1004, 1989.
[52] Olivecrona H and Lysholm E: Die Chirurgische Behandlung der Gehirntumoren: *Eine Klinische Studie* (German Edition). 346, 1927.
[53] Oya S, Kim SH, Sade B and Lee JH: The natural history of intracranial meningiomas. *J Neurosurg* 114: 1250, 2011.
[54] Park CK, Jung HW, Kim JE, Paek SH and Kim DG: The selection of the optimal therapeutic strategy for petroclival meningiomas. *Surg Neurol* 66: 160, 2006.
[55] Perneczky A and Reisch R: Keyhole Approaches in Neurosurgery: Volume 1: *Concept and Surgical Technique*. 301, 2008.
[56] Reuss DE et al. Secretory meningiomas are defined by combined KLF4 K409Q and TRAF7 mutations. *Acta Neuropathol* 125: 351, 2013.
[57] Rhoton ALJ: The temporal bone and transtemporal approaches. *Neurosurgery* 47: S211, 2000.
[58] Roberti F, Sekhar LN, Kalavakonda C and Wright DC: Posterior fossa meningiomas: surgical experience in 161 cases. *Surg Neurol* 56: 8, 2001.
[59] Roche PH, Pellet W, Fuentes S, Thomassin JM and Regis J: Gamma knife radiosurgical management of petroclival meningiomas results and indications. *Acta Neurochir* (Wien) 145: 883, 2003.
[60] Rubin G, Herscovici Z, Laviv Y, Jackson S and Rappaport ZH: Outcome of untreated meningiomas. *Isr Med Assoc J* 13: 157, 2011.
[61] Sahm F et al. AKT1E17K mutations cluster with meningothelial and transitional meningiomas and can be detected by SFRP1 immunohistochemistry. *Acta Neuropathol* 126: 757, 2013.
[62] Samii M, Ammirati M, Mahran A, Bini W and Sepehrnia A: Surgery of petroclival meningiomas: report of 24 cases. *Neurosurgery* 24: 12, 1989.
[63] Samii M and Tatagiba M: Experience with 36 surgical cases of petroclival meningiomas. *Acta Neurochir* (Wien) 118: 27, 1992.
[64] Samii M, Tatagiba M and Carvalho GA: Resection of large petroclival meningiomas by the simple retrosigmoid route. *J Clin Neurosci* 6: 27, 1999.
[65] Seifert V: Clinical management of petroclival meningiomas and the eternal quest for preservation of quality of life: personal experiences over a period of 20 years. *Acta Neurochir* (Wien) 152: 1099, 2010.
[66] Seifert V, Raabe A and Zimmermann M: Conservative (labyrinth-preserving) transpetrosal approach to the clivus and petroclival region--indications, complications, results and lessons learned. *Acta Neurochir* (Wien) 145: 631, 2003.
[67] Sekhar LN, Jannetta PJ, Burkhart LE and Janosky JE: Meningiomas involving the clivus: a six-year experience with 41 patients. *Neurosurgery* 27: 764, 1990.

[68] Sekhar LN, Swamy NK, Jaiswal V, Rubinstein E, Hirsch WEJ and Wright DC: Surgical excision of meningiomas involving the clivus: preoperative and intraoperative features as predictors of postoperative functional deterioration. *J Neurosurg* 81: 860, 1994.

[69] SIMPSON D: The recurrence of intracranial meningiomas after surgical treatment. *J Neurol Neurosurg Psychiatry* 20: 22, 1957.

[70] Spetzler RF, Daspit CP and Pappas CT: The combined supra- and infratentorial approach for lesions of the petrous and clival regions: experience with 46 cases. *J Neurosurg* 76: 588, 1992.

[71] Starke R et al. Stereotactic radiosurgery of petroclival meningiomas: a multicenter study. J Neurooncol 119: 169, 2014.

[72] Starke RM, Williams BJ, Hiles C, Nguyen JH, Elsharkawy MY and Sheehan JP: Gamma knife surgery for skull base meningiomas. *J Neurosurg* 116: 588, 2012.

[73] Stone JL: Sir Charles Ballance: pioneer British neurological surgeon. Neurosurgery 44: 610, 1999.

[74] Subach BR, Lunsford LD, Kondziolka D, Maitz AH and Flickinger JC: Management of petroclival meningiomas by stereotactic radiosurgery. *Neurosurgery* 42: 437, 1998.

[75] Tahara A et al. Petroclival meningiomas: surgical management and common complications. *J Clin Neurosci* 16: 655, 2009.

[76] Tatagiba M, Samii M, Matthies C and Vorkapic P: Management of petroclival meningiomas: a critical analysis of surgical treatment. *Acta Neurochir Suppl* 65: 92, 1996.

[77] Tedeschi H and Rhoton ALJ: Lateral approaches to the petroclival region. *Surg Neurol* 41: 180, 1994.

[78] Ture U and Pamir MN: Small petrosal approach to the middle portion of the mediobasal temporal region: technical case report. *Surg Neurol* 61: 60, 2004.

[79] Van Havenbergh T, Carvalho G, Tatagiba M, Plets C and Samii M: Natural history of petroclival meningiomas. *Neurosurgery* 52: 55, 2003.

[80] Watanabe T, Katayama Y, Fukushima T and Kawamata T: Lateral supracerebellar transtentorial approach for petroclival meningiomas: operative technique and outcome. *J Neurosurg* 115: 49, 2011.

[81] Xiao X et al. Surgical resection of large and giant petroclival meningiomas via a modified anterior transpetrous approach. *Neurosurg Rev* 36: 587, 2013.

[82] Yamakami I, Higuchi Y, Horiguchi K and Saeki N: Treatment policy for petroclival meningioma based on tumor size: aiming radical removal in small tumors for obtaining cure without morbidity. *Neurosurg Rev* 34: 327, 2011.

[83] Yang J et al. Large and giant petroclival meningiomas: therapeutic strategy and the choice of microsurgical approaches - report of the experience with 41 cases. *Br J Neurosurg* 25: 78, 2011.

[84] Yang J, Ma SC, Fang T, Qi JF, Hu YS and Yu CJ: Subtemporal transpetrosal apex approach: study on its use in large and giant petroclival meningiomas. *Chin Med J* (Engl) 124: 49, 2011.

[85] Yaşargil MG, Mortara RW and Curcic M (1980) Meningiomas of basal posterior cranial fossa. In *Advances and technical standards in neurosurgery* (eds pp. 3-115. Springer.

[86] Yaşargil MG: Microneurosurgery IVa-b CNS tumors: surgical anatomy, neuropathology, neuroradiology, neurophysiology, clinical considerations, operability, treatment options. xv, 396, 1994.

[87] Zentner J, Meyer B, Vieweg U, Herberhold C and Schramm J: Petroclival meningiomas: is radical resection always the best option? *J Neurol Neurosurg Psychiatry* 62: 341, 1997.

[88] Zhu W, Mao Y, Zhou LF, Zhang R and Chen L: Keyhole approach surgery for petroclival meningioma. *Chin Med J* (Engl) 119: 1339, 2006.

In: Current Management of Central Nervous System … ISBN: 978-1-63483-856-6
Editors: Steven D. Chang and Anand Veeravagu 

*Chapter 4*

# COMPREHENSIVE TREATMENT OF CAVERNOUS SINUS MENINGIOMAS

***Koray Özduman, MD and M. Necmettin Pamir, MD***
Department of Neurosurgery, Acibadem University, School of Medicine,
Istanbul, Turkey

## ABSTRACT

Cavernous sinus Meningiomas (CSM) are defined as lesions that involve the sinus, originating in the cavernous sinus or from neighboring structures. Meningioma growth within the cavernous sinus can encompass vital structures, including cranial nerves and the internal carotid arteries. This results in a tumor that cannot always be treated definitely with surgery. As the understanding of CSM has progressed, successful treatment strategies have been developed. Gross total resection is achieved in a minority of patients as the degree of resection is dictated by the consistency, vascularity and anatomical extent of the tumor. Additionally, radiosurgical methods have been utilized in the treatment of CSM with significant success. Nevertheless, there is currently no consensus treatment paradigm for CSM. Small CSM with minimal mass effects are usually treated with primary radiosurgery. Encouraged by the satisfactory results of radiosurgery in small CSM, newer treatment strategies for larger CSM with significant mass effects combine maximal resection of the extra-cavernous portion with postoperative radiosurgery. Despite these advancements in CSM management, further quality evidence from prospective randomized controlled studies is among several other factors that are needed to help determine and establish optimal treatment strategies.

## INTRODUCTION

Among intracranial meningiomas, the management of cavernous sinus meningiomas (CSM) deserves special attention due to the complexity of the disease and its treatment. The cavernous sinus (CS) was not recognized as a primary site of origin in Cushing's initial classification of meningiomas [6], despite the long-recognized association of CSM with neurological complications. Other authors, however, such as Simpson, noted the difficulties and dilemmas in the management of CSM [41]. A renewed interest in CSM occurred after the 1980s, when the microsurgical anatomy of the cavernous sinus was studied in greater depth and after surgical approaches to this area were devised by pioneers such as Parkinson and Dolenc. In the last 50 years the understanding and treatment of CSM has undergone a remarkable evolution and is continuing to evolve today. This chapter will underline the fundamental concepts in understanding CSM and will guide the reader through the progression of modern treatment paradigms.

## Definition of CSM

The CS is an innately complex anatomical compartment with important neurovascular structures located within the confines of a few centimeters. It is defined as a parasellar anatomical compartment that is limited on all sides by dura mater. It contains the bilateral internal carotid arteries, the third, fourth, first two divisions of the fifth and sixth cranial nerves, the pericarotid sympathetic plexus, as well as a network of interconnected venous spaces [12]. The inferior and medial walls are formed as a continuum of the periosteal layer of the sellar dura. The superior and lateral walls are formed by fusion of the dural sheaths of the third, fourth and first division of the fifth cranial nerves in the embryological period. The complicated anatomy particular to the CS may be involved by meningiomas in different ways, allowing for its pathoanatomy to serve as the basis for CSM management.

There is a consensus among neurosurgeons to use the anatomical origin of meningiomas for classification [6, 10]. The origin is particularly important from a surgical point of view, as surgical success depends on understanding the pathological anatomy. This is influenced by the tumor's interaction with its surrounding neurovascular structures (impingement, displacement, adherence, encasement, invasion) [10]. The biology and growth pattern of meningiomas are comparable for most cases: Typical meningiomas arise at the dural side of arachnoidal cisterns, underneath the visceral dura, and grow slowly by expansion towards the area of least resistance (towards the parenchyma). The expansion against the surrounding arachnoid creates multiple arachnoidal planes between the tumor and surrounding neurovascular structures. This is to the advantage of the surgeon, as these planes facilitate protection of surrounding neurovascular structures if intra-arachnoidal dissection is used [10]. At this stage of meningioma growth, invasion of the surrounding tissues (e.g., dura, bone) by the meningioma is microscopic. Due to the slow growth of this benign tumor, the consequences of microscopic meningioma invasion become clinically important only after decades of undetected growth or at recurrence. Therefore, the clinical course is primarily dictated by the tumor mass growing at the initial cistern, creating individual anatomo-clinical entities (e.g., tuberculum sella, olfactory groove, cerebellopontine angle (CPA), petrous apex meningiomas with unique behavior, presentation, symptoms, treatments and outcome). With continuous expansile growth, meningiomas eventually grow or break beyond the borders of the initial cistern. At this instance, adherence to surrounding neurovascular structures is inevitable (e.g., distal vascular invasion in a tuberculum sella meningioma) [34]. An analogous situation occurs if the tumor point of origin is located at cisternal boundaries. Here, the relation between the "point of origin" and the individual anatomical variation in "cisternal borders" results in the absence of an arachnoid plane between the tumor and surrounding neurovascular structures. A striking example of this is seen through the behavior of anterior clinoid meningiomas, where orbital- or carotid-invasion is a consequence of the relation between the meningioma's point of origin and the individual variations in cisternal anatomy [10].

The variable nature of meningioma growth and character emphasizes the necessity to individualize the approach to cases. However, certain tendencies have been recognized. Meningiomas of the CS can result from primary CS lesions or they can be the product of invasion of tumors originating in neighboring structures, such as the clinoid or petroclival junction. Primary CSM initially grow within the CS, though they can also spread to surrounding structures. The resulting CS expansion leads to its impingement on the internal carotid artery (ICA) and cranial nerves within and at the walls of the CS. Due to the lack of arachnoidal planes within the CS, attachment to intracavernous structures is inevitable. Secondary CS involvement may be seen in anterior skull base meningiomas, meningiomas of the orbital apex, clinoidal meningiomas (clinocavernous), medial sphenoid wing meningiomas (sphenocavernous, sphenoclinoidocavernous), meningiomas of the middle fossa, including Meckel's cave meningiomas, meningiomas of the tentorial notch, petroclival meningiomas (PCM), CPA meningiomas and sphenopetroclival meningiomas.

The lateral wall of the CS is a strong barrier for meningioma invasion. Meningiomas originating at either side of this dural barrier (CSM and sphenoid wing meningiomas) grow at their site of origin without crossing to the other side in the vast majority of cases. Primary CSM growth within the CS can cause CS expansion but it will not break through the lateral CS wall. With such a strong anatomical barrier laterally, secondary invasion from primary CSM will be towards the orbit and petroclival region but not towards the sphenoid wing. Laterally situated meningiomas (e.g., medial sphenoid wing meningiomas) will typically involve the lateral cavernous component, without entering the medial cavernous component. When a meningioma reaches a particular size after decades of growth, it can be difficult to differentiate subtypes amongst one another. Moreover, distinguishing lesions with overlapping anatomic locations requires knowledge of the behavior that is characteristic to each lesion, as specific indicators will lead the physician to the exact diagnosis. For example, a large sphenopetroclival meningioma may be a primary CSM with secondary petroclival invasion or a primary PCM with secondary CS and sphenoid wing invasion (Figure 1). In this specific case, the potential lesions can be delineated. Primary CSM cannot invade the lateral wall of the CS as the primary PCM can. The primary PCM will invade anterior structures on both sides of the lateral CS wall, including the CS and middle fossa-sphenoid wing. The point of origin will dictate the clinical behavior of meningiomas, thus these subtle differences are of clinical significance.

## INCIDENCE AND CLINICAL PRESENTATION

The most common presenting symptom of a CSM is decreased vision in the ipsilateral eye. The incidence of this symptom varies between 23% and 54% among studies. A classical finding in CSM is disturbance of ocular movements. Proptosis and varying degrees of ocular movement limitations that range from complete opthalmplegia to slight functional disturbances may be observed.

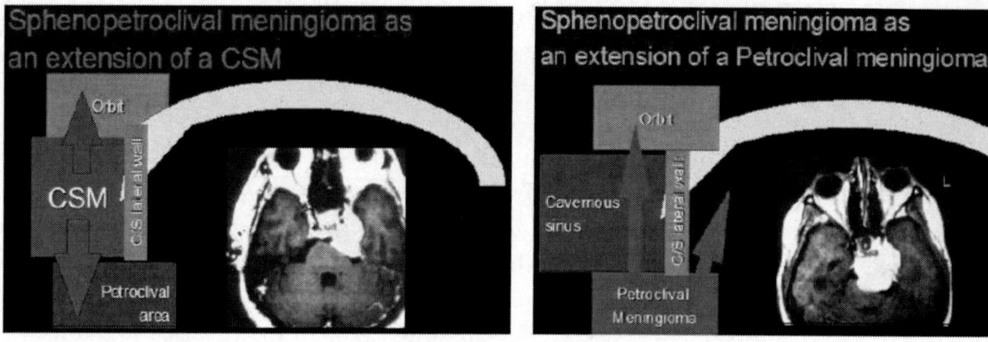


Figure 1. The cavernous sinus can be involved by a primary meningioma or can be secondarily invaded by nearby meningiomas (e.g., anterior clinoidal meningiomas, petroclival meningiomas, orbital meningiomas). In these cases the endpoint will be a sphenopetroclival meningioma. However, the growth pattern of the tumor will be determined by its origin. Pure CSM arise within the cavernous sinus and primarily expand within the cavernous sinus. However, the tumor can extend into the orbit or posterior fossa, but will not transgress the lateral cavernous sinus wall and extend into the sphenoid wing (left). In contrast, primary petroclival meningiomas may invade the cavernous sinus. The tumor will grow on both sides of the lateral cavernous sinus wall and will occupy both the cavernous sinus and the lateral side of the lateral cavernous sinus wall, growing in the sphenoid wing (right).

Trigeminal involvement, resulting in facial pain syndromes or sensory changes, is observed in a minority of patients. Headaches are present in roughly one third of patients. Other findings such as hemiparesis, mental changes or epilepsy are observed in an even smaller minority. Incidental CSM are commonly found during cranial radiological studies. Very few of the clinical studies on CSM treatment report the incidence of asymptomatic cases. Nakamura et al. [27] reported that CSM made up 17% of 41 incidentally found meningiomas. A quick glance at the published series indicates that the symptomatology differs slightly between meningiomas and non-meningial tumors of the CS [31].

The incidence of headache and double vision are higher in non-meningial tumors of the CS [31]. Radiology forms the backbone of diagnosis. MRI and CT are extremely important for both preoperative diagnosis and for surgical planning. Both studies are complementary for the correct diagnosis of skull based lesions. If there is a significant risk of internal carotid involvement, digital subtraction angiography can provide very valuable functional information.

## Surgical Anatomy

Due to the anatomical complexity of the CS and the pathoanatomical complexity of meningiomas in relation to this anatomy, the management of pathologies located within this neurovascular compartment is challenging. Currently there are no standards of care for such lesions and the best treatment paradigm is determined on a patient basis. In the last few decades we have experienced drastic changes in the understanding of the CS as a surgical target. The evolution in managing CSM is the most dramatic example, as CSM were once considered inoperable. With further advancements in anatomical awareness and surgically refined technical advancements, we now approach CSM with the matured understanding that it is surgically curable. Though an optimal treatment strategy for CSM does not exist, current treatment paradigms provide improvement in symptomatology and lasting tumor-growth control in the vast majority of cases without the need for functional sacrifice. However, the management of CSM has not reached its final maturation. A simple example lies in the current inability to reverse neurological deficits in most CSM cases, regardless of the form of treatment. Future strategies will certainly benefit from the growth of several factors such as our understanding of meningioma biology and the accumulation of quality scientific evidence from prospective randomized controlled trials to help guide decision-making. This chapter's aim is to give an overview of the current surgical management of CSM and its results.

## Historical Evolution of the CS Concept and Surgery

The historical evolution of the “cavernous sinus concept" is an excellent guide to understanding the management principles for CSM. The first description of this anatomical compartment was provided by Galen of Pergamon as a “vascular rete around the carotid artery in the neck” [33].

This conclusion was based on comparative anatomy knowledge, gained by dissections on lower vertebrae. Further studies came centuries later, in 1658, when Wepfer described that the carotid artery passed through a deep and conspicuous sinus during its course through the skull base. In 1685 Vieussens described the relation of cranial nerves to the outer walls of this venous compartment and in 1695 Ridley gave the first formally detailed anatomical description. The term “cavernous sinus” was first used by Winslow in 1734, as an analogy to the corpus cavernosum of the penis. In 1896 Krogius performed the first tumor removal from the CS and in 1937 Browder performed the first successful surgical electrocoagulation for a carotico-cavernous fistula [4].

Despite such individual achievements, lesions within the CS were then considered inoperable. The first direct and systematical surgical approach to the CS was performed by Parkinson in 1965 [32]. This was followed by several systematic studies on the microsurgical anatomy of the CS led by Taptas [43], Dolenc [11], Parkinson [32], and Umansky and Nathan [44]. Better appreciation of the microsurgical anatomy led to the description of novel surgical approaches. Hakuba et al. [17] described the combined orbitozygomatic infratemporal epidural and subdural approach in 1982. This was followed by the very popular frontotemporal epidural approach of Dolenc in 1983 [11].

Sekhar and Moller [36] reported the preauricular infratemporal approach in 1986 and Al-Mefty and Smith [2] reported the cranioorbitozygomatic approach and extended middle fossa zygomatic approaches in 1988. These approaches led the way to the popularization of CS surgery, and a new era in surgical treatment of CS lesions began. The start of the skull base era marked the appearance of reports describing high total resection rates and persistent decreases in mortality. With the popularization of MRI in postoperative evaluation, the optimistic findings of the CT era were called into question. It is now recognized that total resection of CSM is possible but that it can rarely be achieved for meningiomas that involve the CS proper.

## Pathological Differential Diagnosis

The CS may be involved by neoplastic, infectious, inflammatory processes and vascular pathologies. In general, roughly two thirds of CS masses are tumors and one fourth are vascular pathologies. Among neoplasias involving the CS, meningioma is the most commonly reported pathology in most modern series and they make up roughly two-thirds of all CS tumors. Meningiomas are followed by invasive pituitary adenomas, schwannomas and chordomas [31].

Sharply defined borders, isointensity both on T1W and T2W images, intense and homogenous contrast enhancement, presence of a dural tail, invasion (of and from) surrounding structures (such as the orbit, Meckel's cave, perimesencephalic cistern and the posterior fossa), hyperostosis of the surrounding bone, bone erosion, calcification within the tumor, encasement or narrowing of the ICA or pseudoaneurysm formation are radiological findings suggestive of a meningioma. As previously mentioned, the CS may be involved by meningiomas primarily or by secondary extension from meningiomas of neighboring structures.

## Therapeutic Decision-Making

There is no current consensus on the optimal management strategy for CSM as several treatment strategies continue to develop. The goal is to maintain or improve patient functionality, while providing long-term control of tumor growth and the clinical outcome of associated problems. Rational strategies are heavily dependent on the precise knowledge of CSM's disease biology, a topic that currently mandates greater understanding. A large proportion of CSM cases present with significant clinical symptomatology such as decreased vision, proptosis and disturbance in conjugated gaze. A significant proportion of cases are incidentally found on radiological studies. Nakamura et al. [27] analyzed 41 meningioma patients with incidentally found meningiomas and this cohort included 7 CSM patients. Patients were observed without interventions for a mean period of 43 months. From serial imaging studies, the authors calculated a mean absolute growth rate of 1.34 $cm^3$/yr and a mean tumor doubling time of 13.6 years. Similarly, to analyze the incidence of growth in incidentally found skull base meningiomas, Bindal et al. [3] observed 40 patients clinically for a mean of 83 months and radiologically for a mean of 76 months. During this follow-up, 7 patients (17%) experienced tumor growth and 11 patients (27.5%) experienced neurologic progression. These studies indicate that a significant proportion of CSM do progress and therefore treatment is recommended.

The treatment approach used is controversial. With the popularization and initial optimism surrounding skull base surgery, radical surgical excision of CSM was widely advocated. In the last decade, conservative approaches have gained popularity. Gamma Knife radiosurgery (GKS) has also emerged as an effective, safe alternative or adjuvant treatment modality. Current treatment options are radical surgical excision, extra-cavernous excisions with or without adjuvant radiosurgery, and primary radiosurgery in small CSM without significant mass effect. The rate of total resection in primary CSM is low. This is dictated by the invasive nature of meningiomas, their vascularity, and the common hard consistency. Attempts at resecting a tumor in such a tight space that contains highly fragile and extremely important neurovascular structure is naturally associated with significant surgical morbidity. Safe resection can be performed in a subset of meningiomas that have a soft consistency and poor vascularity. However, these cases constitute a minority and the information on these tumor characteristics can only be obtained during surgery. In a recent article, Sindou et al. [42] demonstrated that attempts at resection of the intracavernous component are associated with a significantly higher rate of visual impairment and cranial nerve morbidity relative to the resection of the extracavernous portion exclusively. This inspired several authors to plan alternative treatment strategies to achieve maximal safe resection of the tumor outside the CS, with or without adjuvant radiosurgery. The aim of such treatment combinations is to debulk the tumor to a size that can be safely treated with radiosurgery, which is used to obtain long-term tumor growth control. Several publications have indicated that this is an acceptable strategy with good short-term results, while also allowing for the avoidance of high complication rates particular to aggressive surgical treatment strategies. One study in the literature compares the results of aggressive surgical excision to those of maximally safe extracavernous resections combined with GKS [30]. This study concluded that extracavernous resection followed by GKS is as effective as radical surgery and that the third-year tumor volume growth control and cranial nerve outcome are better in the combination treatment group [30].

At our institution GKS became available in 1997 and we have changed our treatment paradigm to the resection of the extracavernous part followed by immediate adjuvant radiosurgery. The study was a retrospective comparison of these two periods when two different management strategies were used in the same clinic.

Other centers have also reported similar experiences [1, 13, 14]. There are varying opinions on the timing of radiosurgery. While some advocate immediate postoperative use, others choose to use it in the case of radiologically documented volumetric growth or symptomatic recurrence. Since the combination of maximally safe surgery with adjuvant radiosurgery is a fairly recent concept, long-term results are still not available. There are no prospective randomized studies to compare the results of maximally safe surgery, thus making it difficult to evaluate the benefits of added adjuvant radiosurgery. Small but symptomatic CSM can be successfully treated with radiosurgery alone, providing adequate short-term tumor growth control and minimal morbidity.

Secondary CS involvement may be seen in the meningiomas of the tuberculum sella, clinoidal, medial sphenoid wing, and sphenopetroclival meningiomas. Secondary CS involvement significantly decreases the chance of good surgical results in such cases unless the invasion is confined to the lateral wall of the CS. Less radical strategies for secondary CS involvement have been reported in recent literature and do not significantly differ from those of primary CSM.

## Surgical Approach

Because of the aforementioned complexities involved with treating lesions of the CS, CSM lack a standardized treatment approach. The choice of approach depends on the nature and biology of the lesion, its extension within and outside the CS, and on the surgical aim.

Lesions located in the anterior compartment of the CS are best treated with the basic frontotemporal extra-intradural approach. The frontotemporal epidural-subdural approach was first described by Dolenc and forms the foundation of all anterolateral approaches to the CS. Modifications and variations on the technique have been devised by several authors, most notably Hakuba, Dolenc and Kawase [11, 17]. For a majority of non-meningeal tumors of the CS, which are located within the lateral wall of the CS, an epidural approach is sufficient (Figure 2).

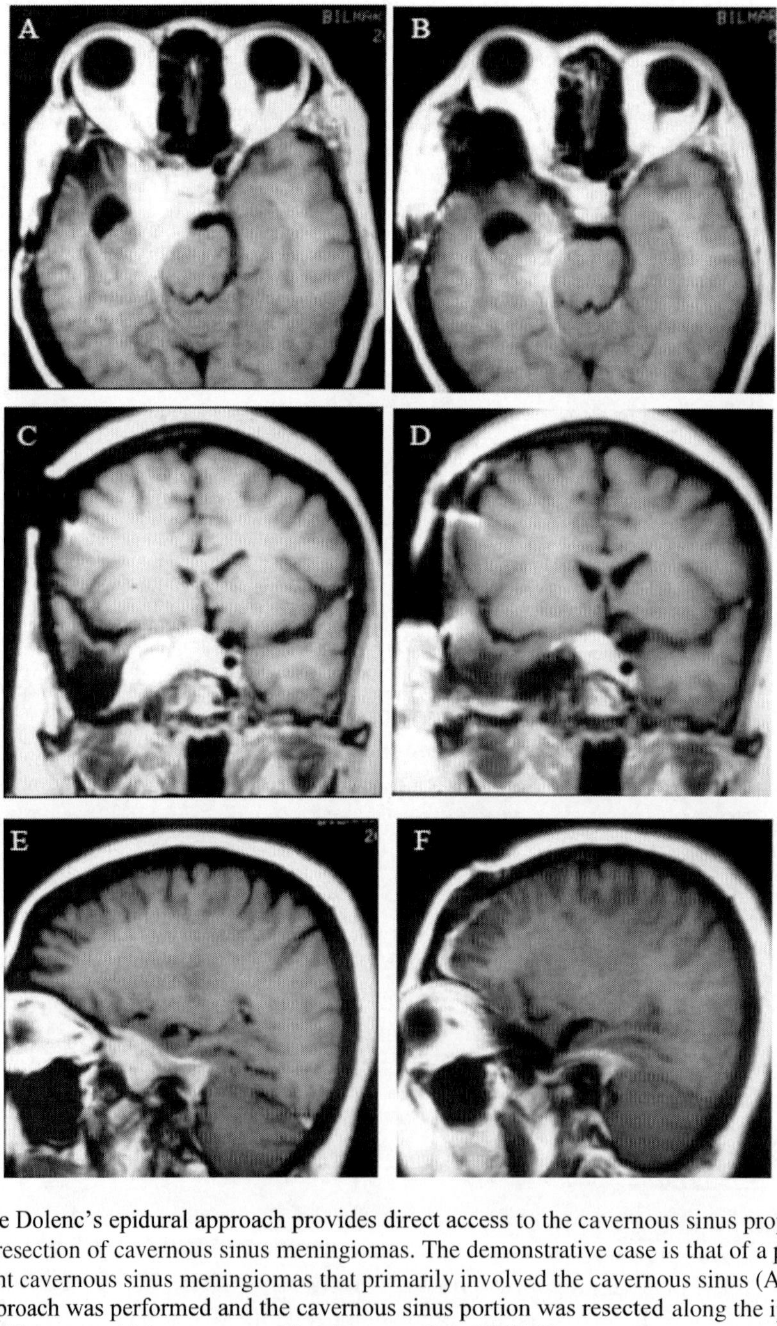


Figure 2. The Dolenc's epidural approach provides direct access to the cavernous sinus proper and is suitable for resection of cavernous sinus meningiomas. The demonstrative case is that of a previously operated right cavernous sinus meningiomas that primarily involved the cavernous sinus (A, B, C). A Dolenc's approach was performed and the cavernous sinus portion was resected along the ipsilateral internal carotid artery, which was trapped for this procedure (D, E, F).

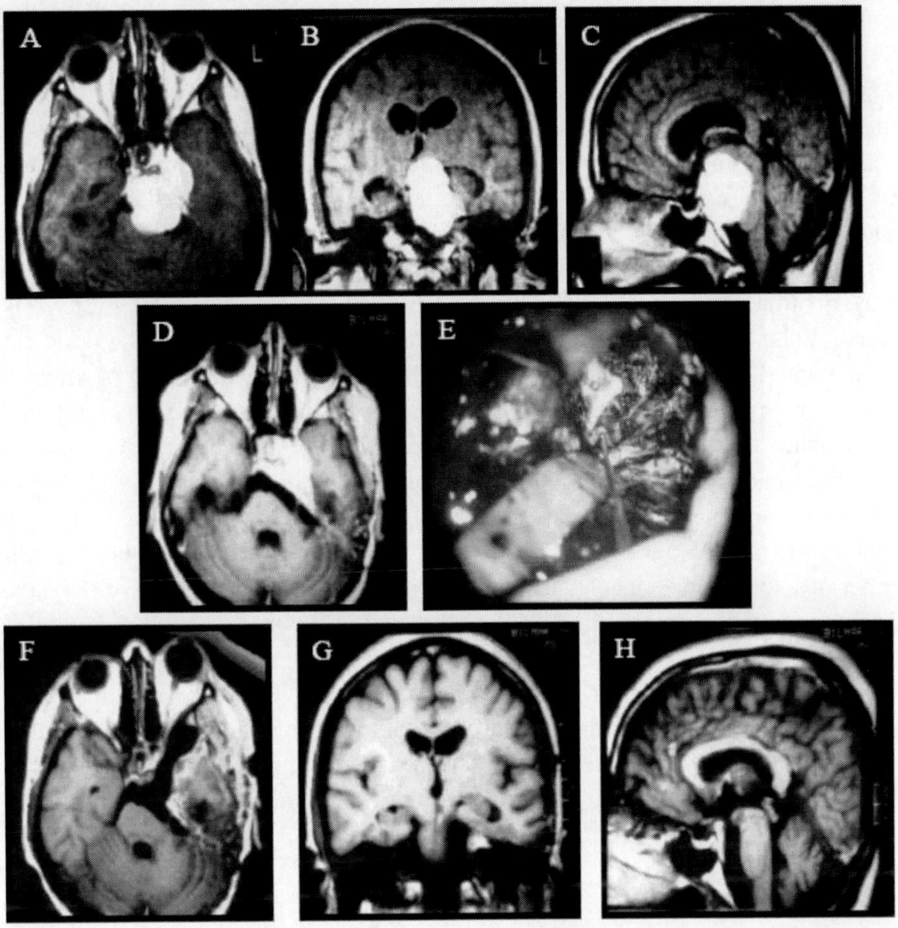


Figure 3. For extensive cavernous sinus meningiomas that involve both the cavernous sinus and surrounding anatomical areas, staged procedures are usually performed. Demonstrated here is a left petroclival meningiomas that secondarily involved the left sided cavernous sinus (A, B, C). Postoperative imaging demonstrated successful resection of the posterior fossa component (D). In a second procedure using a left-sided Dolenc's approach (E) the remaining cavernous sinus component was resected resulting in gross total resection of the entire sphenopetroclival meningioma (F, G, H).

Meningiomas, on the contrary, are frequently located within the CS proper. In these cases, exposure of the CS walls is followed by intradural access through various "safe surgical corridors", called CS triangles. For a description of these CS triangles, the reader can refer to an extensive and systematic review by Fukushima [15]. For meningiomas extending into the petroclival area or the posterior fossa, combined approaches (such as with the transpetrosal approach) are recommended (Figure 3).

The Dolenc approach is a frontotemporal craniotomy, which also combines exposure and splitting of the dura at the superior orbital fissure to gain an epidural access to the lateral wall of the CS. The Hakuba approach similarly exposes the CS purely extradurally while the Kawase approach involves a frontotemporal-orbitozygomatic craniotomy (or alternatively a simple temporal craniotomy). Proposed modifications are based on use of different skin flaps, different scalp flap dissections, and different osteotomies. The core operation can be modified by a combination with a transpetrosal approach for CSM extending posteriorly.

The frontotemporal craniotomy is extended using zygomatic and orbital osteotomies to maximize the low lateral retraction of the temporal muscle, helping gain additional fronto-basal to superior viewing angle. This can be further improved by the removal of the orbital rim. In the basic frontotemporal epidural approach, the craniotomy is followed by drilling of orbital roof and exposing the periorbita. Special attention must be paid to avoid damaging the periorbita. The dorsal surface of the superior orbital fissure is then exposed in its entirety. The dural fold extending from the temporal dura, through the superior orbital fissure to the periorbit is then incised from its lateral aspect. This helps obtain a plane of dissection between the two layers of the lateral wall of the CS, and the dural reflection is peeled posteriorly from cranial nerve V(1). The next step in the CS exploration is the opening of the optic canal by removing the anterior clinoidal process. This can be performed extradurally or after opening the dura and cisternal cerebrospinal fluid (CSF) drainage. Although there is no systematically collected evidence to support either method, anecdotal reports have indicated that injury to the optic nerve can occur in extradural clinoidectomy but not with an intradural approach. In either approach, the anterior clinoidal process is removed using a diamond drill. Drilling starts at the center of the anterior clinoidal process and is performed under constant irrigation for short periods, to minimize mechanical and thermal injury to the optic nerve. Variations on the bony anatomy of the anterior clinoid process are encountered where the internal carotid process is encircled by bone. Therefore the anterior clinoidal process should be skeletonized and be gently broken but never extracted in one piece. Exposure of the optic canal simultaneously exposes the clinoidal and the ophthalmic segments of the ICA and the distal dural ring. The extradural exposure advances with drilling of the temporal bone and further peeling of the CS lateral wall outer leaf, towards the Gasserian ganglion. Cranial nerve V(3) is exposed at the foramen rotundum.

The middle meningeal artery is sectioned and coagulated at the foramen spinosum, which is then plugged. The greater petrosal nerve is exposed and protected to avoid the risk of xeropthalmia.

The majority of meningiomas are not confined to the interdural layer at the lateral wall of the CS. Therefore the pure epidural approach is seldom sufficient for meningioma resection. Extension into surrounding structures such as the optic canal, orbit, sella, Meckel's cave and the posterior fossa are addressed with slight modifications of the basic approach. The hard consistency of meningiomas and their rich vascular supply further complicate the surgery.

Furthermore, meningiomas can encircle, encase and invade the adventitia of the ICA. The ICA can be encased and invaded within the CS, in the C4 segment. Attempts at resection of the intracavernous part are associated with a significant risk of ICA rupture. A postoperative major disabling stroke is reported in roughly 5% of CSM cases [7, 8, 19].

To predict this risk preoperatively, Sekhar and Altschuler classified intracavernous neoplasms into five grades, depending on the number of areas involved and the degree of encasement of the ICA (Hirsch Grade) [38]. If such an intracavernous resection is planned, proximal and distal vascular control is necessary. Proximal control can be obtained by an exposure of the petrous segment of the ICA. This requires the unroofing of the petrous carotid canal posterior to foramen ovale and medial to foramen spinosum. Distal control can be obtained after sylvian dissection, proximal to the posterior communicating artery in the ophthalmic segment.

Preoperative workup with digital subtraction angiography and a balloon occlusion test should be performed in cases with high risk of ICA involvement. The balloon occlusion test can also be combined with SPECT imaging or Xenon blood flow studies to increase its reliability. In the end, patients are stratified to groups of low-intermediate and high risk of neurological complications after a possible carotid takedown.

## Radiosurgery for CSM

GKS has obtained general acceptance in the management of various skull base pathologies in the last 2 decades. The treatment goal of GKS is fundamentally different from that of surgical intervention. In most anatomical locations, surgery alleviates mass effect and decreases tumor burden to decrease the chances of recurrence. On the contrary, the primary aim of radiosurgery is to prevent present and future tumor growth.

For skull base meningiomas, the radiation dose has significant clinical implications. Although high doses provide adequate tumor growth control, the risk of side effects increases with an increasing dose. Conversely, low marginal doses are associated with an increased risk of treatment failures. Initial high doses of 18-20 Gy were in time abandoned and current treatment strategies recommend marginal doses of 14-15 Gy.

Today there is no level-1 evidence to guide the treatment decision for CSM. Most authors agree that small CSM should be treated with radiosurgery once the diagnosis is ascertained to a certain degree. MRI and CT studies provide much of this required evidence. For large CSM or those that involve the CS secondarily, most current treatment strategies favor maximally safe resection combined with adjuvant GKS [42]. Some authors favor waiting after resecting the extra-cavernous portion, and thus postpone adjuvant treatment until documented regrowth [42].

## Clinical Outcomes

### *Surgical Mortality and Morbidity*

With advancements in the last several decades, the mortality associated with CS surgery has decreased significantly (Table 1). Today, CS explorations can be performed with mortality rates comparable to other common neurosurgical procedures. The risk of surgical morbidity in the recent literature is within the range of 5%. However, rates as high as 61% have also been reported. Invasive skull base approaches are associated with significant morbidity.

The most feared adverse events are cerebrovascular. Major disabling strokes due to ICA closure were observed in about 5% of the cases. Venous complications are less predictable and are catastrophic in most cases. In subtemporal approaches, temporal lobe edema or venous infarctions can be life threatening. Hematomas in the surgical cavity or postoperative hydrocephalus are also reported. Diabetes insipidus can be observed after CS surgery but is transient in most cases. CSF leaks are a significant complication of skull base surgery. It is also critically important to the pack the air sinuses with muscle tissue during surgery. CSF leaks can also result after drilling of pneumatized anterior clinoid processes.

### *Vision Outcome*

Preoperative visual deficits are common in CSM. Compromised vision in the ipsilateral eye has been reported in 24-80% of patients with CSM [9, 16, 20, 22, 26, 29]. The deficit is attributed to both physical compression by the large tumor, the impingement of the optic nerve at the falciform ligament, and to vascular compromise. Decompression of the optic nerve may improve vision. Among all cranial nerve functions, optic nerve function stands alone in having possible significant improvement after CS surgery. However, iatrogenic worsening in vision can also be encountered with or without pre-existing and preoperative visual impairment. Injury to the microvasculature around the optic nerve, vasospasm and direct mechanical injury to the optic nerve during anterior clinoid removal have been suspected as the cause. Several studies have drawn attention to heat damage related to the use of a diamond drill [12]. In large tumors, attempts at extradural removal of the anterior clinoid process may put extra tension on the already impinged optic nerve. In a retrospective analysis, Yonekawa et al. [45] found a 10% risk of postoperative visual dysfunction in cases where the anterior clinoid was removed extradurally, while no dysfunction was noted in intradurally resected cases. A comparable rate of postoperative optic nerve damage (7%) was reported in a large series that utilized extradural anterior clinoid removal [28]. Many studies have not reported such dysfunction, as it can be easily missed clinically without dedicated assessment.

### *Cranial Nerve Outcome*

Existing cranial nerve deficits do not improve in the majority of CSM cases regardless of the mode of treatment. Improvement in cranial nerve function is rare after CS exploration and there is a significant risk of transient or permanent cranial nerve morbidity. The most common complication after CS exploration is a cranial nerve VI palsy. Reports indicate that preoperative deficits in abducens nerve function do not improve after surgery. Worsening of cranial nerve VI function, on the contrary, is common and has been reported in up to 76% of patients who did not have preoperative dysfunction. These deficits improved in 50% of patients but persisted in others. Occulomotor nerve palsy also commonly complicates CS exploration.

As in abducens nerve function, preoperative deficits rarely improve after surgery. Novel third nerve deficits are common after CS exploration. Reports have concluded that the severity of this deficit is also predictive of its prognosis. The majority of cases with incomplete third nerve palsies improve in time. Complete deficits are far less likely to improve [23]. Trigeminal nerve dysfunction is also observed after CS surgery and xeropthalmia is the most significant complication. This complication rarely improves over time and must be treated aggressively to prevent corneal ulcerations. The surgical cranial nerve complication rate is not the same in all CS pathologies. The risk of cranial nerve morbidity is higher in meningiomas due to their invasive nature, their frequently hard consistency, and their highly vascular nature.

Improvement in cranial nerve function in CSM is seen after GKS in a small but significant proportion of patients. Kano et al. reported a very large series from the University of Pittsburgh and have shown that the chances of cranial nerve recovery is worse if the patients have had previous surgery. However, this is not unexpected due to the bias in patient selection (larger tumors are selected for surgery, higher doses for patients treated before 1987). It must be kept in mind that new cranial nerve deficits are also not uncommon after radiosurgery (Table 2).

### Table 1. Major surgical series of cavernous sinus meningiomas

| Study | n | Gross total resection (%) | Detection method | Surgical mortality (%) | Cranial nerve morbidity (%) | Surgical morbidity (%) | Vision | CN III | CN IV | CNVI | CNV | Persistent growth or regrowth (%) | Follow-up period |
|---|---|---|---|---|---|---|---|---|---|---|---|---|---|
| Hakuba et al. 1982 [17] | 4 | N/A | Surgeon's impression | 8 | 23 | 8 | | | | | | | |
| Lesoin et al, 1985 [25] | 16 | 0 | | 0 | 25 | 0 | | | | | | | |
| Sekhar and Moller, 1986 [36] | 2 | 100 | Surgeon's impression | 0 | 50 | 0 | | | | | | | |
| Cioffi et al. 1987 [5] | 12 | 8.3 | | 0 | 0 | 25 | | | | | | | |
| Al-Mefty and Smith, 1988 [2] | 14 | 79 | | 6 | 22 | 50 | | | | | | | |
| Hakuba et al. 1989 [18] | 4 | "Extremely radical" | Surgeon's impression | 0 | 50 | 25 | | | | | | | |
| Sepehrnia et al. 1991 [40] | 26 | 69 | | 3.7* | N/A | N/A | | | | | | | |
| Sekhar and Altschuler, 1991 [38] | 45 | 82.2 | Postoperative radiology | 0 | N/A | N/A | N/A | N/A | N/A | N/A | N/A | 8.9 | N/A |
| Sekhar and Altschuler, 1991 [38] | 48 | 89 | | 0 | N/A | 47 | | | | | | | |
| Sekhar, et al. 1993 [39] | 70 | 87 | | 1.5 | 52* | 49* | | | | | | | |
| Risi et al. 1994 [35] | 15 | 27 | | 12 | 32 | 20 | | | | | | | |
| DeMonte et al. 1994 [9] | 41 | 76 | | 7.3 | 18 | 12 | 15% better 85% same | 13% worse 7% better 79% same | 5% worse 91 %same | 11% worse 33% better 56% same | 16% worse | 13.15 | 3.75y |

**Table 1. (Continued)**

| Study | n | Gross total resection (%) | Detection method | Surgical mortality (%) | Cranial nerve morbidity (%) | Surgical morbidity (%) | Vision | CN III | CN IV | CNVI | CNV | Persistent growth or regrowth (%) | Follow-up period |
|---|---|---|---|---|---|---|---|---|---|---|---|---|---|
| Cusimano et al. 1995 [7] | 124 | 80 | | 0 | N/A | 6.5 | | | | | | 10 | 2.42y |
| Larson et al, 1995 [24] | 26 | 63 | | 0 | 5 | 5 | | | | | | | |
| Knosp et al. 1996 [23] | 29 | 21 | | 10 | 41 | 5 | 0% worse | 14% worse 43% better | 58%worse 0% better | 4% worse 50%better | 21%worse 7% better | 11 | 3mo-7y |
| Kim et al. 1996 [21] | 21 | 47 | | 9.5 | 43 | 61 | | | | | | | |
| Sekhar et al. 1996 [37] | 114 | 78 | N/A | 0.8 | N/A | 26 | | | | | | | Median 3.9y |
| De Jesus et al. 1996 [8] | 119 | 61 | | N/A | N/A | N/A | | | | | | 11.76 | Mean 2.82y |
| O'Sullivan et al. 1997 [29] | 39 | 20 | Surgeon's impression | 0 | 17.9 | N/A | 6% worse 24% better | 18% worse 21% better | | | | 10.25 | Mean 2y |
| Klink et al. 2000 [22] | 29 | 3 | | | 27.6 | | 48% worse | 28% worse 4% better | | | | 62 | Mean 13.6 y |
| Dolenc and Rogers, 2003 [12] | 388 | 46 | | 1 | 9 | 5 | | | | | | N/A | N/A |
| Heth et al. 2003 [19] | 163 | 44 | N/A | N/A | N/A | N/A | N/A | N/A | N/A | N/A | N/A | N/A | N/A |
| Abdel-Aziz et al. 2004 [1] | 38 | 63.2 | MRI at 1 month | 0 | 16 | N/A | | | | | | 10.5 | Mean 8y |
| Sindou et al. 2007 [42] | 100 | 12 | Surgeons impression and CT at 3 months | 5 | 33 | 5 | 19% worse 16% better 60% same | 29% worse 6% better 60% same | 15% worse 6% better 74% same | 17% worse 4% better 74% same | 24% worse 7% better 64% same | 13.25 | Mean 8.3y (3-20 y) |

All tumors included in the analysis.

**Table 2. Radiosurgery series on cavernous sinus meningiomas**

| Study | n (primary treatment) | Median peripheral dose | Median follow-up time | Actuarial tumor growth control rates 5 and 10 years | New cranial nerve complication rate |
|---|---|---|---|---|---|
| Morita et al. 1999 | 88 | 16Gy* | 35mo | 95% at 5 years | 10.2% |
| Liscak et al. 1999 | 67 | 12Gy** | 19mo | ? | 3.8% |
| Roche et al. 2000 | 80 | 28Gy** | 30.5mo | 92.8% at 5 years | 5.8% |
| Shin et al. 2001 | 40 | 14Gy | 42mo | 82.3 at 10 years | 20% |
| Spiegelmann 2002 | 36 | 13.5Gy** | 36mo | 97.5% at 5 years | 7.5% |
| Nicolato 2002 | 156 | 14.8Gy* | 48.9mo | 96.5 at 5 years | 1% |
| Lee 2002 | 159 | 26Gy** | 35mo | 93.1% and 93.1% | 9% |
| İwai 2003 | 42 | 11Gy** | 22mo | 92% at 5 years | 4.8% |
| Maruyama et al. 2004 | 40 | 16Gy* | 47mo | 94.1% at 5 years | 13% |
| Pamir et al. 2005 | 26 | 15Gy* | 52mo | 100% at 3 years | 0 |
| Pollock et al. 2005 | 49 | 15.9Gy* | 58mo | 80-85% at 5 years | 10% |
| Kuo et al. 2004 | 57 | 15Gy** | 42mo | 97% at 5 years | 2.2% |
| Hasegawa et al. 2007 | 111 | 13Gy** | 62mo | 87% and 73% | 5% |
| Kimball et al. 2009 | 49 | 14Gy* | 50mo | 100% and 98% | 3.5% |
| Skeie et al. 2010 | 92 | 12Gy* | 82mo | 94% and 91% | 2% |
| Spiegelmann et al. 2010 | 102 | 13.5Gy* | 67mo | 98% at 5 years | 5% |
| Kano et al. 2013 | 303 | 13Gy* | 60mo | 92% and 85% | 14% |
| Dos Santos et al. 2012 | 88 | 14Gy* | 67mo | 92.5% and 82.5% | 12.5% |
| Pollock et al. 2013 | 115 | 16Gy* | 89mo | 99% and 93% | 12% |

*median ** mean.

***Recurrence of CSM***

When compared with meningiomas in other anatomical locations, the recurrence rate reported for CSM is relatively low. Although the follow-up period varies among studies, reported recurrence rates range from 10-13.3% after surgery alone (2-8.3 years mean follow-up period) and 6-13.6% after radiosurgery (1.6-4.12 years mean follow-up period). Sindou et al. [42] compared the recurrence rates after surgery alone to surgery with adjuvant radiotherapy and found no significant difference. There was no statistically significant difference in recurrence between the cases that underwent resection of only the extracavernous portion and those that underwent a subtotal resection of the intracavernous tumor. Meningiomas are known to be slow growing and recurrences of CSM are expected several years after surgical resection [22, 42].

## CONCLUSION

Today, CSM can be surgically resected with an acceptable mortality rate. A Simpson grade I or II resection is not possible. Gross total resection is possible but can only be achieved in a small minority of patients. The degree of resection is dictated by the consistency, vascularity and anatomical extent of the tumor. Preexisting cranial nerve deficits rarely improve after surgery and novel (transient or persistent) cranial nerve morbidity is high. Improvement or stabilization of vision is frequently achieved, especially if it is present in the contralateral eye. Encouraged by the satisfactory results of radiosurgery in small CSM, newer treatment strategies combine maximal resection of the extracavernous portion with postoperative radiosurgery. Quality evidence from prospective randomized controlled studies are needed to determine the optimal treatment strategy.

## REFERENCES

[1] Abdel-Aziz KM et al. Large sphenoid wing meningiomas involving the cavernous sinus: conservative surgical strategies for better functional outcomes. *Neurosurgery* 54: 1375, 2004.

[2] Al-Mefty O and Smith RR: Surgery of tumors invading the cavernous sinus. Surg Neurol 30: 370, 1988.

[3] Bindal R, Goodman JM, Kawasaki A, Purvin V and Kuzma B: The natural history of untreated skull base meningiomas. *Surg Neurol* 59: 87, 2003.

[4] Browder J: Treatment of carotid artery-cavernous sinus fistula. Report of a case. *Arhives of Opthalmology* 37: 95, 1937.

[5] Cioffi FA, Bernini FP, Punzo A, Natale M and Muras I: Cavernous sinus meningiomas. *Neurochirurgia* (Stuttg) 30: 40, 1987.

[6] Cushing H and Eisenhardt L: Meningiomas: Their Classification, Regional Behavior, Life History, and Surgical End Results. 785, 1962.

[7] Cusimano MD et al. The results of surgery for benign tumors of the cavernous sinus. *Neurosurgery* 37: 1, 1995.

[8] De Jesus O, Sekhar LN, Parikh HK, Wright DC and Wagner DP: Long-term follow-up of patients with meningiomas involving the cavernous sinus: recurrence, progression, and quality of life. *Neurosurgery* 39: 915, 1996.

[9] DeMonte F, Smith HK and al-Mefty O: Outcome of aggressive removal of cavernous sinus meningiomas. *J Neurosurg* 81: 245, 1994.

[10] DeMonte F, McDermott MW and Al-Mefty O: *Al-Mefty's Meningiomas*. 448, 2011.

[11] Dolenc V: Direct microsurgical repair of intracavernous vascular lesions. *J Neurosurg* 58: 824, 1983.

[12] Dolenc V and Rogers L: *Microsurgical anatomy and surgery of the central skull base*. 2003.

[13] Duma CM, Lunsford LD, Kondziolka D, Harsh GR and Flickinger JC: Stereotactic radiosurgery of cavernous sinus meningiomas as an addition or alternative to microsurgery. *Neurosurgery* 32: 699, 1993.

[14] Friedlander RM, Ojemann RG and Thornton AF: Management of meningiomas of the cavernous sinus: conservative surgery and adjuvant therapy. *Clin Neurosurg* 45: 279, 1999.

[15] Fukushima T: Direct operative approach to the vascular lesions in the cavernous sinus: summary of 27 cases. *Mt Fuji Workshop on Cerebrovascular Diseases* 6: 169, 1988.

[16] George B, Ferrario CA, Blanquet A and Kolb F: Cavernous sinus exenteration for invasive cranial base tumors. *Neurosurgery* 52: 772, 2003.

[17] Hakuba A, Nishimura S, Shirakata S and Tsukamoto M: [Surgical approaches to the cavernous sinus. Report of 19 cases (author's transl)]. *Neurol Med Chir* (Tokyo) 22: 295, 1982.

[18] Hakuba A, Tanaka K, Suzuki T and Nishimura S: A combined orbitozygomatic infratemporal epidural and subdural approach for lesions involving the entire cavernous sinus. *J Neurosurg* 71: 699, 1989.

[19] Heth JA and Al-Mefty O: Cavernous sinus meningiomas. *Neurosurg* Focus 14: e3, 2003.

[20] Jacob M, Wydh E, Vighetto A and Sindou M: Visual outcome after surgery for cavernous sinus meningioma. *Acta Neurochir* (Wien) 150: 421, 2008.

[21] Kim DK, Grieve J, Archer DJ and Uttley D: Meningiomas in the region of the cavernous sinus: a review of 21 patients. *Br J Neurosurg* 10: 439, 1996.

[22] Klink DF, Sampath P, Miller NR, Brem H and Long DM: Long-term visual outcome after nonradical microsurgery patients with parasellar and cavernous sinus meningiomas. *Neurosurgery* 47: 24, 2000.

[23] Knosp E, Perneczky A, Koos WT, Fries G and Matula C: Meningiomas of the space of the cavernous sinus. *Neurosurgery* 38: 434, 1996.

[24] Larson JJ, van Loveren HR, Balko MG and Tew JMJ: Evidence of meningioma infiltration into cranial nerves: clinical implications for cavernous sinus meningiomas. *J Neurosurg* 83: 596, 1995.

[25] Lesoin F et al. Management of cavernous sinus meningiomas. *Neurochirurgia* (Stuttg) 28: 195, 1985.

[26] Maruyama K, Shin M, Kurita H, Kawahara N, Morita A and Kirino T: Proposed treatment strategy for cavernous sinus meningiomas: a prospective study. *Neurosurgery* 55: 1068, 2004.

[27] Nakamura M, Roser F, Michel J, Jacobs C and Samii M: The natural history of incidental meningiomas. *Neurosurgery* 53: 62, 2003.

[28] Newman S: A prospective study of cavernous sinus surgery for meningiomas and resultant common ophthalmic complications (an American Ophthalmological Society thesis). *Trans Am Ophthalmol Soc* 105: 392, 2007.

[29] O'Sullivan MG, van Loveren HR and Tew JMJ: The surgical resectability of meningiomas of the cavernous sinus. *Neurosurgery* 40: 238, 1997.

[30] Pamir MN, Kilic T, Bayrakli F and Peker S: Changing treatment strategy of cavernous sinus meningiomas: experience of a single institution. *Surg Neurol* 64 Suppl 2: S58, 2005.

[31] Pamir MN, Kilic T, Ozek MM, Ozduman K and Ture U: Non-meningeal tumours of the cavernous sinus: a surgical analysis. *J Clin Neurosci* 13: 626, 2006.

[32] Parkinson D: A surgical approach to the cavernous portion of the carotid artery. Anatomical studies and case report. J Neurosurg 23: 474, 1965.

[33] Parkinson D: Lateral sellar compartment O.T. (cavernous sinus): history, anatomy, terminology. *Anat Rec* 251: 486, 1998.

[34] Peker S, Kurtkaya-Yapicier O, Kilic T and Pamir MN: Microsurgical anatomy of the lateral walls of the pituitary fossa. *Acta Neurochir* (Wien) 147: 641, 2005.

[35] Risi P, Uske A and de Tribolet N: Meningiomas involving the anterior clinoid process. *Br J Neurosurg* 8: 295, 1994.

[36] Sekhar LN and Moller AR: Operative management of tumors involving the cavernous sinus. *J Neurosurg* 64: 879, 1986.

[37] Sekhar LN, Patel S, Cusimano M, Wright DC, Sen CN and Bank WO: Surgical treatment of meningiomas involving the cavernous sinus: evolving ideas based on a ten year experience. *Acta Neurochir Suppl* 65: 58, 1996.

[38] Sekhar LN and Altschuler EM (1991) Meningiomas of the cavernous sinus. In *Meningiomas* (ed O A-M), pp. 445-460. Raven Press, New York.

[39] Sekhar LN, Ross DA and Sen C (1993) Cavernous sinus and sphenocavernous neoplasms. In *Surgery of cranial base tumors.* (eds Sekhar LN and PI J), pp. 521-604. Raven press.

[40] Sepehrnia A, Samii M and Tatagiba M: Management of intracavernous tumours: an 11-year experience. *Acta Neurochir Suppl* (Wien) 53: 122, 1991.

[41] SIMPSON D: The recurrence of intracranial meningiomas after surgical treatment. *J Neurol Neurosurg Psychiatry* 20: 22, 1957.

[42] Sindou M, Wydh E, Jouanneau E, Nebbal M and Lieutaud T: Long-term follow-up of meningiomas of the cavernous sinus after surgical treatment alone. *J Neurosurg* 107: 937, 2007.

[43] Taptas JN: The so-called cavernous sinus: a review of the controversy and its implications for neurosurgeons. *Neurosurgery* 11: 712, 1982.

[44] Umansky F and Nathan H: The lateral wall of the cavernous sinus. With special reference to the nerves related to it. *J Neurosurg* 56: 228, 1982.

[45] Yonekawa Y et al. Selective extradural anterior clinoidectomy for supra- and parasellar processes. Technical note. *J Neurosurg* 87: 636, 1997.

In: Current Management of Central Nervous System … ISBN: 978-1-63483-856-6
Editors: Steven D. Chang and Anand Veeravagu 

*Chapter 5*

# Surgical Management of Planum and Olfactory Groove Meningiomas

***Jayson A. Neil, MD, Marcus D. Mazur, MD and William T. Couldwell, MD, PhD***
Department of Neurosurgery, University of Utah School of Medicine, Salt Lake City, Utah, US

## Abstract

Olfactory groove meningiomas (OGMs) and planum sphenoid meningiomas (PSMs) comprise a significant subset of meningiomas. They encompass the anterior skull base, from the rostral-most portion of the cribriform plate to the posterior aspect of the planum sphenoidale. These lesions present insidiously and are often quite large when discovered. Because of their unique location on the anterior skull base, they can be surgically addressed through multiple access points. From above, smaller or more lateralized lesions may be approached through a unilateral frontal, pterional, or fronto-orbital craniotomy. Larger lesions may be approached through a bifrontal approach, with or without a subcranial component. From below, they can be resected through an expanded endonasal approach. This chapter will discuss OGMs and PSMs with respect to topics such as the removal of these tumors by reviewing their anatomy, some technical and clinical pearls with case presentations, and the associated literature and looking into the future directions of addressing these lesions.

## Introduction

Olfactory groove meningiomas (OGMs) and planum sphenoidale meningiomas (PSMs) share common characteristics that distinguish them from meningiomas originating in other locations. These include an anatomic location on the anterior skull base, the propensity for extended growth prior to symptomatic presentation, and the tendency to displace neurovascular structures superiorly and posteriorly (with the exception of the optic apparatus, which is displaced inferiorly and posteriorly). Despite these shared characteristics, most published clinical series group OGMs and PSMs separately. Most retrospective studies have grouped PSMs with tuberculum sellae meningiomas because of their close proximity to the diaphragma sellae. In part, this inclusion is because PSMs are relatively uncommon tumors. Only a handful of cases have been reported in series that include PSMs. A low sample size precludes drawing evidence-based conclusions on the management and outcomes of patients affected by this type of meningioma. In this chapter, we have included OGM and PSM together based on their anatomical location and propensity to present as large mass lesions [1].

OGMs comprise roughly 10% (8–25%) of all meningiomas, making the olfactory groove the most prevalent location for meningiomas in some studies [2-4]. OGM holds a prominent place in neurosurgery as one of the first intracranial tumors to be successfully resected with a good neurological outcome. In 1885, Francisco Durante successfully resected a left OGM in a 35-year-old woman [5, 6]. However, as a harbinger of the challenges of meningioma surgery, the patient suffered a recurrence 11 years later, which was also successfully resected. Harvey Cushing is well known for his contributions to meningioma surgery and he included 29 cases of OGM in his famous 1938 monograph [7].

The pathologic diagnosis of OGM mirrors that of meningiomas found elsewhere. It is predominantly a World Health Organization (WHO) grade 1 tumor, with the meningothelial variant being most commonly observed [8, 9]. Because of the benign nature of these lesions, complete resection is the primary goal of surgery and is readily obtainable in many cases. These tumors are asymptomatic at early stages and therefore commonly grow to impressive sizes prior to being diagnosed. The most common symptoms observed are apathy, personality changes, or changes in judgment that progress imperceptibly over several years [9]. These mental disturbances can further contribute to the late presentation of these tumors. Anosmia is an early symptom that is commonly overlooked despite being present in at least 50% of diagnosed cases [9].

Seizures are a presenting symptom in up to 20% of cases [9]. Late symptoms include headaches and visual changes (generally inferior visual field loss and changes in acuity). Prior to the development of modern imaging techniques, many of these tumors presented in fulminant features of Foster-Kennedy syndrome with anosmia, unilateral optic atrophy, and contralateral papilledema [7]. Fortunately, this presentation is rare. Although headaches are a late feature of OGM, they are a common finding in the population and account for a larger percentage of the presenting symptoms leading to imaging and the diagnosis [8].

## Surgical Anatomy – Anatomy and Relevant Images

OGMs typically develop in the midline at the frontosphenoid suture on the posterior cribriform plate or from the cribriform plate itself. They may encompass any portion of the midline anterior skull base, from the crista galli to the planum sphenoidale, necessitating a detailed understanding of the anterior skull base anatomy for successful surgical management of these patients (Figure 1). OGMs occasionally enlarge asymmetrically, resulting in a laterality of the tumor. As they grow, they displace the frontal lobes superiorly and

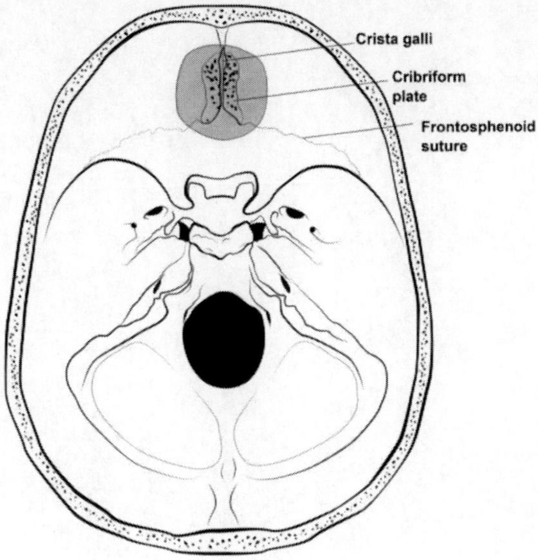


Figure 1. Anterior skull base bony anatomy as viewed from above. The region of OGM growth is shown in pink overlying the crista galli, cribriform plate, and frontosphenoid suture.

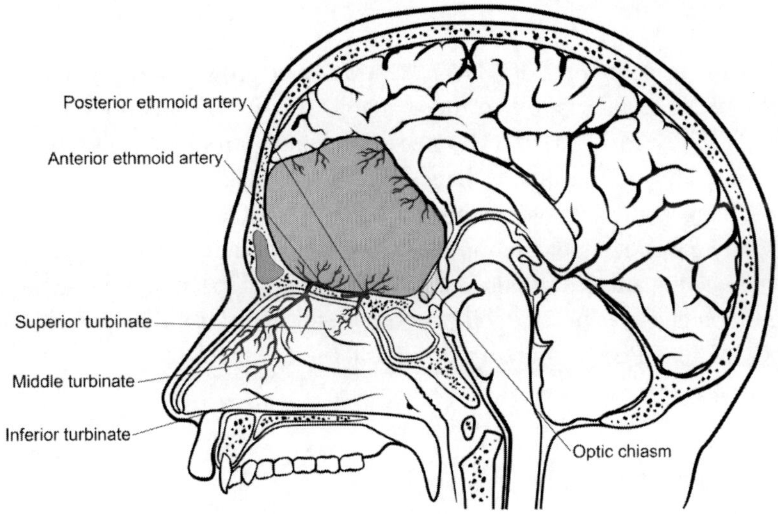


Figure 2. Sagittal midline view with tumor shown in pink. Neurovascular structures are displaced posteriorly and superiorly with the exception of the optic chiasm, in yellow, which is displaced posteriorly and inferiorly. The vascular supply to these tumors may arise from the anterior or posterior ethmoidal arteries, the middle meningeal arteries, the meningeal branches of ophthalmic arteries, the ACA, and the anterior communicating artery branches. Also visualized in this illustration are the paranasal sinuses demonstrating the inferior, middle, and superior turbinates, the sphenoid sinus, and the cribriform plate.

posteriorly, the olfactory nerves laterally, and the anterior cerebral arteries (ACAs) posterosuperiorly and laterally. In large tumors, the optic nerves and chiasm are displaced posteriorly and inferiorly (Figure 2). This serves as a differentiating feature from tuberculum sellae meningiomas, which displace the chiasm superiorly. Although hyperostosis of the

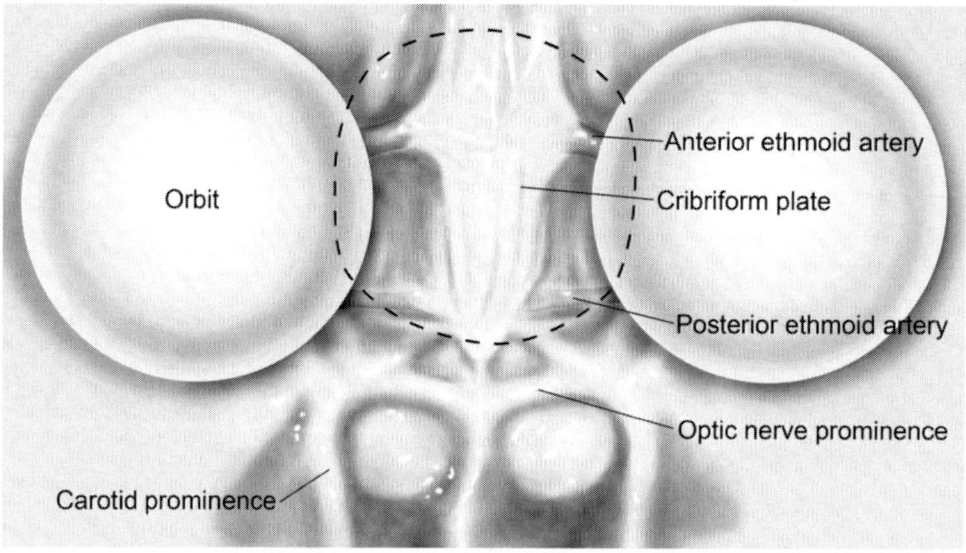


Figure 3. Anterior skull base as viewed from below through an endoscope showing the lamina papyracea bilaterally and bony prominences for the carotid arteries, optic nerves, and anterior and posterior ethmoidal arteries. The tumor is indicated with the dotted line.

anterior skull base is common, OGMs and PSMs may grow inferiorly into the ethmoid sinuses up to 15–30% of the time, into the sphenoid sinuses, or laterally into the orbits [10-15]. The blood supply to OGMs/PSMs is predominantly from the anterior and posterior ethmoidal arteries. They also commonly receive contributions from the anterior branches of the middle meningeal arteries and meningeal branches of the ophthalmic arteries. Large meningiomas may parasitize the cerebral vasculature including branches from the ACAs and anterior communicating arteries (Figure 2). Likewise, an understanding of the anatomy of the nasal passages, paranasal sinuses, and anterior skull base from below is critical when approaching OGMs and PGMs through a transnasal route (Figures 2 and 3).

## Detailed Surgical Management

The first step in the management of OGM and PSM is determining whether the tumor requires treatment. If the patient is asymptomatic, including absence of mental or psychiatric dysfunction, and the lesion is small, then observation with repeat imaging is appropriate given there is no evidence of growth. If the patient is very elderly or at significant risk because of his or her general physical health, then radiosurgery (for tumors <3 cm) or stereotactic radiotherapy can be considered. Likewise, radiation may have a role in treating recurrent lesions or atypical meningiomas (WHO grade II) after resection. If the lesion is large, growing, or symptomatic, surgery may be indicated. Many approaches have been utilized in the resection of OGM and PSM, but we will discuss the techniques for the unilateral frontal, pterional, and fronto-orbital craniotomies, as well as bifrontal and subcranial craniotomies. Lastly, we will discuss the expanded endonasal approach to OGM and PSM. All of these approaches have been employed successfully, although determining the best approach for each tumor and patient is complex. This decision should be based on tumor size, laterality, and infiltration of adjacent structures; patient age, health, and life expectancy; and the surgeon's personal experience with these procedures. Although there have been attempts to define a standardized algorithm for this decision, we will simply discuss the relative merits and drawbacks of each approach because surgeons should provide an individualized approach to each patient [10]. There are many commonalities among these approaches, and judicious use of lumbar puncture, lumbar drain, or external ventricular drain will typically aid both brain relaxation and prevention of postoperative cerebrospinal fluid (CSF) leak.

## Unilateral Frontal, Pterional, and Fronto-Orbital Approaches

The patient is positioned supine with ipsilateral shoulder elevation and the operating table is slightly reflexed, with the head elevated above the right atrium of the heart. The head is fixed in a 3-pin head holder with the single pin located 2 finger breadths above the ipsilateral pinna. The head is rotated 20–30 degrees and slightly extended to place the ipsilateral maxillary process at the highest point. Injection of an anesthetic combined with epinephrine along the planned incision line will assist in hemostasis. The incision follows the standard bicoronal arc behind the hairline from the zygoma and less than one cm anterior to the tragus on the ipsilateral side, but it is often unnecessary to extend it beyond the contralateral superior temporal line (Figure 4).

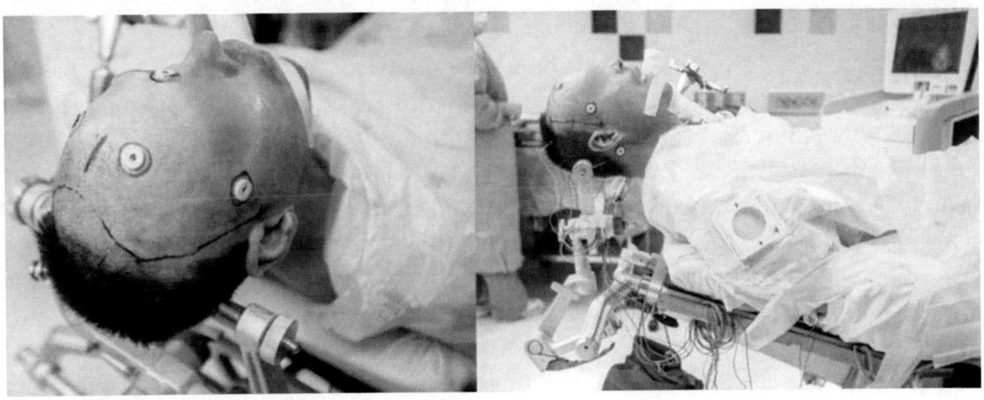

Figure 4. Operative photographs showing patient positioning for bifrontal craniotomy and marked skin incision.

The depth of the incision is to the pericranium medially and the superficial temporal fascia laterally. Care must be taken to avoid injury to the superficial temporal artery. The loose areolar tissue is dissected in the subgaleal space, and the scalp flap is reflected anteriorly. Once the fat pad is reached over the temporalis muscle, subfascial dissection is used to protect the frontalis branch of the facial nerve. In most cases of patients with OGM or PSM, temporal exposure is not required. If the planned craniotomy extends below the superior temporal line, then the temporalis is incised to leave a cuff on the superior temporal line for re-suspension at the end of the case. Elevation of the periosteal layer with the temporalis assists in hemostasis. The surgeon may reflect the temporalis inferiorly or reflect it forward in a single layer with the skin as a musculocutaneous flap. In either case, the temporalis fascia should be dissected from the frontozygomatic process, revealing the suture. Further subgaleal dissection can be performed posteriorly to allow the pericranium to be incised behind the skin incision and reflected forward, which provides for a larger pericranial graft. The supraorbital nerves and arteries are visualized, protected, and elevated from their notch. They can also be freed from their foramen using an osteotome or drill. The pericranial graft can be used to reconstruct the skull base and prevent CSF leak at the end of the case. Care is taken when replacing the bone flap over the graft to ensure adequate blood flow and avoid strangulation of the graft.

## Unilateral Frontal Craniotomy

Unilateral frontal craniotomies with the subfrontal approach are better utilized for small and mid-sized tumors rather than for larger tumors. Their advantage lies in the low complexity with reduced operative time and their sparing of contralateral hemisphere retraction. No superior sagittal sinus ligation is needed and access to the tumor vascular supply early is variable. The frontal sinus may be transgressed providing an opportunity for CSF leak, brain retraction may be necessary, and the exposure is more limited than with a bilateral approach.

The temporalis is incised to the level of the keyhole along the planned craniotomy lines. This allows for closure of the muscle above the craniotomy and a burr hole for improved cosmesis. A burr hole is placed at the keyhole, and, if necessary, further burr holes are placed posterior along the superior temporal line and posteromedially lateral to the superior sagittal sinus. No burr holes are placed in the low frontal region (forehead). The dura is dissected from the calvaria, and the craniotomy is performed with a high-speed drill and footplate. The inferior exposure is limited to one cm above the orbital rim (Figure 5). However, the inferior extent of exposure provides early access to the tumor's vascular supply and minimizes brain retraction. The anteromedial portion of the craniotomy should be carefully inspected. If the frontal sinus is transgressed, it is addressed at this time with the resection of the mucosa and cranialization with the plugging of the nasofrontal duct. All mucosa is also removed with a high-speed drill from the bone flap to avoid the late complication of mucocele development.

The dura is incised in a C-shaped fashion and reflected inferiorly. With arachnoid dissection and gentle elevation of the frontal lobe, the tumor will be visible. The frontal lobe should be sharply dissected from the olfactory bulb and nerve in an effort to preserve olfactory function, when present preoperatively. The tumor resection is performed from anterior to posterior. The basal attachments are coagulated first to devascularize the tumor from its blood supply (anterior and posterior ethmoid arteries and meningeal branches from the middle meningeal and ophthalmic arteries) and prevent excessive blood loss. The tumor may then be debulked, as the capsule is dissected from its surrounding tissue and resected. The ACAs, optic nerves and optic chiasm are the last to be visualized during this approach. Consequently, the surgeon must be vigilant to avoid injury to these structures.

Closure of the dura is performed in a watertight fashion, and a dural graft may be necessary. The skull base is reconstructed using the pericranial graft. The bone is replaced using titanium plates and screws, while avoiding placing any hardware anteriorly over the forehead. Soft tissue closure is performed in the usual fashion.

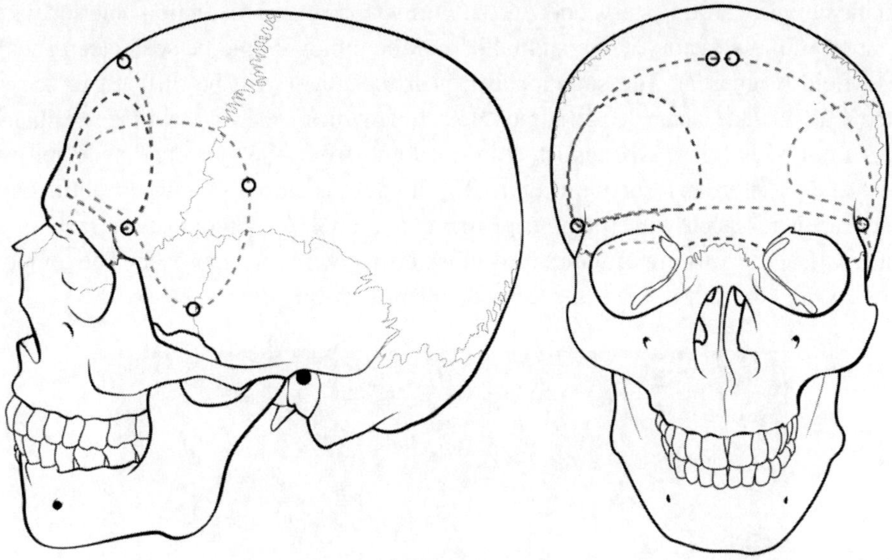

Figure 5. Diagram illustrating craniotomy paths based on operative approach: unilateral frontal (red), pterional (green), and bifrontal (blue) approaches. Additional orbital (orange) and subcranial (purple) cuts may be made.

## Pterional Craniotomy

The frequency with which a pterional craniotomy is used in the resection of OGMs and PSMs has increased over the past few years, with greater advocacy in specific circumstances [10, 16, 17]. The advantages of the pterional approach include its familiarity to most neurosurgeons, early visualization of the optic nerves, optic chiasm and ACAs, and early access to the CSF for brain relaxation. There is less frequent transgression of the frontal sinus, which reduces the likelihood of CSF leak or infection, and no ligation of the superior sagittal sinus. The working distance to the ipsilateral suprasellar space is shortened compared with the unilateral frontal approach, but the working distance to the contralateral aspects of the tumor can be quite long with narrow working angles. If significant drilling of the anterior skull base is necessary or if the tumor invades the ethmoid or sphenoid sinus, requiring anterior skull base reconstruction, this approach may afford less access than a bifrontal approach. This approach is favorable for those tumors in which there is a particular concern for the optic nerves, optic chiasm and ACAs in addition to tumors with less anterior skull base involvement.

After the temporalis muscle is reflected anteriorly or inferiorly, burr holes are placed at the keyhole, low temporal fossa, and posterior aspect of the exposed superior temporal line (Figure 5). The dura is separated from the calvaria, and a craniotomy is performed with a high-speed drill and footplate. The frontal portion of the craniotomy may be customized to the patient's pathology. After bone flap elevation, the middle meningeal artery is sealed using bipolar cautery and the sphenoid wing is removed using bone rongeurs and a high-speed drill (Figure 6). The dura is incised in a C-shaped fashion and reflected anteroinferiorly. Early dissection of the Sylvian fissure allows CSF egress, providing brain relaxation and exposure of the optic nerves, carotid artery, and ACAs. Further arachnoid dissection anteriorly provides visualization of the olfactory nerve and bulb, and the tumor should be seen clearly within the operative field (Figure 7). The superior aspect of the tumor will be difficult to see without brain retraction. Once again, early tumor detachment from the base will devascularize the tumor. Tumor debulking will assist in dissection from the surrounding neurovascular structures and assist in its resection (Figure 8). The dura is closed in a watertight fashion, and the bone flap is replaced with titanium plates and screws. A cranioplasty is fashioned from Medpor to offset the wasting of temporalis muscle seen with this approach. The temporalis is re-suspended and the soft tissue is closed in standard fashion.

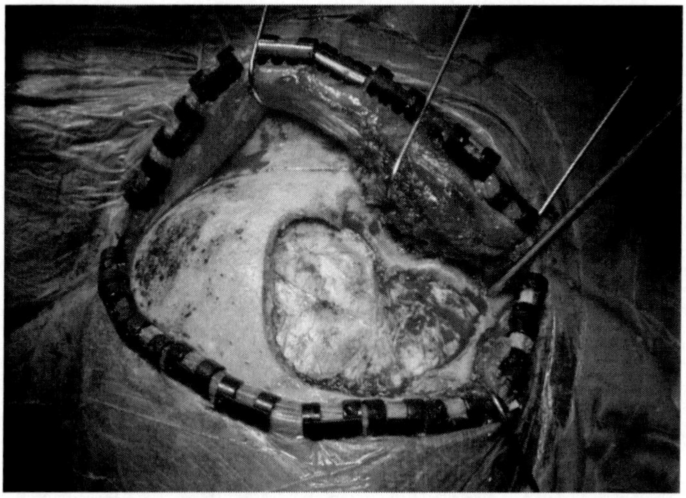

Figure 6. Operative photograph demonstrating skin incision, elevation of musculocutaneous flap, and right pterional craniotomy.

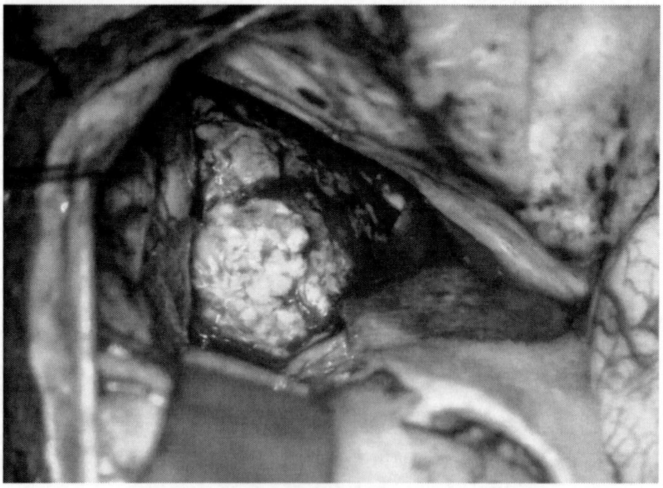

Figure 7. Operative photograph of OGM (just superior to the metal retractor) as viewed through a right pterional approach.

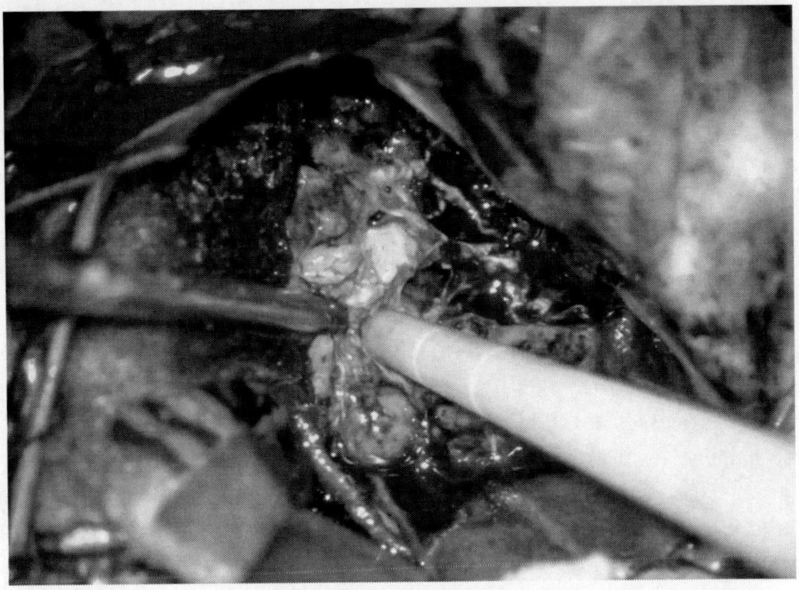

Figure 8. Operative photograph showing debulking of OGM using an ultrasonic aspirator through a right pterional approach.

## Fronto-Orbital Craniotomy

Orbital osteotomies can be added to either the unilateral frontal or pterional craniotomies to provide a fronto-orbital craniotomy. The removal of the orbital roof provides a number of benefits to the surgeon. The approach to the base of the tumor is direct, allowing for excellent exposure to the skull base and vascular supply. The approach offers a lower trajectory, providing tumor access with less brain retraction. After the osteotomy, the ipsilateral anterior, and posterior ethmoid arteries may be coagulated prior to entry into the tumor and tumor dissection [18]. This approach provides greater exposure for drilling or repairing the anterior skull base. However, the frontal sinus will be transgressed in this exposure, which increases the risk of CSF leak. The surgical time will also increase, not only during the osteotomy, but also in the craniofacial reconstruction required for adequate cosmesis.

After the frontal or pterional craniotomy is performed and the frontozygomatic suture is exposed, the periorbita is dissected from the roof and walls of the orbit from the orbital side. With the periorbita dissected and protected, the osteotomies can be performed using an oscillating saw blade or a high-speed drill with a footplate. Before these cuts are made, it is often beneficial to choose the instrumentation planned for reconstruction and drill pilot holes, both of which will facilitate the later reconstruction and cosmesis. Once the orbital roof is removed, the anterior and posterior ethmoid arteries are visualized at approximately 24 mm and 36 mm posterior to the anterior crest of the nasolacrimal duct, respectively. The tumor is then detached from the base, debulked, dissected, and resected.

## Bifrontal and Subcranial Craniotomies

Bifrontal and subcranial craniotomies are best utilized for larger tumors. Their advantage lies in the exquisite exposure provided by these approaches. There is early access to the tumor vascular supply and good visualization of neurovascular structures with little brain retraction. However, the superior sagittal sinus is ligated and the frontal sinus is transgressed. This approach provides excellent exposure for drilling and repair of the anterior skull base. Careful closure is critical to avoid postoperative complications relating to CSF leak.

The patient is positioned supine without head rotation, and the operating table is slightly reflexed with the head elevated above the right atrium. The head is fixed in a 3-pin head holder and slightly extended (to facilitate brain retraction from the tumor). This places the bilateral maxillary processes at the highest point. The incision follows the standard bicoronal arc behind the hairline from zygoma to zygoma less than one cm anterior to the tragus. The injection of an anesthetic combined with epinephrine will assist in hemostasis. The general surgical technique for these approaches is similar to that described in detail under the *Unilateral frontal, pterional, and fronto-orbital approaches* heading. Once the dissection is completed as described above, bilateral burr holes are placed at the keyhole. Further burr holes are placed posterior along the superior temporal line and posteromedially lateral to the superior sagittal sinus. Care is taken to dissect the region of the superior sagittal sinus. If the superior sagittal sinus proves to be significantly adherent, a Kerrison punch may be used across this region or a trough can be drilled using a diamond bit. No burr holes are placed over the forehead. The dura is dissected from the calvaria, and the craniotomy is performed with a high-speed drill and footplate. The frontal sinus can now be exenterated and cranialized by removing the posterior wall with rongeurs and a high-speed drill. The frontal sinus mucosa may be removed using pituitary forceps and high-speed drills. The base of the posterior wall is drilled flush using a diamond bit. The frontonasal ducts are plugged with temporalis muscle and fascia.

If a subcranial approach is needed, then after the bifrontal craniotomy is performed and the frontozygomatic suture is exposed, the periorbita is dissected from the roof and walls of the orbit from the orbital side. Before the osteotomies are performed, it is often beneficial to choose the instrumentation to be used for reconstruction and drill pilot holes. Both will facilitate the later reconstruction and cosmesis. With the periorbita dissected and protected, the lateral osteotomies just lateral to the frontozygomatic suture can be performed using an oscillating saw blade or high-speed drill with a footplate. Using the drill with the straight collar, intracranial cuts are made on the medial aspect of the orbit, anterolateral to the crista galli and into the ethmoid sinuses. Extracranially, a cut is made horizontally superior to the frontonasal suture. This allows for complete elevation of the bilateral orbital roof complex. Following removal of the orbital roof, the anterior and posterior ethmoid arteries are visualized at 24 and 36 mm posterior to the anterior crest of the nasolacrimal duct, respectively.

The dura is opened on either side of the superior sagittal sinus as anteriorly as is afforded by the pathology (generally well within the anterior third of the sinus and just above the crista galli). The sinus is tied off with two double loops of 2-0 silk suture though the falx and is incised between these sutures. The tumor resection is performed from anterior to posterior. The basal attachments are coagulated first to devascularize the tumor from its blood supply (anterior and posterior ethmoid arteries and meningeal branches from the middle meningeal and ophthalmic arteries) and prevent excessive blood loss. The tumor may then be debulked using microsurgical techniques and the ultrasonic aspirator; the capsule will be dissected from surrounding tissue and resected. The ACAs, optic nerves, and optic chiasm are visualized posterolateral to the tumor. The surgeon must be vigilant to avoid injury to these structures.

Closure of the dura is performed in a watertight fashion, and a dural graft may be necessary. The anterior skull base may be packed with fat to further prevent CSF leak, and fascia may be harvested from the same site for use as the dural graft. The skull base is further reconstructed using the pericranial graft. The bone is replaced using titanium plates and screws, while avoiding placing any hardware anteriorly over the forehead. Care is taken when replacing the bone flap over the graft to ensure adequate blood flow to the pericranium and to avoid strangulation of the graft. Soft tissue closure is performed in the usual fashion. CSF diversion may be considered to assist in CSF leak prevention.

## Expanded Endonasal Approach

The expanded endonasal approach is best utilized for small to medium-sized tumors and tumors that grow inferiorly into the ethmoid and sphenoid sinus. The advantages include the lack of ligation of the superior sagittal sinus, minimal to no brain manipulation, early access to tumor vascular supply, and excellent visualization in smaller tumors. The disadvantages are the late visualization of neurovascular structures, higher rates of CSF leak, higher rate of anosmia postoperatively, and potentially lower rates of gross total resection if the tumor extends laterally. In particular, the approach is hindered in tumors that extend laterally over the orbits, superiorly and anteriorly against the frontal sinus, or above medial carotid arteries posteriorly. Tumors with a dural tail extending beyond the skull base opening are particularly challenging. In addition, olfaction must be considered. If olfaction is present preoperatively, the endonasal approach is not chosen because the approach will most likely sacrifice this nerve function. A cranial approach can be chosen to preserve at least one olfactory nerve.

The endoscopic approach will be discussed, although an operative microscope and nasal speculum may be used in adjunct. Just prior to surgery, the patient is given a decongestant nasal spray. The patient is positioned supine on the operating table, and after intubation, the tube is taped to the left side. The head is extended to facilitate access to the anterior skull base. The nasal cavities are packed with decongestant-soaked pledgets. The table is manipulated to position the patient's head above the right atrium of the heart. The patient is placed in a 3-pin head holder, and the head is very slightly laterally extended to the left and rotated to the right. This allows the surgeon standing to the right of the patient to have a neutral view of the head (Figure 9). Neuronavigation is registered, and the monitors for navigation and the endoscope are placed at the head of the bed. The right lower quadrant of the abdomen or right lateral thigh is prepped for fat or fascia graft harvesting. A $4^{th}$-generation cephalosporin is given as prophylaxis and the patient is draped in the usual fashion.

The packing pledgets are removed, and the nostrils are entered using a zero-degree endoscope. The anatomy is visualized including the inferior, middle, and superior turbinates, choana, septum, and sphenoid ostium (Figures 2 and 3).

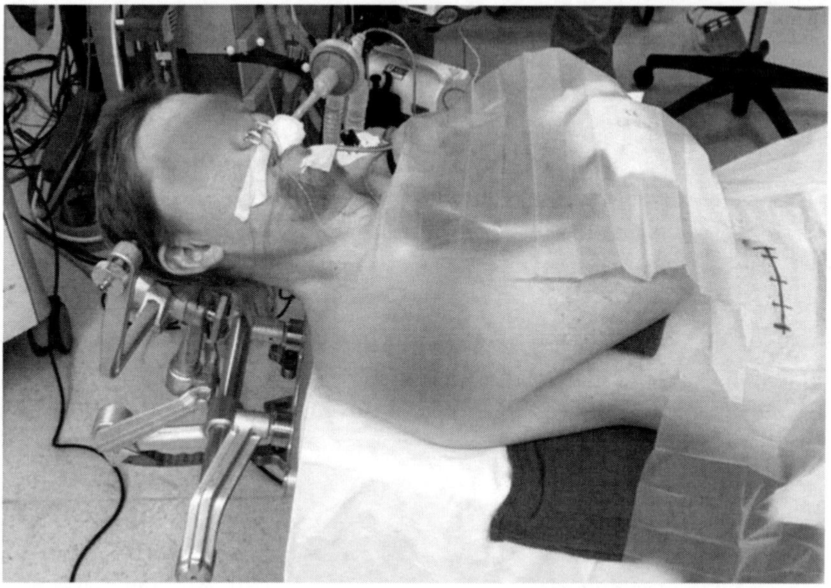

Figure 9. Operative photograph of patient positioned for transnasal endoscopic approach. The head is fixed in a 3-pin head holder. The head is extended very slightly laterally to the left and rotated to the right.

Anesthetic with epinephrine may be infiltrated into the nasal mucosa as needed for hemostasis. In most cases, the right middle turbinate will be resected and the left middle turbinate will be lateralized. Throughout the procedure, the endoscope is maintained at the top of the operative field. The suction will generally be at the bottom of the field entering through the right nostril. The various operative tools may enter either nostril between the endoscope and suction. Depending on the anterior or posterior position of the tumor, an anterior sphenoidectomy and 1- to 2-cm posterior/superior septectomy will be performed. The bullae ethmoidalis and the anterior and posterior ethmoid cells are opened. The anterior and posterior ethmoid arteries are visualized and coagulated, which aids in hemostasis and devascularizes the tumor. The lamina papyracea may be removed to gain lateral exposure but care should be taken to respect the periorbita unless it is involved with tumor. The nasal mucosa and olfactory epithelium are cauterized and removed, and the cribriform plate is resected using a high-speed drill. The dura is coagulated and opened, and internal debulking is performed in standard neurosurgical fashion using ultrasonic aspiration, cautery, and microsurgical techniques. Care should be taken to avoid undue traction on the tumor. The neurovascular structures are the last to be seen and caution should be taken as the capsule is dissected from them, usually with sharp dissection.

Closure is meticulous in these cases because of the risk of CSF leak. The dead space from tumor removal is occasionally packed with fat or Gelfoam. Our preference is for the autologous fascia graft to be tucked underneath the dural edges. In large defects, this is reinforced with the autologous vomer or septal bone covered with a vascularized nasoseptal flap. This may be reinforced with a sealant or fat. The nostrils are then packed with expandable foam that has been sutured into the cut finger of a surgical glove. CSF diversion using either an external ventricular drain or lumbar drain is routinely utilized.

## Illustrative Cases

### *Case 1*

A 31-year-old man presented with headaches, vision loss, anosmia, a decreased sense of taste, and seizures. Direct funduscopic examination revealed bilateral papilledema. MRI showed a 10-cm OGM with erosion of the cribriform plate into the ethmoid sinus. The mass abutted the sella turcica, encroached on the left orbital apex, and caused marked mass effect on the frontal lobes (Figure 10).

A bifrontal craniotomy was performed with preservation of the pericranium. The brain was under significant pressure despite administration of 50 g of mannitol. The dura was opened and the superior sagittal sinus was ligated. A small corticectomy was made in the right frontal lobe to access the tumor, and the tumor was debulked from its core outward using an ultrasonic aspirator.

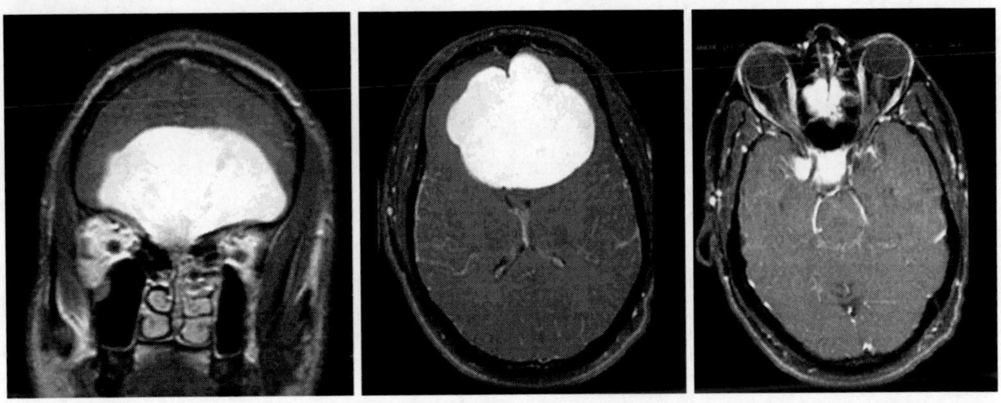

Figure 10. Case 1. Preoperative contrast-enhanced T1-weighted images of a 10-cm OGM. The meningioma invaded through the cribriform plate with involvement of the ethmoid and sphenoid bones and extension into the sella region. There is marked mass effect on the frontal lobes.

The tumor attachment at the crista galli was cauterized and the involved dura was excised. A diamond burr was used to drill out the bony infiltration of the meningioma into the cribriform plate, and the tumor was resected from portions of the ethmoid and sphenoid bones. A gross total resection was achieved. The anterior skull base was repaired with a fascia lata and fat graft, and a pericranium flap was used to cover the dural defect. Postoperative MRI demonstrated no residual tumor. The patient was discharged after an uneventful hospital course. MRI obtained at 8-year follow-up showed no evidence of recurrence (Figure 11). The patient still requires antiepileptic medications for seizure management.

### *Case 2*

A 56-year-old man presented with a 5-year history of anosmia. He denied having headaches or vision loss. Contrast-enhanced T1-weighted MRI demonstrated a 4-cm OGM without extension into the nasal cavity (Figure 12A). A unilateral right frontal craniotomy was performed. After the bone flap was elevated and the dura opened, a subfrontal brain retractor was placed. An arachnoid layer separated the pia from the meningioma, which facilitated dissection of the tumor from the brain. The meningioma was first debulked internally using an ultrasonic aspirator.

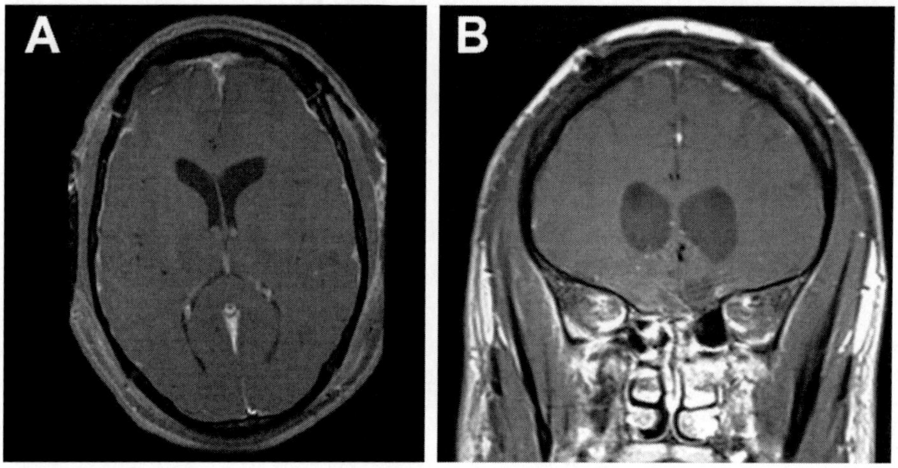


Figure 11. Case1. Postoperative axial MRI on day 1 (A) reveals improvement of mass effect and expected postsurgical changes related to ligature of the superior sagittal sinus. Coronal MRI at 8 years (B) reveals no evidence of meningioma recurrence.

A portion of the falx was removed to aid in the visualization of the tumor crossing to the contralateral side. The attachment to the cribriform plate was then cauterized. A dural margin of approximately one cm was excised. The anterior skull base was then drilled with a diamond burr to remove all hyperostotic bone. A fascia lata and fat graft was used to repair the anterior skull base and was tacked to the remaining dura with sutures and fibrin glue. A lumbar drain was placed for CSF diversion and continued for three days. After an uneventful hospital course, the patient was discharged home with no evidence of a CSF leak. Follow-up MRI at three years demonstrated no evidence of recurrent disease (Figure 12B).

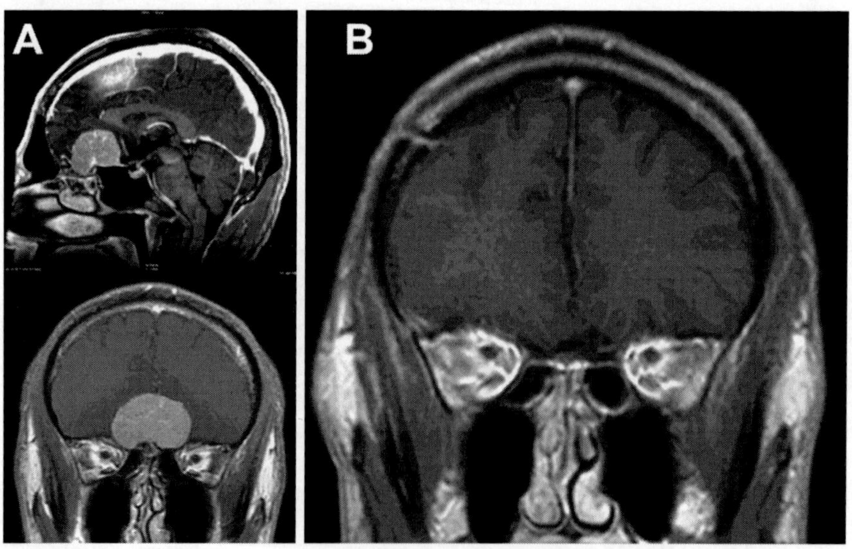


Figure 12. Case 2. (A) Preoperative contrast-enhanced sagittal (top) and coronal (bottom) T1-weighted MRIs demonstrate a 4-cm OGM. (B) Postoperative contrast-enhanced coronal T1-weighted MRI demonstrates no evidence of recurrence at 3 years.

*Case 3*

A previously healthy, 66-year-old woman underwent a surgical resection of a large right-sided petroclival meningioma with brainstem compression. Pathological analysis was consistent with WHO Grade I meningioma. After an uneventful hospital course, the patient was discharged home. At 1-year follow-up, MRI showed a complete resection of the lesion. Five years later, a routine surveillance MRI demonstrated a new 1.4-cm OGM that had not been present on previous imaging (Figure 13A). The patient had no new complaints or symptoms; she elected to have the OGM treated with stereotactic radiosurgery. A dose of 1500 cGy was administered.

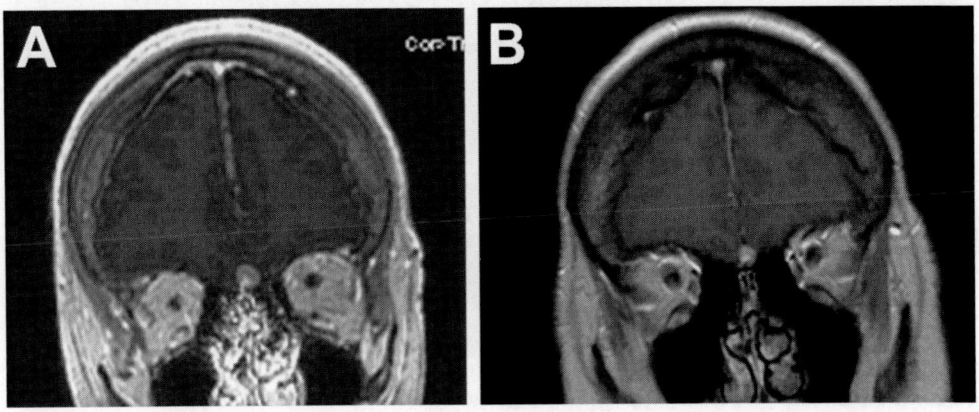


Figure 13. Case 3. (A) Pre-treatment and (B) 5-year post-treatment axial MRIs demonstrating unchanged appearance of a small OGM treated with radiosurgery.

Six months after radiosurgery, MRI demonstrated that the OGM had decreased to 7 mm in size. Five years later, the tumor remained unchanged and the patient did not develop any new or worsening symptoms (Figure 13B).

*Case 4*

After suffering a right thalamic stroke, a 66-year-old man was diagnosed with a 2-cm PSM that was visualized on MRI. The meningioma was not thought to be associated with the patient's stroke. A surveillance MRI obtained two years later demonstrated interval enlargement of the meningioma. (Figure 14) It was eccentric to the right with mild compression of the right frontal lobe and in contact with the optic chiasm.

A right pterional craniotomy was performed. After the bone flap was elevated and the dura opened, the right frontal lobe was retracted so that the base of the tumor and its dural attachment could be seen. The meningioma was adherent to the right olfactory nerve, which was sacrificed. Dissection was performed in an arachnoid plane that separated the tumor from the brain. The tumor was excised *en bloc* along with its dural base. The dural defect was repaired by suturing a small piece of dural graft substitute. The patient was discharged home after an uneventful hospital course. An MRI obtained four years later showed no evidence of tumor recurrence (Figure 15).

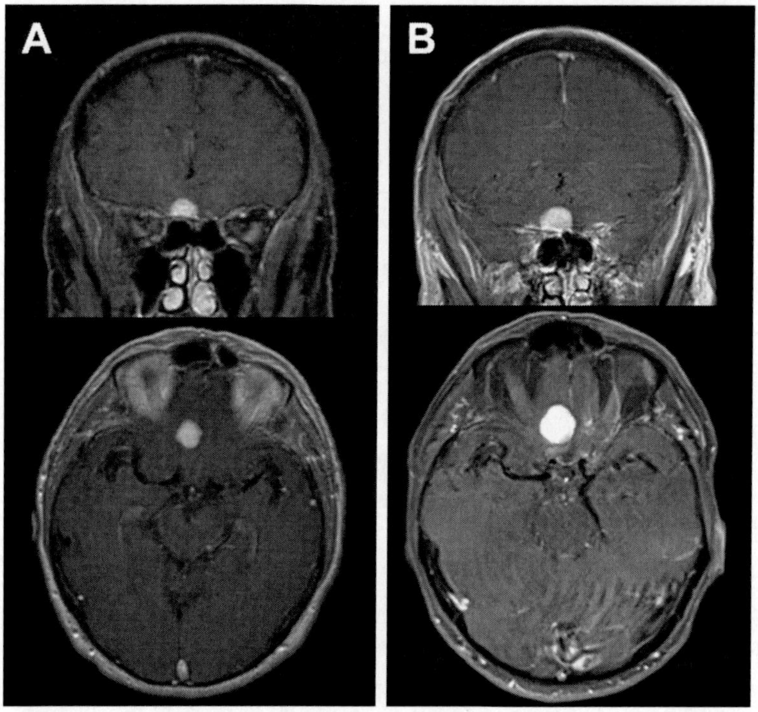


Figure 14. Case 4. (A, B) Contrast-enhanced coronal (top) and axial (bottom) T1-weighted images taken 1 year apart demonstrate an enlarging PSM.

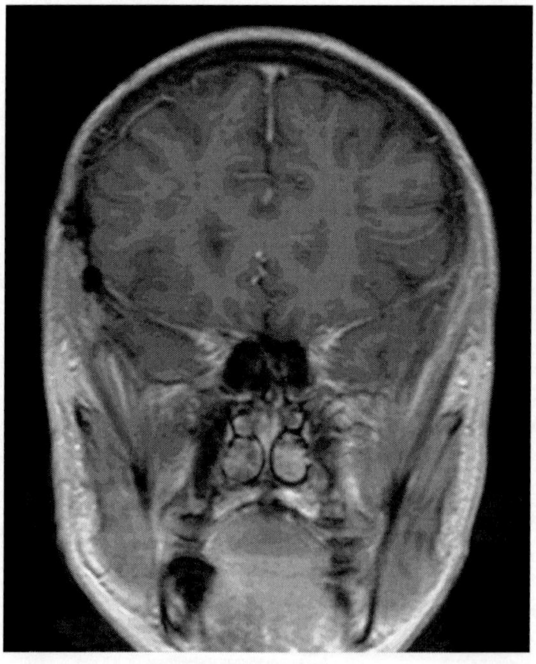

Figure 15. Case 4. Coronal contrast-enhanced T1-weighted MRI taken 4 years after a right pterional craniotomy for resection demonstrates no evidence of residual or recurrent disease.

***Case 5***

A 64-year-old woman was found to have a 2-cm PSM during an evaluation for new-onset seizure (Figure 16A). The tumor partially encased the right supraclinoid internal carotid artery without occlusion or narrowing. The meningioma was not thought to be the cause of the patient's seizure. She underwent a surgical resection of the tumor via a transsphenoidal approach. The sphenoid bone was hyperostotic and required drilling with a diamond burr to access the suprasellar region. The dura overlying the meningioma was incised, and the carotid arteries were visualized. An endoscope was used to identify the extent of the tumor. It abutted the optic chiasm, prechiasmatic optic nerves, anterior communicating artery, and proximal portions of the anterior cerebral arteries. A gross total resection was achieved. The dural defect was repaired with a fat and fascia graft obtained through an abdominal incision. The repair was bolstered using BioGlue. Postoperatively, the patient did not develop any endocrinopathy and was discharged after an uneventful course. An MRI obtained at two-year follow-up demonstrated no evidence of residual disease or recurrence (Figure 16B).

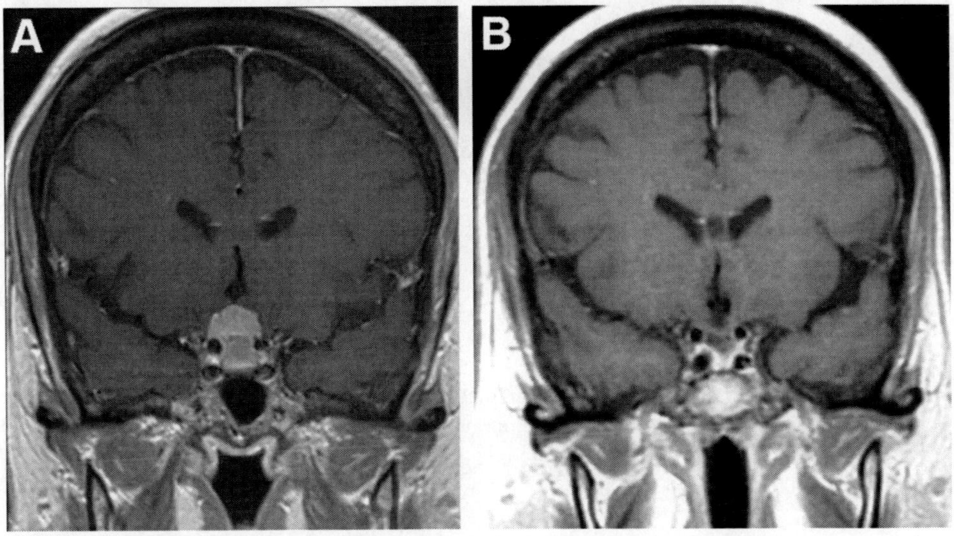


Figure 16. Case 5. (A) Contrast-enhanced T1-weighted MRI demonstrates a PSM with partial encasement of the right internal carotid artery. (B) Two years after resection via a transsphenoidal approach, there is no residual meningioma or recurrence.

***Case 6***

Thirty-five years after a undergoing a bifrontal craniotomy for a resection of a meningioma involving the anterior skull base, a 54-year-old woman presented with decreased vision and partial palsies of left eye cranial nerves III and VI. MRI demonstrated multiple meningiomas, the largest of which was 4 cm in diameter based at the planum sphenoidale. It extended into the cribriform plate and further into the ethmoid sinus (Figure 17A). Posteriorly, the mass also entered the sella turcica, extended into the left optic canal and compressed the optic nerve. A 1.7-cm parafalcine meningioma was identified as well as multiple smaller meningiomas along the convexity of the right sphenoid wing.

A revision bifrontal craniotomy was performed. The dura was opened at the frontobasal portion and the anterior aspect of the superior sagittal sinus was ligated. The parafalcine meningioma was resected and the falx was cut to assist in visualization of the skull base.

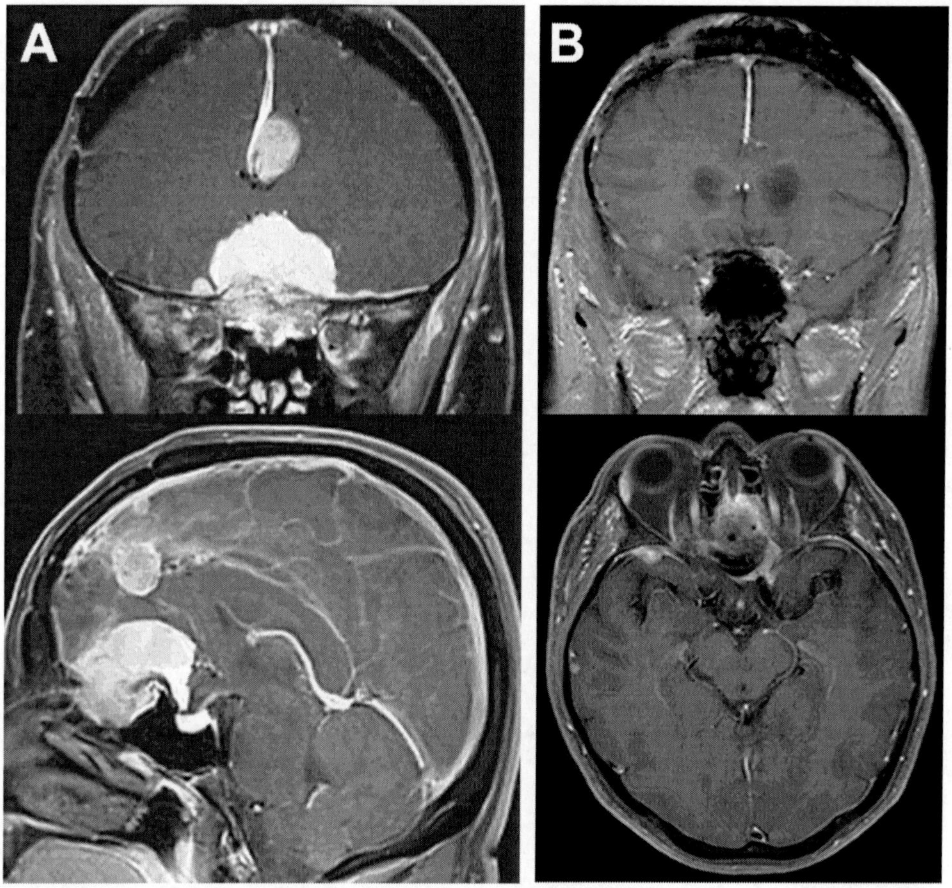


Figure 17. Case 6. (A) Contrast-enhanced T1-weighted MRI demonstrates a large meningioma based at the cribriform plate and planum sphenoidale. Meningiomas at the falx and right sphenoid wing are also seen. (B) Postoperative contrast-enhanced T1-weighted MRI at 6 years demonstrates residual enhancement along the cribriform plate, left anterior clinoid process, and right sphenoid wing.

The PSM was identified and resected using a bipolar electrocautery and an ultrasonic aspirator. Dissection was carried to the planum sphenoidale and the cribriform plate. The hyperostotic bone was drilled out with a diamond burr, but an extensive resection of the ethmoid bones was not performed. The meningioma was then tracked into the left optic canal. The roof of the optic canal was removed and tumor was carefully dissected off of the optic nerve. Several small dural-based tumors were resected during the operation. A pericranium flap was used to cover the defect in the anterior skull base and suturing a dural graft substitute repaired the dural defect.

Postoperatively, the patient's vision remained stable. She underwent stereotactic radiosurgery for the remaining lesions at the cribriform plate, anterior falx, right sphenoid wing, and convexity. A dose of 1500 cGy was administered to each of the five lesions. An MRI obtained after three years demonstrated stable disease without any new enhancing lesions or evidence of progression (Figure 17B).

# DISCUSSION

OGM and PSM share common characteristics that distinguish them from meningiomas originating in other locations. They are located relatively far from critical neural structures that may be sensitive to the pressure of mass effect, such as the brainstem or optic chiasm. Often, this distance enables OGM and PSM to grow large before they become symptomatic and are diagnosed. They also have a general tendency to displace neurovascular structures superiorly and posteriorly, although the optic apparatus are displaced inferiorly and posteriorly.

## Literature Review

Our literature review comprises 16 clinical series published between 1999 and 2014 that are representative of the current OGM surgical management. Each of these is a retrospective cohort study. Sample sizes ranged from 13 to 82 patients, with a mean follow-up time ranging from 2.0 to 10.2 years.

Fifteen articles focused solely on OGM (646 patients) and 1 article included 18 patients with PSM. Articles that included PSM among tuberculum sellae meningiomas were excluded because the sample sizes of PSM in these series were too small to identify trends. This literature review provides a basis for understanding several important points related to the management of OGM, such as common presentation, trends in surgical management, clinical outcomes and complications, and recurrence rates.

## Presentation

One of the distinguishing characteristics of OGM and PSM is their large size found at presentation. Many authors have reported series in which more than half of patients had OGM greater than 5 cm in size [17, 19]. Symptomatic patients may demonstrate personality changes, headaches, and decreased visual acuity or visual field deficits. In contrast to tuberculum sellae meningiomas, which frequently cause bitemporal hemianopsia as the tumor causes mass effect from below the optic chiasm, an inferior visual field deficit is more common with OGM and PSM because the tumor compresses the optic nerves and chiasm from above. Diminished sense of smell is common, although it is not typically a primary complaint [19]. Foster-Kennedy syndrome (unilateral optic atrophy and contralateral papilledema) was first described in OGM, but is not frequently observed [20].

## Paranasal Sinus Involvement

Although it is uncommon for a meningioma to have predominant involvement of the ethmoidal bones, caudal extension of OGM into the paranasal sinuses occurs in 3–67% of reported cases (mean 19%) (Table 1). The management of meningiomas with extension into the paranasal sinuses is controversial. Some surgeons prefer a conservative approach, in which only the tumor that is visible and accessible is removed, only the superficial hyperostotic bone is drilled, and/or the dural attachment is coagulated. However, such a subtotal resection increases the risk for recurrence. Published series of cases with a high incidence of paranasal sinus involvement often also demonstrate high recurrence rates [8, 21]. It is unclear whether recurrence is due to residual disease left behind to preserve the integrity of the anterior skull base and decrease the risk of a CSF fistula from developing or to unrecognized bone invasion. Given the indolent growth of many OGMs, paranasal sinus involvement may reflect extensive spread of tumor at the time of diagnosis.

For an increased likelihood of obtaining definitive treatment, an aggressive resection of all tumor, including removal of all hyperostotic ethmoidal bone, if present, and reconstruction of the anterior skull base, is advocated. Many surgeons who favor a radical resection have a preference towards transnasal operations for OGMs with paranasal sinus involvement. Current trends have focused on aggressive removal with drilling of involved bone in the paranasal sinuses extending into the cranial floor. However, extensive removal of ethmoidal bones and drilling of the cribriform plate often creates a large osteodural defect and a risk of CSF fistula if the anterior fossa floor is not appropriately repaired.

## Management

Surgical management of OGMs is most commonly performed via an open craniotomy. Several authors have published series of patients with OGMs resected using either a bifrontal or unilateral craniotomy with good results. The choice of surgical approach does not appear to affect the extent of resection (Table 1). The surgical approach appears to be frequently based on the senior author's preference or familiarity, but many surgeons tailor the operative approach according to the tumor size, location, and involvement of the paranasal sinuses. Large tumors are frequently approached using a bifrontal craniotomy, which enables the most operative exposure and access to tumor margins with the least frontal lobe retraction. Small tumors may be accessed via a unilateral subfrontal or supraorbital "keyhole" approach. Pterional approaches enable early visualization of the neurovascular structures. Orbital osteotomies are used in combination with various craniotomies to increase the operative exposure, decrease working distance, and reduce the amount of frontal lobe retraction. Transnasal approaches are often employed when the aim of the operation is to resect tumors with a large presence in the paranasal sinuses.

Because OGMs typically present as large tumors, radiosurgery is usually not recommended as a primary treatment strategy. However, radiosurgery may be appropriate for small tumors, in older patients, or in poor surgical candidates. For recurrent disease, radiosurgery may be employed for tumor control. It may be a useful adjunct for patients who undergo subtotal resection for the preservation of critical neurovascular structures.

## Outcomes

Surgical resection of OGMs and PSMs can be challenging because of their larger size. Despite this, outcomes tend to be good, with most retrospective series reporting a gross total resection in the majority of patients (Table 1). In all of the series reviewed, a complete or Simpson grade 1 or grade 2 resection was reported in 585 of 664 patients (88%).

Symptom improvement is frequently observed after surgical resection. Several authors have reported improvement in vision and restoration of mental status in the majority of patients after surgery [17, 19]. Patients who present with seizures are often seizure-free postoperatively and do not require antiepileptic medications [9]. Anosmia, however, does not typically improve after surgery except in rare instances [22, 23].

Because of the attachment of these tumors to the cribriform plate and their frequent invasion of the paranasal sinuses and involvement of the ethmoidal bones, the osteodural defect resulting from surgical resection increases the risk of a CSF fistula developing. Identification of the CSF leak intraoperatively and performing an adequate reconstruction of the floor of the anterior fossa are critical to preventing CSF fistula formation. If CSF rhinorrhea arises postoperatively, CSF diversion via a lumbar drain is usually sufficient to stop the leak in most cases. In cases of refractory CSF rhinorrhea, reoperation may be needed. In our review of 14 publications reporting data on postoperative CSF leaks, 48 out of 602 (8%) patients developed CSF leaks, of which 35 (78%) resolved with lumbar drainage, 9 (19%) required reoperation, and 1 resolved spontaneously. The management of the CSF leak in 3 patients was not described in detail. Patients with CSF leaks are at risk for meningitis, which occurs much more frequently after a surgical resection of an OGM than postoperative wound infections [24]. With modern microsurgical technique, the risk of a major postoperative complication is low and dissection is aided by the frequent presence of an arachnoid membrane that separates the tumor from neurovascular structures. But meningiomas encasing the internal carotid arteries, ACAs, or the anterior communicating artery must be treated carefully. Artery encasement with tumor has been identified as a risk factor for morbidity [1]. The ACAs can be hidden behind the tumor and may not be visualized until late during the resection. Deaths from vascular injury have been reported [25]. Because of these risks, many authors recommend performing a subtotal resection in cases where the OGM is adherent to critical vascular structures.

Patients who undergo a craniotomy for resection of an OGM are at risk for postoperative cerebral edema. Retraction on the frontal lobes, such as during a bilateral subfrontal approach, can cause intraparenchymal contusions and brain swelling. Cerebral edema may also be precipitated if the anterior portions of the superior sagittal sinus or its draining veins are sacrificed during the surgical approach. The tendency of OGMs to present at large size may increase the risk for a perioperative complication. Large lesions are more cumbersome—their size often obscures visualization, inadvertent injury to the venous sinus or draining veins may occur, and more brain retraction may be required during the dissection.

## Recurrence

Although several authors have reported complete resection of OGM in the majority of patients, recurrence rates have been as high as 41% historically [2]. More recent studies that reflect modern microsurgical techniques report much lower recurrence rates, ranging from 0 to 17% (mean 6%) (Table 1). It is generally believed that a subtotal resection increases the risk for recurrence [26, 27]. A complete resection requires drilling of all involved bone at the

**Table 1. Clinical characteristics of patients with olfactory groove meningiomas**

| Series | Sample size (n) | Follow-up (y) | Approach (n) | Paranasal sinus involvement (%) | Gross total resection (Simpson Grade I or II) (%) | WHO Grade (n) | CSF leak (%) | Recurrence rate (%) |
|---|---|---|---|---|---|---|---|---|
| Turazzi et al. 1999 [17] | 37 | 4.0 | Pterional (37) | 1 (3) | 37 (100) | NR | 0 | 0 |
| Hentschel and DeMonte 2003 [19] | 13 | 2.0 | Bifrontal (13) | 6 (46) | 11 (85) | NR | 0 | 0 |
| Obeid and Al-Mefty 2003 [27] | 15 | 3.7 | Supraorbital, subfrontal, unilateral or bilateral (15) | 10 (67) | 14 (93) | Grade I (15) | 3 (20) | 0 |
| Spektor et al. 2005 [10] | 80 | 5.9 | Bifrontal (35)<br>Unilateral subfrontal (8)<br>Pterional (18)<br>Fronto-orbital (7)<br>Subcranial (12) | 21 (26) | 72 (90) | Grade I (78)<br>Grade II (2) | 10 (13) | 2 (3) |
| Tuna et al. 2005 [35] | 25 | 4.9 | Bifrontal (19)<br>Pterional (6) | 3 (12) | 25(100) | NR | 4 (16) | 0 (0) |
| Bassiouni et al. 2007 [22] | 56 | 5.6 | Bifrontal (36)<br>Pterional (13)<br>Frontolateral (4)<br>Supraorbital (3) | 5 (9) | 56(100) | Grade I (55)<br>Grade II (1) | 3 (5) | 5 (9) |
| Nakamura et al. 2007 [9] | 82 | 5.3 | Bifrontal (46)<br>Frontolateral (34)<br>Pterional (2) | 16 (20) | 75 (93) | Grade I (82) | 1 (1) | 4 (5) |
| Gazzeri et al. 2008 [40] | 36 | 9.3 | Bifrontal (35)<br>Frontotemporal (10 | 1 (3) | 31 (86) | Grade I (36) | 2 (6) | 2 (6) |
| Chen et al. 2009 [41] | 35 | 5.3 | Bifrontal (21)<br>Bifronto-orbital (6)<br>Bifronto-interhemispheric (5)<br>Unilateral subfrontal (6)<br>Pterional (1) | 0 | 29 (83) | NR | 4 (10) | 3 (9) |

| Series | Sample size (n) | Follow-up (y) | Approach (n) | Paranasal sinus involvement (%) | Gross total resection (Simpson Grade I or II) (%) | WHO Grade (n) | CSF leak (%) | Recurrence rate (%) |
|---|---|---|---|---|---|---|---|---|
| El Bahy et al. 2009 [25] | 18 | 2.6 | Frontolateral (18) | 3 (17) | 14 (78) | Grade I (18) | 3 (17) | 0 |
| Romani et al. 2009 [42] | 66 | 3.8 | Lateral supraorbital (66) | 25 (38) | 60 (91) | Grade I (58)<br>Grade II (8) | 6 (9) | 4 (6) |
| Pepper et al. 2011 [8] | 19 | 3.4 | Bifrontal subcranial (19) | 12 (63) | 12 (63) | Grade I (15)<br>Grade II (1)<br>Grade III (3) | 3 (16) | 3 (16) |
| Tomasello et al. 2011 [5] | 18 | 7.8 | Pterional craniotomy (18) | 0 | 17 (94) | Grade I (18) | NR | 3 (17) |
| Ciurea et al. 2012 [21] | 59 | 7.0 | Bilateral subfrontal (38)<br>Unilateral subfrontal (12)<br>Pterional (9) | 14 (24) | 52 (88) | Grade I (56)<br>Grade II (3) | 7 (12) | 6 (10) |
| Bitter et al. 2013 [43] | 61 | 10.2 | Pterional craniotomy (61) | 3 (5) | 60 (98) | Grade I (55)<br>Grade II (3)<br>Grade III (2) | 2 (3) | 3 (5) |
| Zygourakis et al. 2014 [1] | 44 | 2.0 | Unilateral craniotomy (10)<br>Bifrontal craniotomy (26)<br>Gamma knife (5)<br>Observation (3) | 7 (16) | 20 (46) | Grade I (27)<br>Grade II (9) | NR | 4 (9) |

NR, not reported.

cribriform plate, ethmoidal bones, and/or planum sphenoidale. Hyperostosis is common and is due to tumor infiltration of bony interstices, rather than a reactive inflammatory process from adjacent disease [28]. The literature on recurrence after resection of OGM and PSM must be interpreted cautiously. Most published articles on OGM recurrence are limited by their retrospective design, small sample size, and variable length of follow-up. Recurrence rates have been noted to be higher in studies with longer follow-up periods than in those with short follow-up periods, which frequently report no tumor recurrence [2, 11, 22, 25, 27, 29].

Histological subtype also is expected to affect recurrence rates. The incidence of atypical and anaplastic OGM is varied in the published series. Series consisting of a large proportion of patients with OGM involving the paranasal sinuses and those with atypical and anaplastic subtypes have reported high recurrence rates [8]. Tumors that recur in the nasal cavity without significant intracranial regrowth may be obscured by nasal mucosa on contrast-enhanced MRI [22].Therefore, they may be underreported.

# FUTURE DIRECTIONS

## Endoscopic Approach

An anterior endoscopic endonasal trans-cribriform approach may confer advantages to OGM management for certain tumors, based on size and location. Namely, the OGM can be accessed directly, complete resection of hyperostotic bone of the olfactory groove is more easily accomplished, and manipulation of neurovascular structures and brain retraction on the frontal lobes to increase exposure is avoided [30, 31]. In an endoscopic approach, the craniotomy through the cribriform plate is made directly over the basal dural attachment at the anterior skull base. The meningioma can be devascularized early during the operation to decrease blood loss and facilitate tumor removal. Complete removal of all bone that has become hyperostotic from tumor infiltration facilitates a Simpson Grade I resection. An OGM that has recurred or extends into the paranasal sinuses may be suitable for an endoscopic approach.

Disadvantages of the endonasal endoscopic approach stem from the inherent limitations of its midline exposure [32]. Tumors with extension beyond the medial orbital wall, or over the superior orbital roof, and those with dural attachments extending lateral to the optic canal, or into the sphenoid wing, are difficult to access from a midline endonasal approach. They may be better approached through an open transcranial technique. Cranial nerves and vascular structures are identified later in the dissection during an endonasal endoscopic technique and may be prone to injury if manipulated. Tumors encasing the internal carotid or anterior cerebral arteries should be approached by an open technique for more complete visualization and to avoid vascular injury. Large tumors can be challenging to manage endoscopically. They must be sufficiently debulked before they can be delivered through the small bony opening created through an endoscopic approach. If the OGM has a large dural attachment, complete dural resection with a margin of normal dura (Simpson Grade 0 [33]) may not be possible using an endonasal technique. Furthermore, current evidence regarding the effectiveness of endoscopic approaches for management of OGM is limited by the studies' retrospective design, limited follow-up time, and small sample sizes. High-quality studies examining the extent of resection, recurrence rates, and complications are currently lacking.

CSF leaks requiring endonasal exploration for repair may be more common with endoscopic surgery. The osteodural defect is larger when created by an approach from below than when created by a Simpson Grade I resection with a transcranial approach from above. Approaching an OGM may require resection of bone and dura extending from the posterior wall of the frontal sinus to the planum sphenoidale [31]. Resection of the hyperostotic endonasal bones and entering the paranasal sinuses further increases the risk of a CSF leak developing. One case series reported that 4 of 15 patients with OGM treated endoscopically had persistent CSF leaks requiring additional surgical repair despite lumbar drainage [34]. In contrast, other authors have reported that CSF leaks after craniotomy can typically be managed with lumbar drain for CSF diversion [10, 35]. Because of the risk of a CSF fistula, many surgeons prefer a conservative approach. They accept a subtotal resection by coagulating the dural base and monitor patients postoperatively with routine imaging surveillance [36].

In doing so, these surgeons accept a higher OGM recurrence rate, which has been reported to range from 23% to 41% [2, 27]. Modern surgical techniques, such as the use of vascularized nasoseptal mucosal flaps and allogenic acellular dermal allograft (AlloDerm), may decrease the rate of CSF leaks without the need for lumbar drainage. This may grant surgeons the confidence to perform a more complete surgical resection [31, 34, 37-39]. However, prospective trials evaluating the effectiveness of these newer techniques have not yet been published.

## Conclusion

Historically, OGMs and PSMs hold a significant place in neurosurgery because an OGM was one of the first successfully resected intracranial tumors. Nevertheless, they remain a significant challenge and there is no current consensus on surgical strategy.

Here we discuss multiple surgical strategies for treatment, any of which must be tailored to the individual tumor and patient. As is evident in the literature, the traditional approaches are very much still in use. However, the minimally invasive techniques, including expanded endonasal routes, are becoming more widespread and many of their limitations are being overcome with improved tools and techniques. These lesions continue to have excellent surgical outcomes when treated by surgeons with knowledge of the anatomy who can tailor the approaches for their patients.

## References

[1] Zygourakis CC, Sughrue ME, Cabero AB, Parsa AT, Berger MS, McDermott MW. Management of planum/olfactory meningiomas: predicting symptoms and postoperative complications. *World Neurosurg*. 2014 Dec;82(6):1216-23.

[2] Mirimanoff RO, Dosoretz DE, Linggood RM, Ojemann RG, Martuza RL. Meningioma: analysis of recurrence and progression following neurosurgical resection. *J Neurosurg.* 1985 Jan;62(1):18-24.

[3] Mezue WC, Ohaegbulam SC, Ndubuisi CC, Chikani MC, Achebe DS. Intracranial meningiomas managed at Memfys hospital for neurosurgery in Enugu, Nigeria. *J Neurosci Rural Pract.* 2012 Sep;3(3):320-3.

[4] Chan RC, Thompson GB. Morbidity, mortality, and quality of life following surgery for intracranial meningiomas. A retrospective study in 257 cases. *J Neurosurg.* 1984 Jan;60(1):52-60.

[5] Tomasello F, Germano A. Francesco Durante: the history of intracranial meningiomas and beyond. *Neurosurgery.* 2006 Aug;59(2):389-96; discussion -96.

[6] Cushing H, Eisenhardt L. Notes on the first reasonably successful removal of an intracranial tumor. *Bull Los Angeles Neurol* Soc. 1938;3:95-8.

[7] Cushing H, Eisenhardt L. *Meningiomas: Their Classification, Regional Behavior, Life History, and Surgical End Results.* Springfield, IL: Charles C Thomas; 1938.

[8] Pepper JP, Hecht SL, Gebarski SS, Lin EM, Sullivan SE, Marentette LJ. Olfactory groove meningioma: discussion of clinical presentation and surgical outcomes following excision via the subcranial approach. *Laryngoscope.* 2011 Nov;121 (11):2282-9.

[9] Nakamura M, Struck M, Roser F, Vorkapic P, Samii M. Olfactory groove meningiomas: clinical outcome and recurrence rates after tumor removal through the frontolateral and bifrontal approach. *Neurosurgery.* 2007 May;60(5):844-52; discussion -52.

[10] Spektor S, Valarezo J, Fliss DM, Gil Z, Cohen J, Goldman J, et al. Olfactory groove meningiomas from neurosurgical and ear, nose, and throat perspectives: approaches, techniques, and outcomes. *Neurosurgery.* 2005 Oct;57(4 Suppl):268-80; discussion -80.

[11] Solero CL, Giombini S, Morello G. Suprasellar and olfactory meningiomas. Report on a series of 153 personal cases. *Acta Neurochir* (Wien). 1983;67(3-4):181-94.

[12] Maiuri F, Salzano FA, Motta S, Colella G, Sardo L. Olfactory groove meningioma with paranasal sinus and nasal cavity extension: removal by combined subfrontal and nasal approach. *J Craniomaxillofac Surg.* 1998 Oct;26(5):314-7.

[13] Derome PJ, Guiot G. Bone problems in meningiomas invading the base of the skull. *Clin Neurosurg.* 1978;25:435-51.

[14] Bonfils P, Brasnu D, Roux FX, Laccourreye H. [Olfactory meningioma with ethmoido-orbital extension. Diagnostic and therapeutic problems. Apropos of a case]. *Ann Otolaryngol Chir Cervicofac.* 1988;105(3):179-81.

[15] Bakay L, Cares HL. Olfactory meningiomas. Report on a series of twenty-five cases. *Acta Neurochir* (Wien). 1972;26(1):1-12.

[16] Hassler W, Zentner J. Pterional approach for surgical treatment of olfactory groove meningiomas. *Neurosurgery.* 1989 Dec;25(6):942-5; discussion -45-7.

[17] Turazzi S, Cristofori L, Gambin R, Bricolo A. The pterional approach for the microsurgical removal of olfactory groove meningiomas. *Neurosurgery.* 1999 Oct;45(4):821-5; discussion -25-6.

[18] McDermott MW, Rootman J, Durity FA. Subperiosteal, subperiorbital dissection and division of the anterior and posterior ethmoid arteries for meningiomas of the

cribriform plate and planum sphenoidale: technical note. *Neurosurgery.* 1995 Jun;36(6):1215-8; discussion -18-9.

[19] Hentschel SJ, DeMonte F. Olfactory groove meningiomas. *Neurosurg Focus.* 2003 Jun 15;14(6):e4.

[20] Kennedy F. Retrobulbar neuritis as an exact diagnostic sign of certain tumors and abscesses in the frontal lobes. *Am J Med Sci.* 1911;142:355-68.

[21] Ciurea AV, Iencean SM, Rizea RE, Brehar FM. Olfactory groove meningiomas: a retrospective study on 59 surgical cases. *Neurosurg Rev.* 2012 Apr;35(2):195-202; discussion

[22] Bassiouni H, Asgari S, Stolke D. Olfactory groove meningiomas: functional outcome in a series treated microsurgically. *Acta Neurochir* (Wien). 2007 Feb;149(2):109-21; discussion -21.

[23] Gerber M, Vishteh AG, Spetzler RF. Return of olfaction after gross total resection of an olfactory groove meningioma: case report. *Skull Base Surg.* 1998;8(4):229-31.

[24] Coppens J, Couldwell W. Olfactory groove meningiomas. In: Pamir M, Black P, Fahlbusch R, editors. *Meningiomas: A Comprehensive Text.* Philadelphia: Elsevier; 2010.

[25] El-Bahy K. Validity of the frontolateral approach as a minimally invasive corridor for olfactory groove meningiomas. *Acta Neurochir* (Wien). 2009 Oct;151(10):1197-205.

[26] Mathiesen T, Lindquist C, Kihlstrom L, Karlsson B. Recurrence of cranial base meningiomas. *Neurosurgery.* 1996 Jul;39(1):2-7; discussion 8-9.

[27] Obeid F, Al-Mefty O. Recurrence of olfactory groove meningiomas. *Neurosurgery.* 2003 Sep;53(3):534-42; discussion -42-3.

[28] Poppen JL. Operative techniques for removal of olfactory groove and suprasellar meningiomas. *Clin Neurosurg.* 1964;11:1-7.

[29] Tsikoudas A, Martin-Hirsch DP. Olfactory groove meningiomas. *Clin Otolaryngol Allied Sci.* 1999 Dec;24(6):507-9.

[30] Adappa ND, Lee JY, Chiu AG, Palmer JN. Olfactory groove meningioma. *Otolaryngol Clin North Am.* 2011 Aug;44(4):965-80, ix.

[31] Liu JK, Christiano LD, Patel SK, Tubbs RS, Eloy JA. Surgical nuances for removal of olfactory groove meningiomas using the endoscopic endonasal transcribriform approach. *Neurosurg Focus.* 2011 May;30(5):E3.

[32] Couldwell WT, Heros R, Dolenc V. Skull base meningiomas. *Neurosurg Focus.* 2011 May;30(5):1p prior to E.

[33] Kinjo T, al-Mefty O, Kanaan I. Grade zero removal of supratentorial convexity meningiomas. *Neurosurgery.* 1993 Sep;33(3):394-9; discussion -99.

[34] Gardner PA, Kassam AB, Thomas A, Snyderman CH, Carrau RL, Mintz AH, et al. Endoscopic endonasal resection of anterior cranial base meningiomas. *Neurosurgery.* 2008 Jul;63(1):36-52; discussion -54.

[35] Tuna H, Bozkurt M, Ayten M, Erdogan A, Deda H. Olfactory groove meningiomas. *J Clin Neurosci.* 2005 Aug;12(6):664-8.

[36] Snyder WE, Shah MV, Weisberger EC, Campbell RL. Presentation and patterns of late recurrence of olfactory groove meningiomas. *Skull Base Surg.* 2000;10(3):131-9.

[37] Hadad G, Bassagasteguy L, Carrau RL, Mataza JC, Kassam A, Snyderman CH, et al. A novel reconstructive technique after endoscopic expanded endonasal approaches: vascular pedicle nasoseptal flap. *Laryngoscope.* 2006 Oct;116(10):1882-6.

[38] Eloy JA, Kuperan AB, Choudhry OJ, Harirchian S, Liu JK. Efficacy of the pedicled nasoseptal flap without cerebrospinal fluid (CSF) diversion for repair of skull base defects: incidence of postoperative CSF leaks. *Int Forum Allergy Rhinol.* 2012 Sep-Oct;2(5):397-401.

[39] Kassam AB, Thomas A, Carrau RL, Snyderman CH, Vescan A, Prevedello D, et al. Endoscopic reconstruction of the cranial base using a pedicled nasoseptal flap. *Neurosurgery.* 2008 Jul;63(1 Suppl 1):ONS44-52; discussion -ONS-53.

[40] Gazzeri R, Galarza M, Gazzeri G. Giant olfactory groove meningioma: ophthalmological and cognitive outcome after bifrontal microsurgical approach. *Acta Neurochir* (Wien). 2008 Nov;150(11):1117-25; discussion -26.

[41] Chen S-M, Wei K-C, Lee S-T, Lui T-N, Hsu Y-H, Lin T-K, et al. Olfactory groove meningiomas: surgical experience from 35 cases. *J Chin Oncol Soc.* 2009;25(1):38-48.

[42] Romani R, Lehecka M, Gaal E, Toninelli S, Celik O, Niemela M, et al. Lateral supraorbital approach applied to olfactory groove meningiomas: experience with 66 consecutive patients. *Neurosurgery.* 2009 Jul;65(1):39-52; discussion -53.

[43] Bitter AD, Stavrinou LC, Ntoulias G, Petridis AK, Dukagjin M, Scholz M, et al. The role of the pterional approach in the surgical treatment of olfactory groove meningiomas: A 20-year experience. *J Neurol Surg B Skull Base.* 2013 Apr;74(2):97-102.

In: Current Management of Central Nervous System … ISBN: 978-1-63483-856-6
Editors: Steven D. Chang and Anand Veeravagu 

*Chapter 6*

# SPHENOID WING MENINGIOMAS

***John Henry Cain*[1]*, MD, Daniel Klinger*[1]*, MD***
***and Samuel Barnett*[1]*, MD***
[1]University of Texas Southwestern Medical Center,
Dallas, Texas, US

## ABSTRACT

Meningiomas arising from the region of the sphenoid wing comprise a significant portion of intracranial and skull base meningiomas and present a diverse array of clinical challenges. These tumors can either be focal (globoid) or diffuse (en plaque) in morphology and present a variety of distinct clinical concerns and surgical challenges depending on the location of the tumor along the sphenoid wing. Clinical presentation is variable but visual symptoms are a prominent concern and a frequent driver of clinical decision-making in the management of these tumors. Surgical resection is the most effective treatment of these lesions and a clear understanding of the relevant surgical anatomy of the sphenoid wing is necessary to minimize surgical morbidity. The frontotemporal craniotomy in combination with an interfascial extracranial dissection technique provides excellent surgical exposure for the resection of most sphenoid wing meningiomas. Lateral sphenoid wing meningiomas are the most readily accessible, but can present challenges related to extracranial tumor invasion or with involvement of the sylvian fissure. Medial or clinoidal tumors are generally more challenging to resect, given their location deep on the sphenoid wing and close association with the optic nerve and the internal carotid artery.

The anterior clinoidectomy, via either extradural or intradural approach, is an essential step in safely resecting many of these tumors. En plaque, or spheno-orbital, meningiomas are a unique entity given their diffuse nature, tendency to induce a marked hyperostostic reaction, and frequent extension into the orbit. Resection of spheno-orbital meningiomas can be difficult due to the extent of bony resection often required as well as the management of reconstruction following resection. Radiosurgery can be an important adjuvant treatment modality for these tumors when complete resection is not possible or would result in excessive morbidity.

Surgical outcomes for resection of sphenoid wing meningiomas are historically poor, but have improved markedly in recent years with improvement in skull base dissection techniques.

**Keywords**: pterional meningioma, clinoidal meningioma, spheno-orbital meningioma, en plaque meningioma, sphenoid wing, optic canal, orbit, superior orbital fissure, cavernous sinus, interfascial dissection, anterior clinoid process, anterior clinoidectomy, sylvian fissure, hyperostosis

## INTRODUCTION

Approximately 20% of all intracranial meningiomas, and about 50% of all skull base meningiomas, arise from the region of the sphenoid wing. The first detailed description of sphenoid wing meningiomas was provided by Cushing and Eisenhardt in 1938 [1]. This early series proposed the classification of these tumors into two broad categories on the basis of tumor morphology: en plaque (also known as spheno-orbital meningiomas), and globoid. The en plaque meningiomas were tumors that spread along the sphenoid wing in a carpet-like manner with a high rate of reactive hyperostosis and frequent orbital involvement. The globoid meningiomas were nodular lesions arising from a dural base along the sphenoid wing, and were further divided by their location along the sphenoid wing into lateral (pterional), middle (alar), and medial (clinoidal) groups. This remains the predominant manner for the classification of sphenoid wing meningiomas today, although the middle and lateral globoid sphenoid wing meningiomas are frequently grouped together as the surgical technique for their resection is similar [2, 3].

## SURGICAL ANATOMY

The sphenoid wing is a term which refers to the crest of the sphenoid bone that divides the anterior from the middle cranial fossa floor along the skull base (Figure 1). The greater wing of the sphenoid bone composes the outer third of the sphenoid ridge, which overlies the sylvian fissure and the adjacent frontal operculum and temporal cortex. The greater wing joins the frontal, squamous temporal, and parietal bones at the pterion. The anterior portion of the greater wing also forms the posterolateral orbit. The inner two-thirds of the sphenoid ridge is formed by the lesser wing of the sphenoid bone, ultimately terminating in the anterior clinoid process. The relevant surgical anatomy becomes more complex as one moves medially down the sphenoid ridge towards the anterior clinoid, which is closely associated with both the optic nerve as well as the internal carotid artery.

Furthermore, tumors of the medial sphenoid wing may also extend to the orbit via involvement of the superior orbital fissure, the optic canal, and the cavernous sinus.

A number of neurologic and vascular structures are associated with the sphenoid wing and its foramina, and may be at risk in the exposure and resection of tumors of the sphenoid wing. These include cranial nerves III, IV, $V_1$, and VI, which traverse the superior orbital fissure, cranial nerves $V_2$ and $V_3$, which traverse foramen rotundum and ovale, respectively, the optic nerve and ophthalmic artery, which traverse the optic canal, and the internal carotid artery, which enters the skull base at the carotid canal. The surgical exposure and resection of globoid sphenoid wing tumors frequently requires dissection of the tumor capsule away from the sylvian fissure.

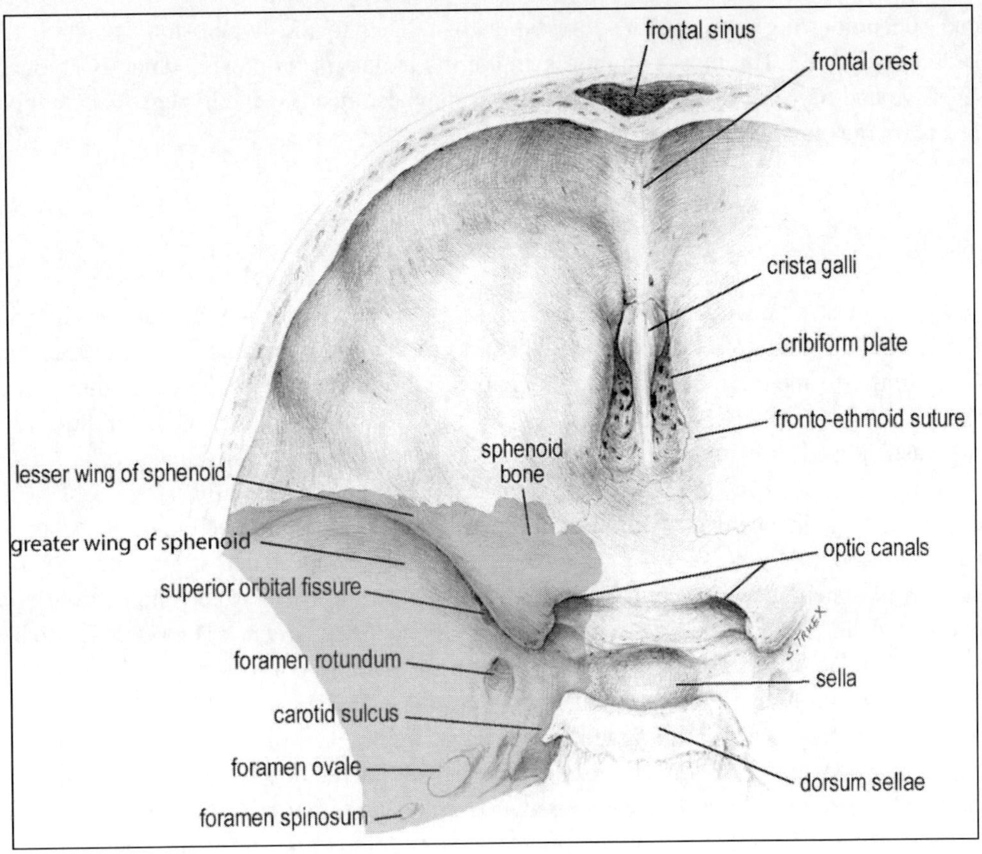


Figure 1. The sphenoid ridge is formed by the junction of the lesser wing (red) and greater wing (blue) and terminates at the anterior clinoid process overlying the optic canal.

Microsurgical dissection of the sylvian fissure may be necessary to protect the sylvian vessels from injury during the resection of larger tumors. The sella lies at the medial limit of the sphenoid ridge, and large medial tumors can compromise the pituitary axis as well.

## Surgical Management

### Presentation

The clinical presentation of sphenoid wing meningiomas is variable and predominantly reflects the location of the individual tumor. The lateral sphenoid wing overlies frontal and temporal cortex which is relatively tolerant of mass effect and as such, these tumors typically present late, as larger tumors. Presenting symptoms commonly include headache, nausea, papilledema, seizure, or hemiparesis. Dominant hemisphere tumors may also induce aphasia. In contrast, medial sphenoid wing meningiomas frequently present with visual field and/or visual acuity deficits, given the close relationship between the medial sphenoid wing and the optic nerve. These tumors may also present with oculomotor palsies and facial sensory deficits secondary to involvement of the cavernous sinus. The presenting symptoms of en plaque sphenoid wing meningiomas are typically related to the hyperostotic reaction that these tumors induce. The most common symptom is unilateral proptosis, which is gradually progressive and may become painful. Visual loss may also result if the hyperostosis involves and narrows the optic canal.

## Imaging

As with most other intracranial tumors, contrast-enhanced magnetic resonance imaging (MRI) is now the study of choice for visualization of the tumor volume. The appearance on MRI is similar to meningiomas in other locations: a homogenously enhancing, dural-based mass. The tumor is usually isointense on both T1- and T2-weighted sequences. In the case of highly vascularized tumors, flow voids may be seen within the tumor parenchyma. MRI is also the best study for evaluating for associated cortical edema. Careful assessment of the extent of dural enhancement is important to ensure that all involved dura is resected. Computed tomography (CT) imaging is also of critical importance in the preoperative evaluation of sphenoid wing meningiomas, as it provides the best visualization of the bone structure and allows one to assess the extent of bone involvement. This is of particular importance in the case of en plaque sphenoid wing meningiomas, where the amount of reactive hyperostosis can be much greater the dural-based tumor component. Depending on the location of the tumor, angiographic sequences (either CT or MRI) can be useful to determine the location of the major intracranial vessels in relation to the tumor. There has been some interest in preoperative catheter angiography and tumor embolization for reduction in intraoperative blood loss. However, in most cases, preoperative tumor embolization is unnecessary and likely not indicated given the rate of complications due to the embolization procedure [4].

## Differential

Globoid sphenoid wing meningiomas are typically well-characterized on standard MRI sequences and the diagnosis of these lesions is usually clear after imaging is completed. However, careful attention to should be paid to the bone-window CT scan, as the presence of bony erosion rather than the expected reactive hyperostosis can indicate a metastatic lesion or other type of osteolytic malignant tumor rather than a meningioma. The diagnosis of en plaque sphenoid wing meningiomas can be more difficult, as the most prominent abnormality is frequently the reactive hyperostosis, which can also result from other pathologies including fibrous dysplasia, sarcoidosis, hyperostosis frontalis interna, Paget's disease, and primary or metastatic tumors of the bone.

## Surgical Indications

Surgical resection is the most effective treatment for sphenoid wing meningiomas. Surgery should be discussed when a patient presents with symptoms referable to the lesion, particularly in the case of progressive neurologic or visual symptoms. However, as the utilization of medical imaging increases, these tumors are increasingly found as incidental lesions. In the case of an asymptomatic tumor, indications for resection include progressive tumor enlargement on serial imaging, the presence of peri-lesional edema in the adjacent brain tissue, and large tumor volume. Tumors that threaten the optic apparatus may also be considered for resection prior to the onset of symptoms, as they may be more safely treated if operated on earlier. As with all neurosurgical procedures, surgical indications need to be individualized, taking into account each patient's age, health status, the surgeon's experience, and the expected risks associated with resection of the patient's tumor. For patients who are not good candidates for surgical resection, radiotherapy can be an alternative option.

### Preoperative Workup

As with any craniotomy, patients should undergo general preoperative medical evaluation in accordance with their age and health status. As discussed, all patients should have preoperative imaging which includes a contrast-enhanced MRI study as well as bone-window CT scan. Vascular imaging should be considered for tumors which are suspected to involve or displace any of the major intracranial vessels. CT- or MR- angiography is generally adequate for this purpose, though catheter angiography can be considered in select cases. For tumors with a significant amount of hyperostosis, the use of three-dimensional reconstructions can be helpful to visualize the extent of involvement and plan for reconstruction after resection. The use of an intraoperative image-guidance system, if available, can also aid in identifying and resecting all of the involved bone.

A full preoperative ophthalmologic evaluation, including dilated fundoscopic examination and formal visual field assessment, should be performed for sphenoorbital tumors as well as medial sphenoid wing meningiomas which threaten the optic pathways. Endocrinologic evaluation to assess the function of the pituitary axis should be performed if there is evidence of sellar or parasellar extension of the tumor.

## Surgical Management

### General Principles

Given the complexity of the anatomy of the sphenoid ridge, particularly along its medial extent, as well as the frequent extension of these tumors into adjacent compartments such as the cavernous sinus and orbit, a comprehensive surgical strategy is elusive [5]. Each tumor must be carefully evaluated on an individual basis to determine the relevant structures at risk in each particular case and the surgical plan must be modified accordingly. However, there are a number of general principles which are relevant for most cases. More specific techniques and operative nuances pertaining to the major sub-classes of sphenoid wing meningiomas will be discussed subsequently.

*Operating Room Preparation:* General anesthesia is administered for the duration of the procedure. Corticosteroid is administered preoperatively. Standard perioperative antibiotic prophylaxis is administered. After induction of anesthesia, the patient is positioned supine on the operating table with the head fixed in a skull clamp. The head is rotated toward the side opposite the tumor with gentle neck extension. For medial tumors, approximately 30 degrees of rotation is ideal. For lateral tumors, a greater amount of rotation will provide better exposure.

*Skin Incision:* A standard frontotemporal skin incision is usually adequate, beginning anterior to the tragus at the root of the zygomatic arch and extending in a gentle curve toward the midline in the superior-anterior direction. Keeping the anterior limb of the incision behind the hairline, if possible, will improve the cosmetic result.

*Extracranial Dissection:* Extracranial dissection technique can be modified based on the location of the tumor. For lateral tumors, the scalp and temporalis muscle can typically be elevated together in a single myocutaneous flap which is reflected anteriorly. This method is efficient and avoids injury to the frontotemporal branch of the facial nerve. The disadvantage to this technique is that the bulk of reflected scalp and temporalis muscle can limit the angle of approach and block visualization of deeper structures when attempting to resect more medial tumors. In certain cases, tumor can extend through the bone into the temporalis muscle tissue. In these cases the scalp needs be dissected separately in order to allow for adequate inspection and resection of the involved muscle. An alternative approach using an interfascial dissection technique is preferable in these situations. In the interfascial approach, the scalp is first dissected away from the temporalis fascia and pericranium and reflected anteriorly until the fat pad which contains the frontotemporal branch of the facial nerve is identified. This fat pad lies between the superficial and deep layers of the temporalis fascia. The two layers of the temporalis fascia are then sectioned posterior to the fat pad, allowing the fat pad and its enveloping fascia to be mobilized anteriorly with the scalp flap. The temporalis muscle can then be safely mobilized and reflected inferiorly over the zygomatic arch. Allowing the scalp and the temporalis muscle to be mobilized in different directions allows for a more direct angle of view down the sphenoid wing, facilitating the resection of deeper tumors. In select cases, mobilization of the zygomatic arch inferolaterally along with the temporalis muscle may be helpful to achieve a more favorable angle of approach along the skull base to the medial aspect of the middle cranial fossa [6].

*Craniotomy:* After the extracranial dissection is completed, the craniotomy can be performed. If the frontotemporal skull is not involved by the tumor, then a standard pterional craniotomy often provides adequate exposure for tumor resection. However, if hyperostosis is present or tumor invasion of the frontotemporal skull is observed, the craniotomy may need to be widened to provide an adequate margin of resection around the involved bone. If extensive hyperostosis is present, craniectomy may be necessary.

*Tumor Resection:* After completion of the craniotomy and resection of the involved bone, the dural component of the tumor can then be resected. The general principles of meningioma surgery also apply to lesions of the sphenoid wing. Early interruption of the blood supply to the tumor is accomplished via the extracranial and epidural dissection. The tumor mass is then internally debulked with the aid of bipolar coagulation, scissors, ultrasonic aspiration, or other instruments depending on the consistency of the tumor. After the tumor is adequately debulked, the tumor capsule may then be carefully dissected away from the surface of the adjacent brain, cranial nerves, and intracranial arteries. The preoperative imaging studies should be reviewed carefully and all of the enhancing dura and hyperostotic bone should be resected, if possible.

*Closure/Reconstruction:* After the resection is complete, dural closure and reconstruction of the skull must be performed. There are a number of options for dural closure. Historically, watertight dural closure using either autologous fascial grafts or a dural substitute product has been advocated. However, good results have also been achieved using dural regeneration matrix onlays without watertight dural repair. If the skull flap was not involved with the tumor, then it may be replaced in standard fashion. When craniectomy must be performed due to bony involvement, reconstruction of the frontotemporal skull contour using titanium mesh, methyl methacrylate, or other material may be required.

## Lateral Sphenoid Wing Meningiomas

Lateral tumors are the most accessible of the sphenoid wing meningiomas. However, they can present a number of particular challenges which the surgeon must be prepared to manage [7]. As discussed previously, tumors of the lateral sphenoid wing are generally better exposed with the head positioned with a greater degree of lateral rotation, which brings the mass of the tumor to the top of the operative field. The bone-window CT scan should be reviewed preoperatively to assess the extent of tumor invasion. Lateral sphenoid wing meningiomas may invade the pterional skull and in some cases can extend to involve the temporalis muscle. In these cases, the extracranial dissection should be performed using the interfascial technique, allowing the temporalis muscle to be inspected and all involved tumor to be resected.

After the temporalis is addressed, the craniotomy can be performed. The size of the craniotomy should be modified to include any region of infiltrated bone along with a margin of normal bone. The underlying tumor may be adherent to the bone flap, in which case the tumor may need to be divided in order to elevate the flap. After the craniotomy flap is elevated, it should be carefully inspected and all abnormal bone should be resected. In some cases in which there is prominent hyperostosis of the frontotemporal skull, the bone may be too thick to allow for the creation of flap using a standard craniotome. In these cases, the margins of the skull flap may need to be developed using the high-speed drill. The hyperostotic bone often has a rich vascular supply and significant bleeding is can be encountered when drilling the hyperostotic skull.

After the craniotomy is complete and extradural hemostasis is achieved, the bulk of the tumor can be addressed. If the tumor is sufficiently lateral and presents beneath the bone flap, then debulking of the tumor can be started directly via the exposed portion of the tumor. If the tumor is deeper along the lateral sphenoid wing and not immediately exposed, then the dura can be opened in a semilunar fashion and flapped anteriorly. Careful arachnoid dissection is then performed to allow the frontal and temporal lobes to be gently mobilized. For deeper tumors, opening the sylvian fissure may be necessary to expose the tumor without excessive brain retraction. If the tumor displaces the middle cerebral artery or its branches, these should be carefully identified and protected as the tumor resection proceeds from superficial to deep.

Once the tumor is debulked, all involved dura should be resected. The preoperative MRI study should be carefully reviewed to ensure that all of the enhancing dura is removed. The bony structures should also be re-inspected and any residual hyperostosis should be removed with the drill. At this point, the tumor resection is complete and the surgeon can proceed with dural closure and skull reconstruction as discussed previously.

## Case Presentation

A 44-year-old man presented with one month of progressive headaches and recurrent episodes of transient right eye visual loss. Initial evaluation was remarkable for papilledema. His neurologic examination was otherwise normal. Magnetic resonance imaging demonstrated a large enhancing dural-based mass centered over the right pterion with extensive abnormal FLAIR signal in the adjacent right frontal lobe (Figure 2).

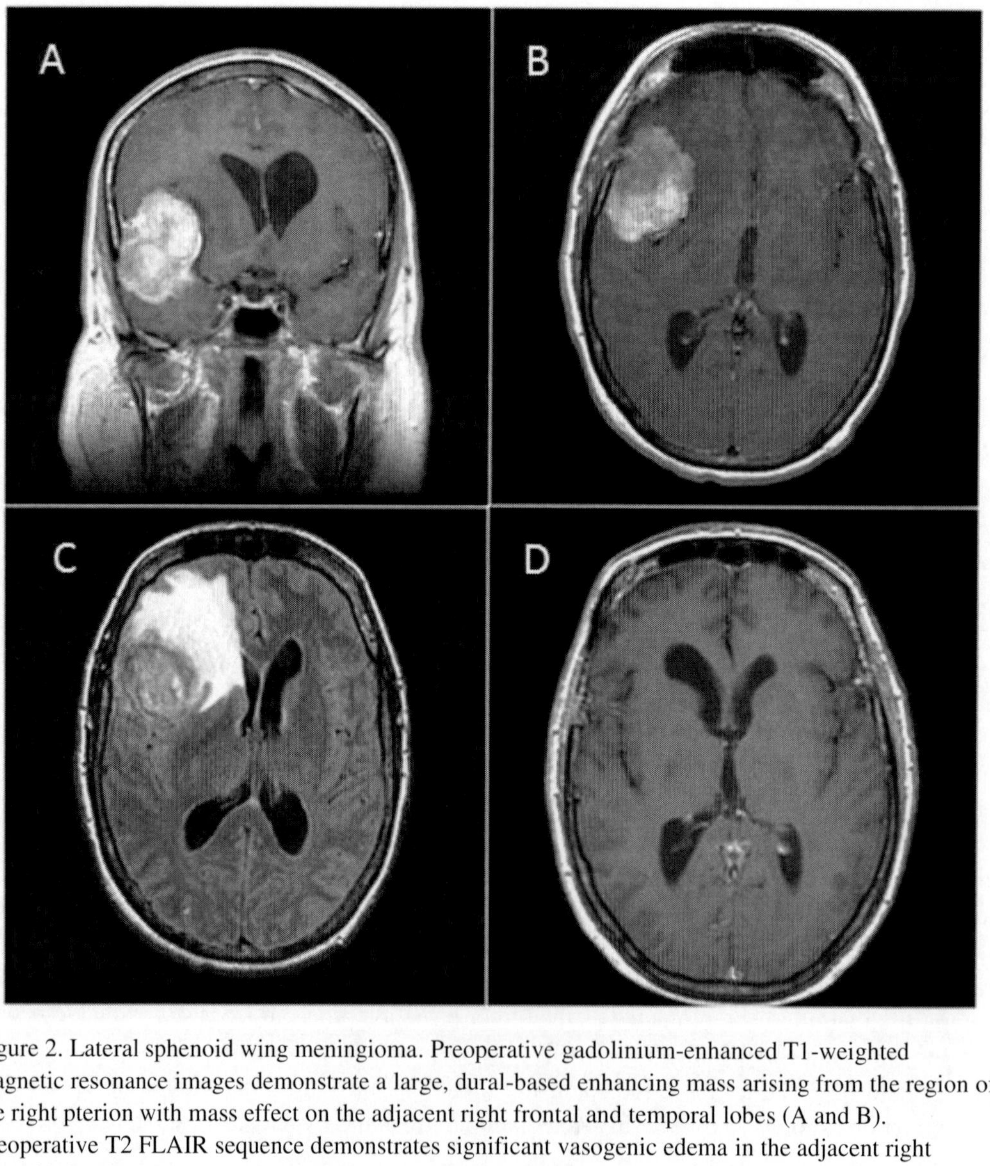


Figure 2. Lateral sphenoid wing meningioma. Preoperative gadolinium-enhanced T1-weighted magnetic resonance images demonstrate a large, dural-based enhancing mass arising from the region of the right pterion with mass effect on the adjacent right frontal and temporal lobes (A and B). Preoperative T2 FLAIR sequence demonstrates significant vasogenic edema in the adjacent right frontal lobe (C). Three-month posteroperative imaging demonstrates no residual tumor (D).

He was treated with intravenous corticosteroids for several days prior to resection of the tumor. Resection was performed via right frontotemporal craniotomy. The scalp and temporalis were reflected in a single myocutaneous flap and a frontotemporal bone flap was fashioned. The lateral sphenoid wing was drilled flat to facilitate access to the tumor. The dura was then opened circumferentially around the base of the tumor. The tumor was then internally debulked and gently mobilized off of the underlying brain. The tumor and dural base were removed in total. Surgical pathology demonstrated WHO grade 2 atypical meningioma. The patient did well after surgery with improvement in his headaches and preoperative visual symptoms.

## Medial (Clinoidal) Sphenoid Wing Meningiomas

Medial, or clinoidal, sphenoid wing meningiomas arise from the dura covering the anterior clinoid process. As with meningiomas elsewhere, they demonstrate variety in their extent and dural involvement. Some of these lesions are isolated to the clinoid itself. Others have a dural base or tumor projection that involves the adjacent lateral sphenoid wing, the medial cavernous sinus, the orbital roof or the tuberculum sellae. For especially large tumors, the precise dural base of the tumor may be difficult to distinguish on preoperative magnetic resonance imaging.

Clinoidal meningiomas are more likely to present with monocular visual loss given the close association of the lesion with the optic nerve. As these tumors enlarge they may displace or encircle the ipsilateral optic nerve, internal carotid artery, its branches or the oculomotor nerve. Other common clinical findings include headache, papilledema, seizure, and contralateral hemiparesis. Patients with extensive cavernous sinus involvement may also develop ophthalmoplegia.

The initial exposure and dissection in clinoidal meningiomas proceeds similarly to that described for the lateral sphenoid wing meningioma. After a frontotemporal incision, frontotemporal craniotomy and lateral sphenoid wing drilling are completed, attention is then turned to removing the anterior clinoid process extradurally. Extradural anterior clinoidectomy proceeds under microscopic visualization with the use of a 4mm diamond drill bit and continuous irrigation to avoid thermal injury to the optic nerve. Extradural dissection is carried to the orbitotemporal periosteal fold, which is then coagulated and cut, along with the orbitomeningeal artery, which travels within this fold. By sectioning this dural fold, a cleavage plane can be developed between the temporal fossa dura and the dura that is continuous with the lateral wall of the cavernous sinus. Extradural dissection continues until there is sufficient visualization of the anterior clinoid process and optic canal. Early extradural removal of the anterior clinoid process is helpful in clinoidal meningiomas for a number of reasons. It allows early devascularization of the tumor base, including the orbitomeningeal artery. In addition, the optic nerve is identified and the optic canal decompressed at an early stage, allowing identification of this critical structure to prevent subsequent injury, minimizing the risk of further nerve compression or injury during tumor debulking and resection, and facilitating a more complete removal of all tumor-involved dura and bone at the skull base. In rare cases, with extremely large tumors and poor brain relaxation, extradural clinoidectomy may be challenging given constraints of brain relaxation.

In these instances, a strategy of later intradural clinoidectomy after sufficient tumor debulking and cerebrospinal fluid (CSF) egress may be preferable. In general, however, intradural clinoidectomy more readily provides access on the proximal internal carotid artery during cerebrovascular aneurysm surgery than in meningioma surgery.

Drilling begins at the posterolateral orbital wall, decompressing the superior orbital fissure. Next, the roof of the optic canal is drilled until "egg-shell" thin and then removed piecemeal. With the optic nerve defined within the optic canal, what remains to be drilled is the anterior clinoid process itself. This is carefully hollowed out with the diamond drill until the dura surrounding it can be carefully dissected with a microdissector and the clinoid can be detached from the optic strut. Once the bone is thin enough, it may be carefully fractured from its connection to the optic strut and removed with a Lempert rongeur or microdecker rongeur. Some surgeons advocate completing the clinoidectomy with the ultrasonic bone curette although there is little data that indicates that this results in less thermal injury to nearby structures. When preparing to complete a clinoidectomy, whether extra- or intra-dural, it is important to take note of the appearance of the anterior clinoid process on preoperative imaging, particularly CT scan when available. With clinoidal meningiomas, the bone may be significantly hyperostotic, requiring much more extensive drilling. In addition, it may be pneumatized, putting the patient at high risk of CSF rhinorrhea through the sphenoid sinus if not repaired intraoperatively.

Once extradural clinoidectomy has been completed, surgical resection proceeds in a similar fashion to all sphenoid wing meningiomas. A general strategy of early dural detachment and devascularization followed by tumor debulking should facilitate careful microdissection of the capsule from the surrounding arachnoid adhesions of the basal cisterns and the pia of the frontal and temporal lobes. It is prudent to exercise care when tumor is densely adherent to the optic nerve, oculomotor nerve or small vessels of the supraclinoid internal carotid or middle cerebral artery. Morbidity can occur when small-vessel (or perforator) sacrifice or manipulation-related vasospasm results in an ischemic insult. In cases of vessel engulfment or encroachment, some surgeons advocate opening of the sylvian fissure to identify branches of the middle cerebral artery early in the resection. Once the tumor is as completely removed as possible, the resection or coagulation of all involved dura is the final objective. Given the high likelihood of residual microscopic disease at the dural base of these lesions, adjuvant radiosurgery for residual or recurrent disease or when the pathology is atypical (grade II) is increasingly the accepted practice. Closure techniques vary from institution to institution but should always entertain the possibility that the patient may require further resection for recurrence at a future time point.

## Case Presentation

A 66-year-old woman presented with subtle memory deficits as well as a single episode of transient speech difficulty which prompted a neurologic workup. Her neurologic examination was normal, including cranial nerve and visual function. Imaging evaluation with computed tomography and magnetic resonance imaging demonstrated a 4cm, enhancing globoid tumor arising from the left medial sphenoid wing (Figure 3). There was some associated hyperostosis of the left anterior clinoid process. There was significant associated abnormal FLAIR signal in the left temporal lobe.

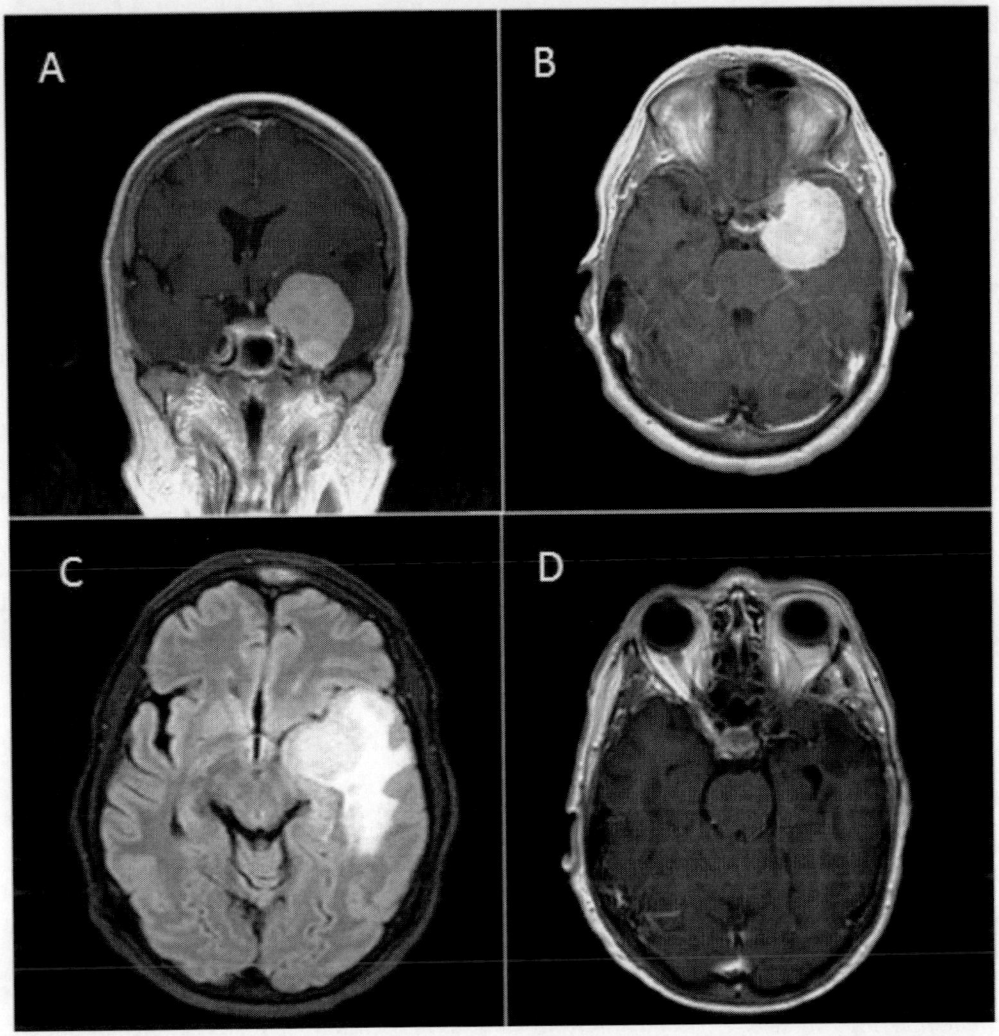


Figure 3. Medial sphenoid wing (clinoidal) meningioma. Preoperative gadolinium-enhanced T1-weighted magnetic resonance images demonstrate a large, dural-based enhancing mass arising from the region of the right anterior clinoid process with mass effect on the adjacent right temporal lobe (A and B). Preoperative T2 FLAIR sequence demonstrates significant vasogenic edema in the adjacent right temporal lobe (C). 2-year postoperative imaging demonstrates no residual tumor (D).

Resection of the tumor was performed via a left frontotemporal craniotomy using the interfascial extracranial dissection technique. After removing the frontotemporal bone flap, the sphenoid wing was drilled flush with the anterior limit of the middle cranial fossa. The medial sphenoid wing was then drilled to the level of the anterior clinoid process and the lateral wall of the cavernous sinus was mobilized. The roof of the optic canal was opened and the anterior clinoid process was removed. The dura was then opened and the tumor was internally debulked until it could be gently mobilized away from the temporal lobe. The tumor was adherent to the underlying left internal carotid artery, sylvian fissure vessels, and third cranial nerve. The tumor was dissected free of these structures and removed. The dural base of the tumor was cauterized. Surgical pathology confirmed WHO-grade 1 meningioma.

The patient did well after surgery with preservation of normal cranial nerve and visual function and improvement in her preoperative memory deficits.

## En Plaque (Spheno-Orbital) Menigiomas

Spheno-orbital meningioma is a term which refers to hyperostosing tumors of the sphenoid wing which have a characteristic tendency to invade the orbit. These tumors can present a number of unique challenges in regard to both surgical resection and reconstruction. Spheno-orbital meningiomas were referred to as "en plaque" meningiomas in Cushing and Eisenhardt's original description [1], though they may also have a globoid tumor component or extend into the cavernous sinus as with clinoidal meningiomas. Extracranial extension into the temporalis muscle, as with lateral sphenoid wing meningiomas, can also occur. The reactive hyperostosis, thought to be secondary to tumor invasion of the bone, is a defining characteristic of these tumors. The degree of hyperostosis is not well correlated with the amount of extra-osseous tumor. As a result of the tendency of these tumors to spread extensively within the bones of the sphenoid ridge, orbit, and on occasion into the paranasal sinuses, achieving complete resection can be challenging. Historically, recurrence rates for these tumors have been high, though improvements in preoperative imaging modalities, surgical techniques, and intraoperative neuronavigation have contributed to improvements in surgical outcomes.

Patients with these tumors may present with a variety of symptoms, related to either the soft tissue component of the tumor or the reactive hyperostosis [8–10]. The most common symptoms relate to vision, and can include proptosis, double vision, and loss of visual acuity. The double vision associated with spheno-orbital meningiomas can be secondary to cranial nerve palsy, rectus muscle entrapment, or exophthalmos from the mass effect of the tumor. Facial sensation can be affected by tumor involvement of the middle fossa floor or cavernous sinus ($V_2$, $V_3$ distributions) or the superior orbital fissure ($V_1$ distribution). Headaches are also a common symptom, and are frequently retro-orbital in location. A small number of patients present with seizures.

The preoperative physical examination should accordingly pay particular attention to the structure and function of the orbital region. A detailed cranial nerve examination is essential, particularly in regard to visual acuity and field testing, ocular movement, and the presence of proptosis. A comprehensive baseline ophthalmologic examination including dilated fundus examination and formal visual field testing should be completed for all patients diagnosed with spheno-orbital meningiomas, as any evidence of compromise of visual function can have implication in the discussion of surgical indications.

Preoperative imaging assessment of patients with spheno-orbital meningiomas should include a thin-cut bone windowed CT scan to identify the extent of the hyperostosis. Careful attention should be paid to the paranasal sinuses as they are a frequent site of extension of these tumors. Gadolinium-enhanced MRI should also be obtained to evaluate the soft tissue component and the extent of dural enhancement. A fat-suppressed T1 sequence must be obtained as part of the study to evaluate for tumor within the orbit.

As for other sphenoid wing meningiomas, patient positioning is supine with the head in a three-pin headholder. The head should be rotated approximately 30 degrees to the contralateral side. A curvilinear frontotemporal incision generally gives adequate exposure. Mobilization of the scalp and the temporalis in separate layers with interfascial dissection technique allows for full inspection of the temporalis and removal of any tumor that has invaded the extracranial tissues. The interfascial technique also allows for better angles of visualization down the sphenoid wing and facilitates the removal of tumor from the medial sphenoid wing structures. The pterional skull is frequently hypertrophied and in many cases it is not possible to perform a standard craniotomy. In these cases, the thickened skull may need to be drilled away in order to expose the frontotemporal dura. Bleeding from the hyperostotic skull during drilling can be profuse. A ready supply of bone wax and other hemostatic agents should be kept on hand to manage the bleeding while the drilling of the skull continues.

After the pterional flap is removed, either via craniotomy or craniectomy, the drilling of the sphenoid wing may commence. All of the hyperostotic bone of the sphenoid wing and the lateral orbit should be removed. The exact extent of bony removal will be guided by the preoperative imaging. Care should be taken to avoid entering the paranasal sinuses unless necessary, as inadvertent opening of the sinuses can result in problems with CSF leak. Intraoperative neuronavigation registered to a high-resolution CT scan can be very helpful in guiding the extent of bony resection. As the drilling of the sphenoid wing proceeds, the frontotemporal dura is carefully dissected and reflected away. Ultimately, mobilization of the dura will be limited by the meningo-orbital band as the dura traverses the superior orbital fissure to become the periorbita. Once adequately exposed, the meningo-orbital band can be divided allowing the temporal dura to be further mobilized and expose the middle fossa floor. When necessary, the drilling can be carried down to the middle fossa floor to decompress the basilar foramina if they are involved with the tumor. For tumors which involve the medial sphenoid wing, it may be necessary to carry the drilling to the anterior clinoid and decompress the optic canal, as with clinoidal meningiomas. All hyperostotic bone should be drilled from the lateral orbital wall and then the orbital roof carefully thinned until the periorbita is exposed. The bony resection is carried to the superior orbital fissure to allow for decompression of the fissure and removal of any traversing soft tissue tumor. Once the bony resection is complete, the orbital component of the tumor can be carefully mobilized from the periorbita. Attempt should be made to preserve the integrity of the periorbita, as violation of the periorbita can increase the risk of postoperative enophthalmos. However, this is not always possible. Orbital exenteration can be considered in cases with nonfunctional vision when there is an extensive orbital tumor component. The key step in exenteration of the orbit is the identification and ligation of the ophthalmic artery at the base of the orbit. Once the ophthalmic artery is controlled, the orbital contents can be freely dissected and removed.

After the bony and orbital components of the tumor are resected, the dura may be opened and any intradural component resected. Reconstruction can pose a particular challenge after the resection of spheno-orbital meningiomas, particularly when there is extensive orbital or sinus involvement. Resection of a single wall of the orbit generally does not require a primary reconstruction, particularly if the periorbita is not violated. However, more extensive orbital resection, particularly if the orbital floor is involved, may require reconstruction to prevent postoperative enophthalmos [11].

Reconstruction needs should be anticipated prior to operation. Some cases may require the harvest of a free muscle flap to fill the craniofacial defect and consultation with colleagues in otolaryngology, plastic surgery, or others with experience in craniofacial reconstruction may be required.

## Case Presentation

A 33-year-old woman presented with 9 months of gradually progressive right frontal headache and bulging of the right eye. Her physical examination was notable for proptosis of the right eye. Her neurologic examination was normal, with intact cranial nerve function and no visual deficits. Imaging workup with computed tomography and magnetic resonance imaging demonstrated a homogenously enhancing dural-based mass overlying the right sphenoid wing (Figure 4). There was marked hyperostosis of the sphenoid wing, lateral orbit, and orbital roof with compression of the orbital contents. Resection of the tumor was performed via a right frontotemporal craniotomy using the interfascial extracranial dissection technique.

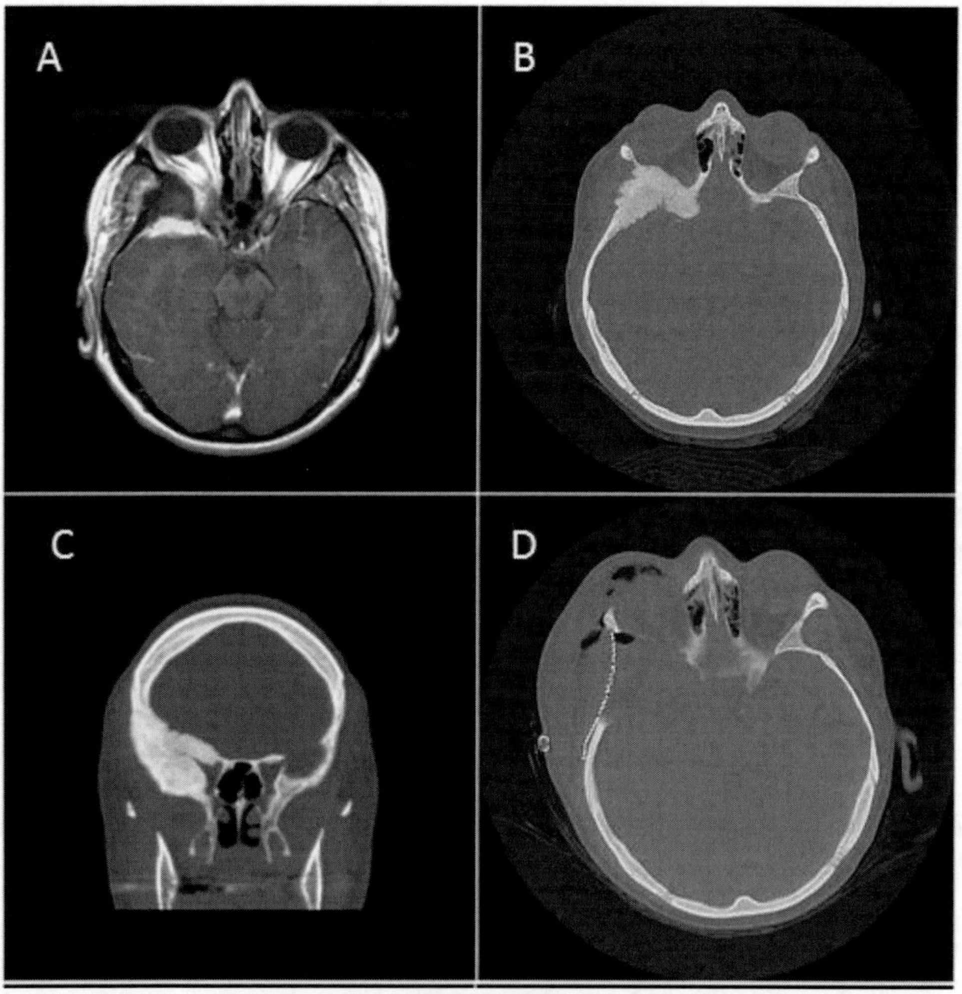


Figure 4. En plaque sphenoid wing (spheno-orbital) meningioma. Preoperative gadolinium-enhanced T1-weighted magnetic resonance imaging demonstrates a plaque-like dural-based enhancing mass overlying the right sphenoid wing and extending into the right lateral orbit (A). Preoperative computed tomography demonstrates significant hyperostosis of the adjacent sphenoid wing and orbital walls (B and C). Postoperative scan demonstrates the extent of bony resection with titanium mesh cranioplasty (D).

The hyperostotic bone was resected using the high-speed drill with the use of frameless stereotactic image guidance to delineate the margins of bony resection. Extradural anterior clinoidectomy was performed to facilitate decompression of the optic nerve. After the bony resection was completed, the involved dura was resected circumferentially using microscissors allowing the soft tissue component of the tumor to be resected en bloc. The dural defect was repaired using an onlay graft. The skull defect was repaired with titanium mesh. Surgical pathology confirmed WHO grade 1 meningioma. The patient recovered well after surgery without neurologic deficit.

## DISCUSSION

Sphenoid wing meningiomas are diverse in their presentation and their best management. Surgical goals and outcomes vary significantly depending on the location and other anatomical characteristics of the tumor. In some cases, more often with lateral tumors, gross total resection can be achieved in a safe and straightforward manner. Medial sphenoid wing and spheno-orbital meningiomas typically present more surgical challenges in comparison with lateral tumors. Medial tumors characteristically envelope the internal carotid artery and compress the optic nerve. In addition, extradural extension of these tumors into the cavernous sinus is common. In these cases and in other instances, such as when the tumor exhibits extensive vascular encasement or adherence to cranial nerves or other critical structures, planned subtotal resection may yield better functional outcomes. In the case of spheno-orbital tumors, the osseous involvement can be extensive and it can be a challenge to identify and remove all of the involved bone at the time of the operation.

The analysis of outcomes data is complicated by the variance in the classification schemes that have been favored over time, though most recent series have favored a three-group classification scheme similar to what is presented in this chapter (lateral globoid/pterional, medial globoid/clinoidal, and en plaque/spheno-orbital). Most of the available case series focus on either medial [3, 12–15] or en plaque [10, 16–18] tumors, as these are considered to be the most surgically challenging. There is a relative paucity of data specific to lateral sphenoid wing meningiomas, though there is at least one recent study that addresses these as well [2].

As one would expect, surgical outcomes for lateral sphenoid wing meningiomas are the most favorable. Sughrue et al. [2] describe a achieving gross total resection in 69% of patients with no new postoperative deficits in a series of 16 patients with lateral-third sphenoid wing meningiomas and 71% rate of gross total resection in 21 patients with middle-third sphenoid wing meningiomas, with one incidence of new postoperative oculomotor palsy and one instance of new postoperative aphasia.

More data has been reported regarding the outcomes of medial or clinoidal sphenoid wing meningiomas. Early series documented relatively poor results for these tumors, with rates of gross total resection under 50% and operative mortality rates as high as 43% [1, 19, 20]. More modern series have demonstrated improved outcomes, likely reflecting improvements in skull base operative techniques. The morbidity of surgery for clinoidal meningiomas has improved as well, though it remains substantially greater than with lateral tumors. In 1990, Al-Mefty reported a series of 24 patients with clinoidal meningiomas. Gross total resection was achieved in 83% of the patients. A number of other case series have since been published which also documented improved rates of gross total resection (55-86%) [2, 3, 12, 14, 21, 22]. Extension of tumor into the cavernous sinus is the most common reason for inability to achieve gross total resection of these tumors [3, 12, 23], and it has been recognized that in many cases, leaving residual tumor in the cavernous sinus may yield a better long-term functional outcome for the patient in comparison to a more radical resection. Visual outcomes are variable, with reported rates of improvement in preoperative visual symptoms ranging from 25-75% [12, 13, 22]. Visual outcomes have been observed to be less favorable in cases with cavernous sinus extension as well as when operating on recurrent tumor. In cases of complete preoperative blindness, visual function typically does not improve after resection. The extent of removal of these lesions depends strongly on their pattern of growth and more specifically whether there is intracavernous tumor extension or tumor adhesion to critical neurovascular structures such as the internal carotid artery or optic nerve. In most modern series, rates of complete resection range from 40-80% of cases. Given these concerns, close and continued post-operative follow-up is advised in these patients, and post-operative adjuvant fractionated radiotherapy or radiosurgery remain viable second-line treatment options.

Similarly, early surgical experiences with spheno-orbital meningiomas resulted high rates of perioperative morbidity and mortality [24]. However, improvements in surgical technique and perioperative care have significantly improved surgical safety, with most recent series reporting mortality rates of 1% or less [8, 10, 17, 18, 25]. There is particular interest in visual outcomes after spheno-orbital meningioma resection. Proptosis is the most common presenting symptom for these tumors, and is difficult to fully resolve even with aggressive surgical resection. Modern series report improvement in proptosis in greater than 70% of patients [9, 10, 17, 18]. The improvement in the proptosis helps with postoperative cosmesis, however subtle residual differences in globe position can result in persistent diplopia despite the measurable improvement. Loss in visual acuity is also a common symptom for patients with spheno-orbital meningiomas. Surgery has been fairly successful in improving visual deficits, with reported rates of postoperative improvement in visual acuity ranging from 64-87% [10, 17, 18, 25]. Patients with complete loss of functional vision preoperatively typically do not improve, even with aggressive decompression of the optic nerve. Diplopia secondary to cranial neuropathy does not improve in most cases, as this typically results from invasion of the cavernous sinus with tumor. Diplopia secondary to extraocular muscle restriction is more likely to improve after surgery [25].

## CONCLUSION

The sphenoid wing is an anatomically complex region and a common site for the development of meningiomas. These tumors are notable for their ability to compromise the optic apparatus as well as their propensity to induce marked hyperostosis of the adjacent skull. Surgical outcomes have improved dramatically with the refinement of skull base resection techniques and advances in surgical technology, however these tumors remain challenging to treat. Gross total surgical resection is the ideal treatment when it can be safely accomplished, though this is not possible in all cases. Tumors involving the cavernous sinus are a particular challenge, and the ideal extent of resection of tumors which extend in to the cavernous sinus remains a point of debate. Stereotactic radiotherapy is an important adjuvant treatment modality for the treatment of residual tumor.

## REFERENCES


[1] Cushing H., Eisenhardt L. Meningiomas: Their classification, regional behaviour, life history, and surgical end results. Thomas C. C., editor. Springfield, IL; 1938.

[2] Sughrue M. E., Rutkowski M. J., Chen C. J., Shangari G., Kane A. J., Parsa A. T., et al. Modern surgical outcomes following surgery for sphenoid wing meningiomas. *J. Neurosurg.,* [Internet]. 2013 Jul; 119(1): 86–93. Available from: http://www.ncbi.nlm.nih.gov/pubmed/23432379

[3] Russell S. M., Benjamin V. Medial sphenoid ridge meningiomas: classification, microsurgical anatomy, operative nuances, and long-term surgical outcome in 35 consecutive patients. *Neurosurgery,* [Internet]. 2008 Mar. [cited 2014 Sep 5];62 (3 Suppl. 1):38–50; discussion 50. Available from: http://www.ncbi.nlm.nih.gov/pubmed/18424966

[4] Shah A. H., Patel N., Raper D. M. S., Bregy A., Ashour R., Elhammady M. S., et al. The role of preoperative embolization for intracranial meningiomas. *J. Neurosurg.,* [Internet]. 2013; 119(2): 364–72. Available from: http://www.ncbi.nlm.nih.gov/pubmed/23581584

[5] MacCarty C. S. Meningiomas of the sphenoidal ridge. *J. Neurosurg.,* [Internet]. 1972 Jan. [cited 2014 Sep. 10];36(1): 114–20. Available from: http://www.ncbi.nlm.nih.gov/pubmed/5007268

[6] Mickey B., Close L., Schaefer S., Samson D. A combined frontotemporal and lateral infratemporal fossa approach to the skull base. *J. Neurosurg.,* [Internet]. 1988 May; 68(5): 678–83. Available from: http://www.ncbi.nlm.nih.gov/pubmed/2833586

[7] Pirotte B., Brotchi J. Lateral and Middle Sphenoid Wing Meningiomas. In: Lee J. H., editor. Meningiomas: Diagnosis, Treatment, and Outcome [Internet]. London: Springer London; 2009 [cited 2014 Sep 5]. p. 371–8. Available from: http://link.springer.com/chapter/10.1007/978-1-84628-784-8_39

[8] Roser F., Nakamura M., Jacobs C., Vorkapic P., Samii M. Sphenoid wing meningiomas with osseous involvement. *Surg. Neurol.,* [Internet]. 2005 Jul. [cited 2014 Sep. 11]; 64(1): 37–43; discussion 43. Available from: http://www.ncbi.nlm.nih.gov/pubmed/15993178

[9] Oya S., Sade B., Lee J. H. Sphenoorbital meningioma: surgical technique and outcome. *J. Neurosurg.,* [Internet]. 2011 May [cited 2014 Sep. 5]; 114(5):1241–9. Available from: http://www.ncbi.nlm.nih.gov/ pubmed/21184631

[10] Bikmaz K., Mrak R., Al-Mefty O. Management of bone-invasive, hyperostotic sphenoid wing meningiomas. *J. Neurosurg.,* [Internet]. 2007 Nov. [cited 2014 Aug. 7]; 107(5): 905–12. Available from: http:// www.ncbi.nlm.nih.gov/pubmed/17977259

[11] DeMonte F., Tabrizi P., Culpepper S. A., Abi-Said D., Soparkar C. N., Patrinely J. R. Ophthalmological outcome following orbital resection in anterior and anterolateral skull

base surgery. *Neurosurg. Focus,* [Internet]. 2001 Jan. [cited 2014 Nov. 5]; 10(5): E4. Available from: http://thejns.org/doi/abs/10.3171/foc.2001.10.5.5

[12] Nakamura M., Roser F., Jacobs C., Vorkapic P., Samii M. Medial sphenoid wing meningiomas: clinical outcome and recurrence rate. *Neurosurgery,* [Internet]. 2006 Apr. [cited 2014 Aug. 7];58(4): 626–39, discussion 626–39. Available from: http://www.ncbi.nlm.nih.gov/ pubmed/16575326

[13] Al-Mefty O. Clinoidal meningiomas. *J. Neurosurg.,* [Internet]. 1990 Dec.; 73(6): 840–9. Available from: http://www.ncbi.nlm.nih.gov/ pubmed/2230967

[14] Tobias S., Kim C.-H., Kosmorsky G., Lee J. H. Management of surgical clinoidal meningiomas. *Neurosurg. Focus,* [Internet]. 2003 Jun. 15; 14(6): e5. Available from: http://www.ncbi.nlm.nih.gov/ pubmed/18037043

[15] Bassiouni H., Asgari S., Sandalcioglu I. E., Seifert V., Stolke D., Marquardt G. Anterior clinoidal meningiomas: functional outcome after microsurgical resection in a consecutive series of 106 patients. Clinical article. *J. Neurosurg.,* [Internet]. 2009 Nov. [cited 2014 Sep. 5]; 111(5): 1078–90. Available from: http://www.ncbi.nlm.nih.gov/ pubmed/ 19374499

[16] Mirone G., Chibbaro S., Schiabello L., Tola S., George B. En plaque sphenoid wing meningiomas: recurrence factors and surgical strategy in a series of 71 patients. *Neurosurgery,* [Internet]. 2009 Dec. [cited 2014 Aug. 7]; 65(6 Suppl.): 100–8; discussion 108–9. Available from: http:// www.ncbi.nlm.nih.gov/pubmed/19934984

[17] Schick U., Bleyen J., Bani A., Hassler W. Management of meningiomas en plaque of the sphenoid wing. *J. Neurosurg.,* [Internet]. 2006 Feb.; 104(2): 208–14. Available from: http://www.ncbi.nlm.nih.gov/ pubmed/16509494

[18] Ringel F., Cedzich C., Schramm J. Microsurgical technique and results of a series of 63 spheno-orbital meningiomas. *Neurosurgery,* [Internet]. 2007 Apr. [cited 2014 Aug. 7]; 60 (4 Suppl. 2):214–21; discussion 221–2. Available from: http:// www.ncbi.nlm.nih.gov/pubmed/17415156

[19] Pompili A., Derome P. J., Visot A., Guiot G. Hyperostosing meningiomas of the sphenoid ridge—Clinical features, surgical therapy, and long-term observations: Review of 49 cases. *Surg. Neurol.,* [Internet]. 1982 Jun. [cited 2014 Sep. 11]; 17(6): 411–6. Available from: http://linkinghub.elsevier.com/retrieve/pii/S0090301982800062

[20] Bonnal J., Thibaut A., Brotchi J., Born J. Invading meningiomas of the sphenoid ridge. *J. Neurosurg.,* [Internet]. 1980 Nov.; 53(5): 587–99. Available from: http://www.ncbi.nlm.nih.gov/pubmed/7431070

[21] Puzzilli F., Ruggeri A., Mastronardi L., Agrillo A., Ferrante L. Anterior clinoidal meningiomas: report of a series of 33 patients operated on through the pterional approach. *Neuro. Oncol.*, [Internet]. 1999 Jul. [cited 2014 Sep. 16]; 1(3): 188–95. Available from: http:// www.pubmedcentral.nih.gov/articlerender.fcgi?artid=1920748 andtool=pmcentrezandrendertype=abstract

[22] Risi P., Uske A., de Tribolet N. Meningiomas involving the anterior clinoid process. *Br. J. Neurosurg.*, [Internet]. 1994 Jan. [cited 2014 Sep. 16]; 8(3): 295–305. Available from: http://www.ncbi.nlm.nih.gov/ pubmed/7946018

[23] Abdel Aziz K. M., Froelich S. C., Dagnew E., Jean W., Breneman J. C., Zuccarello M., et al. Large Sphenoid Wing Meningiomas Involving the Cavernous Sinus: Conservative Surgical Strategies for Better Functional Outcomes. *Neurosurgery,* [Internet]. 2004 Jun.

[cited 2014 Aug 7]; 54(6): 1375–84. Available from: http://content.wkhealth.com/linkback/openurl?sid=WKPTLP:landingpageandan=00006123-200406000-00012

[24] Castellano F., Guidetti B., Olivecrona H. Pterional meningiomas en plaque. *J. Neurosurg.*, [Internet]. 1952 Mar. [cited 2014 Nov 5]; 9(2): 188–96. Available from: http://www.ncbi.nlm.nih.gov/pubmed/ 14908653

[25] Shrivastava R. K., Sen C., Costantino P. D., Della Rocca R. Sphenoorbital meningiomas: surgical limitations and lessons learned in their long-term management. *J. Neurosurg.,* [Internet]. 2005 Sep.; 103(3): 491–7. Available from: http://www.ncbi.nlm.nih.gov/pubmed/ 16235682

In: Current Management of Central Nervous System …
ISBN: 978-1-63483-856-6
Editors: Steven D. Chang and Anand Veeravagu


*Chapter 7*

# MENINGIOMAS OF THE PETROUS BONE

***Nataly Raviv, BA, Gabriel A. Smith, MD***
***and Nicholas C. Bambakidis, MD***
Department of Neurological Surgery,
University Hospitals Case Medical Center, Cleveland,
Ohio, US

## ABSTRACT

Meningiomas that originate from the petrous bone are amongst the most challenging lesions that a neurosurgeon may encounter. The surgical decision-making process is difficult and must be approached on a case-by-case basis. Mass effects causing cranial neuropathies, hydrocephalus, or brainstem compression indicate surgical resection due to resulting stigmata such as ataxia, spastic paresis, or somatosensory findings. The tumor's rostral and caudal extension, dural attachment, relation to the internal acoustic canal and size, and the patient's hearing status must all be considered when choosing a surgical approach to achieve maximal safe resection. Stereotactic radiosurgery should be reserved for adjuvant therapy in the cases of residual tumors that demonstrate signs of recurrence or growth as well as for patients who are poor surgical candidates.

**Keywords:** combined transpetrosal approach, gross total resection, GTR: see gross total resection, retrolabyrinthine approach, retrosigmoid approach, petroclival meningioma, petrous meningioma, SRS: see stereotactic radiosurgery, stereotactic radiosurgery, STR: see subtotal resection, subtotal resection, surgical indications, transcochlear approach, translabyrinthine approach, transpetrosal approach

## INTRODUCTION

Petrous meningiomas are a heterogeneous group of posterior fossa tumors. In most classification schemes, they are divided into broad categories based on their dural attachment site in relation to the intracranial nerves and the internal acoustic canal (IAC). Meningiomas of the cerebellopontine angle (CPA) have historically been considered as CPA meningiomas, irrespective to the site of origin and with the majority of these lesions arising from the posterior aspect of the petrous bone [1]. Al-Mefty termed this subcategory of CPA meningiomas "petrosal meningiomas" and further subdivided them into anterior or posterior petrous meningiomas, based on their dural attachment site in relation to the IAC [2, 3]. Bricolo and Turazzi [4] presented a similar anatomical classification scheme. They derived their categorization from the regional topography and associated seventh and eighth cranial nerve displacement patterns of these tumors. Posterior displacement traditionally occurred with anterior petrous tumors and anterior displacement with lesions arising posterior to the IAC [3]. Desgeorges and colleagues [5] further modified this categorization and developed the A-M-P classification in which an additional M subdivision is used to describe rare meningiomas with dural attachment around the porous acousticus of the IAC. The A and P anterior and posterior subdivisions remain as previously outlined. The displacement of the acousticofacial bundle is less predictable with Type M meningiomas. This is due to its dependence on the site of attachment along the margin of the porous and the tumor growth pattern [6]. Tumors meeting the exclusive criteria of origination at the petrous bone, lateral and posterior to the petro-occipital sulcus, will be labeled as "true" petrous meningiomas in this chapter [7]. Posterior fossa meningiomas account for approximately 10% [8] of intracranial meningiomas, and true petrous meningiomas constitute 42% [9] of these lesions.

A broader definition of petrous meningiomas follows the classification system established by Sekhar and other colleagues for posterior fossa meningiomas [10, 11]. These tumors may be included under Types II, III, and IV [12]. Type II CPA meningiomas are defined as lesions arising from the lateral petrous ridge dura mater. They are posterior to the IAC and often extend into the meatus. Type III meningiomas are those that arise in the jugular foramen region or from the cerebellomedullary angle, which may also involve extracranial regions. Type IV petroclival meningiomas originate from the dura of the petrous apex, medial petrosal ridge, or upper two thirds of the clivus, with possible infiltration into the cavernous sinus or Meckel's cave [11].

Petroclival meningiomas are rare, accounting for 3% to 10% of posterior fossa meningiomas [52] and less than 0.15% of intracranial tumors overall, yet are one of the most daunting meningiomas to treat [8, 14]. Petroclival lesions pose a technical challenge. Surgical management has historically been associated with high morbidity and mortality rates, given the contiguity of these lesions with the brainstem and essential neurovascular structures [15, 16]. Prior to 1970, surgical resection of these tumors was associated with greater than 50% mortality [17]. However with the emergence of microsurgical technique, Yasargil [18] reported mortality rates at 10% in 1980 [8]. The refinement of skull base approaches and advances in microsurgical technique, neuroimaging modalities, and intraoperative neurophysiological monitoring have since led to further reductions in surgical morbidity and mortality rendering mortality as a rarity and severe morbidity as uncommon [14, 19].

In this chapter, we will discuss petrous meningiomas using a broader designation that encompasses tumors included under Sekhar's criteria. We will not use Sekhar's specific subtypes and will instead address these tumors according to their diverse origins and associated risks and outcomes. They will be referred to as follows: "true" petrous meningiomas, as defined above with anterior and posterior subtypes, and petroclival meningiomas, which are defined as tumors arising in the upper two thirds of the clivus at the petroclival junction and medial to the fifth cranial nerve [2, 20, 21]. We will discuss the critical points in surgical decision making, anatomy, and approaches related to these tumors with the goal of achieving excellent outcomes and enhancing the care of this unique patient population.

## SURGICAL ANATOMY

Knowledge of the CPA and posterior skull base anatomy is essential in the surgical management of these tumors. The CPA is the triangular potential space in the posterior fossa. It is demarcated by the pons medially, posterior petrous ridge anterolaterally, cerebellum posteriorly, and tentorium superiorly. It is continuous inferiorly with the lateral cerebellomedullary cistern, which may permit lesions from the CPA to extend into the foramen magnum [12, 22]. The contents of the CPA include the posterior circulation, supplying the brainstem and cerebellum, along with cranial nerves V through XI. The fifth nerve crosses over the superior aspect of the CPA cistern, while the seventh and eighth cranial nerves course through it anteriorly and laterally from the ventral aspect of the pontomedullary junction of the brainstem to the IAC. The lower cranial nerves, IX through XI, run through the inferior aspect of the cistern [6, 23].

True petrous meningiomas arise from the dura, overlying the posterior aspect of the petrous bone lateral and posterior to the petro-occipital sulcus [12]. These lesions are located lateral to the skull base foramina of the fifth through eleventh cranial nerves, within a region demarcated by the superior petrosal sinus, inferior petrosal sinus, and the sigmoid sinus. Together with the cavernous sinus, these venous structures form a ring encasing the posterior aspect of the petrous bone [6, 12]. Despite the close proximity of cranial nerves V, VII, and VIII to developing meningiomas in this region, these nerves are protected within their arachnoid sheaths and are preserved with the growth of large tumors. Knowledge of tumor origin and nerve displacement is critical in surgical planning, as excellent functional outcomes can be achieved if care is taken intraoperatively [6].

The displacement patterns of cranial nerves caused by these tumors are dependent on their dural attachment sites. Posterior petrous meningiomas are lateral to the cranial nerve foramina and posterior to the IAC. Thus, the fifth through eighth cranial nerves are displaced anteriorly with caudal displacement of the lower cranial nerves. Likewise, anterior petrous meningiomas arise lateral to the foramina. However, they differ in position relative to the IAC and therefore displace the seventh and eighth cranial nerves posteriorly, the fifth nerve anterosuperiorly, and the ninth to eleventh cranial nerves caudally [19]. These are only the classic displacement patterns and divergence in large broad-based tumors involving multiple sections of the posterior petrous bone can occur. Posterior petrous meningiomas are typically supplied by branches of the ascending pharyngeal artery, occipital artery, vertebral artery, subarcuate artery branch of anterior inferior cerebellar artery AICA, and the middle meningeal artery. There exists some contribution from the pial branches of AICA and the superior cerebellar artery in larger tumors [3]. The petroclival region is a surgical rather than anatomical space, set deeply below the base of the cerebral cortex and positioned in the anterior portion of the posterior fossa. It involves the superior portion of the clivus anteriorly, is laterally bound by the petrous pyramid anterior to the IAC, and is located medial to the fifth cranial nerve. This region is delineated by an elaborate osteomeningeal complex that opens superiorly into the supratentorial space, inferiorly into the peribulbar area, and posteriorly into the CPA [21, 22]. Petroclival meningiomas arise medial to the fifth through eleventh cranial nerve foramina and they tend to displace these nerves posteriorly or laterally. They displace the brainstem and basilar artery posteriorly and contralaterally. Such an occurrence may involve structures such as the IAC, jugular foramen, Meckel's cave, Dorello's canal, and the ipsilateral cavernous sinus, with the latter resulting in contralateral cranial neuropathies [14]. Petroclival meningiomas have attachment patterns that position the ipsilateral cranial nerves into the surgical working corridor. This accounts for the significantly greater morbidity associated with the surgical approach to these lesions, including injury to the third, fourth, and fifth cranial nerves, which are less likely to be injured during resection of true petrous meningiomas [3, 24]. Petroclival meningiomas generally recruit branches from the intracavernous portion of the internal carotid artery, the posterior branch of the middle meningeal artery, the meningeal branch of the vertebral artery, the petrosal branches of the meningeal arteries, and the ascending pharyngeal branches of the external carotid artery [8].

## Clinical Assessment, Surgical Decision Making and Preoperative Workup

Patients with petrous and clival meningiomas present over a broad range of ages, with mean and median ages reported in the middle 40s to 50s [14, 19, 24-26]. The classic presentation is insidious in onset, with clinical manifestations associated with neuropathies of the fifth through eleventh cranial nerves, mass effect on the cerebellum, brainstem compression, and obstructive hydrocephalus [21].

Approximately 80% to 92% of meningiomas are benign, and petrous meningiomas have similar rates of low-grade pathology [12, 27]. The histological profiles of anterior and posterior petrous meningiomas differ, as the former are largely of meningothelial histology and the latter predominantly of the fibrous subtype. This distinction has been cited as evidence for the separate lineages and genetic profiles of these tumor subdivisions [12]. With the vast majority of these tumors being benign, the goals of surgery include the prevention of cranial neuropathy progression, alleviation of brainstem compression, and the maximal safe resection of the tumor. Thus, deciding when to operate largely depends upon tumor growth, cranial neuropathies, hydrocephalus, and somatosensory or motor symptoms.

## Clinical Presentation

The frequency of cranial neuropathies varies according to the site of tumor origin and degree of growth. For example, tumors arising near the IAC are associated with hearing loss, tinnitus, and disequilibrium. Posterior petrous meningiomas often extend into the CPA, and most commonly present with cerebellar dysfunction and gait ataxia [3]. The most common complaints regarding anterior petrous tumor cases involve cranial nerves V, VII and VIII, and present with hearing loss, trigeminal neuralgia, facial hypoesthesia, and facial or abducens nerve palsies. Late-stage petrous meningiomas may compress the cerebellum or obstruct the fourth ventricle, as indicated by the development of diplopia, ataxia, papilledema, or hydrocephalus [3, 19, 24]. Petrous meningiomas, with attachment above the IAC, often manifest clinically with facial pain associated with the fifth cranial nerve prior to the development of eight nerve cranial neuropathies. Those located below the meatus may grow inferiorly toward the jugular foramen and involve the lower cranial nerves, presenting with hoarseness and dysphagia [3]. Cerebellar signs are the most common clinical exam findings associated with petroclival meningiomas, occurring in approximately 70% of cases, while headache is the most frequent chief complaint. Spastic paresis and somatosensory deficits consistent with brain stem compression occurs variably and are respectively reported in 15% to 57% and 15% to 20% of patients [80]. Neuropathy associated with petroclival tumors most frequently involves cranial nerves V and VIII. Cranial nerve VII involvement occurs in half of affected patients, while the lower nerves are involved in a third of cases. Cranial nerves III, IV, and VI neuropathies are present in fewer than half of cases [21].

## CLINICAL EXAMINATION

A comprehensive preoperative evaluation is essential to assess the status of the patient and the extent of tumor involvement. It is also imperative for determining the most appropriate treatment method and surgical approach if surgical management is undertaken. Complete clinical, neurologic, audiologic, and neuroophthalmologic examinations are performed [13]. A standard history and physical examination is performed on every patient, with an emphasis on the neurologic exam as well as particular attention to cranial nerve and cerebellar function. Facial nerve function should be assessed both pre- and postoperatively using the House and Brackmann Scale [24]. The eighth cranial nerve is frequently affected in petrous tumors, with neuropathy affecting 23% to 70% of patients with true petrous meningiomas [7, 9, 24] and up to 75% of petroclival tumor patients [14]. If the tumor is to be observed and to help guide surgical approach selection, audiograms are administered to determine baseline hearing, assess the extent of hearing loss, and establish a baseline for future serial examinations [14]. The classification developed by the American Academy of Otololaryngologists and Head and Neck Surgery is often used in studies [24].

A thorough neuro-ophthalmologic examination is essential, as petroclival meningiomas that infiltrate the cavernous sinus may be associated with extraocular motor neuropathies and papilledema may be an indication of increased intracranial pressure [8, 13]. The lower cranial nerves should also be assessed as they may be displaced or infiltrated by petrous meningiomas that extend into the inferior aspect of the CPA. Our institution elects to obtain an otolaryngology consult both pre-and postoperatively for a formal lower cranial nerve assessment. This includes the direct visualization of the oropharyngeal musculature with laryngoscopy.

## NEUROIMAGING

Neuroimaging is essential in the evaluation and treatment of petrous meningiomas. Multimodality imaging techniques are employed to assess tumor location, size, consistency, vascularity, extension, and the relative locations of surrounding neurovascular structures [8].

Magnetic resonance imaging (MRI) is the modality of choice in the preoperative evaluation of these tumors. It best demonstrates the tumor anatomy, extension, and relative position to surrounding neurovascular structures, in addition to the presence of peritumorial edema and hydrocephalus [13]. T1-weighted sequences reveal hypointense to isointense masses that enhance homogenously after IV gadolinium administration. A dural tail may be visualized, though this feature may also be seen in schwannomas and metastases that infiltrate or undergo reactive changes [3]. MRI T2-weighted images including FLAIR sequences are useful in the assessment of peritumoral edema, tumor infiltration, and in the evaluation of the arachnoid plane between tumor and critical structures, such as cranial nerves and the posterior circulatory vasculature. The absence of a defined arachnoid cleavage plane between the tumor and brainstem suggests a brainstem pial invasion, which stands as one of the most formidable obstacles to the safe resection of these tumors. T2-weighted MRI imaging can also be used to predict tumor consistency. A hyperintense tumor on a T2-weighted image indicates a soft tumor with high water content that is usually more amenable to resection. Moreover, surrounding edema of the brainstem is suggestive of a more aggressive pathology [19].

Standard T2-weighted MRI may provide adequate visualization of larger cranial nerves only. Thus, steady-state free precession (SSFP) sequences are frequently used to examine cranial nerve anatomy and assess for abnormalities as all twelve cranial nerves and their cisternal segments may be demonstrated through this imaging technique. These sequences may be used in the evaluation of the CPA and inner ear. They allow for distinction between branches of the facial and vestibulocochlear nerves and can demonstrate small masses within the CPA and IAC [28]. Our institution employs the fast imaging employing steady-state acquisition (FIESTA) SSFP sequence.

Computed tomography (CT) of the temporal bone is useful in identifying tumor location and involvement of the temporal bone. It may help to determine a diagnosis prior to surgery, as hyperostosis of the temporal bone is seen in bony invasion related to meningioma extension. Whereas, IAC expansion is associated with schwannomas. In cases for which transpetrosal approaches are considered, CT may also be employed to assess the inner ear, its relation to the jugular bulb, as well as the degree of pneumatization of the mastoid bone [8, 13].

Understanding cerebral vasculature in relation to the tumor is crucial in surgical planning [13]. Preoperative diagnostic cerebral angiography of all six vessels is of paramount importance to understanding the vascular supply to the meningioma and the relationship of the posterior circulation to the lesion. A detailed understanding of the blood supply allows surgeons to remove contributing perforating vessels while also preserving displaced vasculature [21]. Magnetic resonance angiography (MRA) and magnetic resonance venography (MRV) are the imaging modalities of choice, as the use of conventional angiography is now largely limited to the further investigation of abnormalities found on MRA and MRV [13, 21]. MRA may demonstrate the blood supply to the tumor in addition to any mass effect on the vertebrobasilar system and its branches [8]. Angiographic evaluation of the basilar artery is essential. Generally, the basilar artery is displaced by the tumor dorsally and to the contralateral side. Dorsal displacement without a lateral component may occur when the tumor arises ventral to the basilar trunk, along the clivus. Absence of displacement may occur if the artery courses along the anterior aspect of the tumor or is encased in the tumor bed. A visualized narrowing of the artery in the area of tumor involvement is suggestive of the latter case. The posterior cerebral artery and superior cerebellar artery are frequently elevated on the ipsilateral side of the tumor and may become splayed with involvement of the tentorial incisura [13]. Displacement of the posterior inferior cerebellar artery and AICA is largely dependent on tumor origin. Tumors originating medially displace these vessels dorsolaterally, whereas laterally placed tumors produce medial displacement.

Angiography is sometimes used in the management of intracranial meningiomas for preoperative tumor embolization to reduce surgical blood loss. However, embolization is rarely beneficial for petrous meningiomas and other lesions of the posterior fossa, as the risk of brain swelling with consequent herniation is substantial in this region [8].

Knowledge of the venous anatomy is as necessary as arterial anatomy in planning the surgical approach and in the reduction of operative complications. MRV can be used to demonstrate the structure of the torcula and the size and patency of the transverse and sigmoid sinuses. Information on the vein of Labbé and its drainage may prove useful if a sigmoid sinus needs to be divided intraoperatively [8]. The sigmoid sinus may spontaneously thrombose following transpetrosal skull base approaches. In which case, a patient's contralateral venous system is required to avoid a catastrophic venous complication.

## SURGICAL APPROACHES AND CLINICAL CASE PRESENTATIONS

Once surgery has been recommended, choosing a surgical approach to limit morbidity, mortality, and enhance access for surgical resection is critical. The surgical anatomy previously discussed is crucial when determining the appropriate approach. At our institution, a retrosigmoid or combined transpetrosal approach are the workhorses for all CPA meningiomas. An orbitozygomatic approach is rarely used if access to the cavernous sinus or supratentorial extension is a goal of the surgery. A subtemporal, transpetrosal, or combined transpetrosal presigmoid and retrosigmoid craniotomy can be used in extenuating circumstances in the presence of larger tumors for the enhancement of access to these lesions (Figure 1). The extent of resection attained is defined by the Simpson Grading System. Grade I and II resections are considered to be gross total resections (GTR) while grades III, IV, and V correspond to subtotal resections (STR).

### Retrosigmoid Approach

The retrosigmoid approach is the pathway most often used to address lesions within the CPA, including petrous meningiomas (Figure 2). This approach allows direct access to the IAC and cranial nerves V, VII, and VIII while also preserving hearing during exposure.

We prefer to use a modified park-bench position at our institution, with the head fixed in a Mayfield headholder and slightly flexed, body bumped with a gel roll, and arm placed across the chest in a near true lateral position. The skin incision varies according to the size and location of the tumor, location of the transverse and sigmoid sinuses, and the extent of the access required.

Generally, a linear incision is made two fingerbreadths behind the external auditory meatus over the asterion.

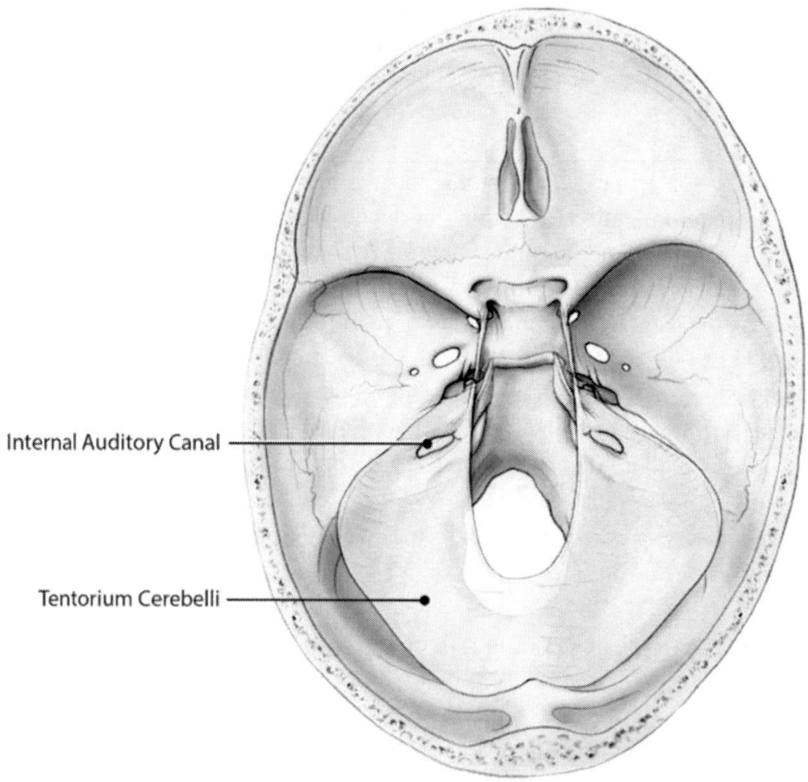


Figure 1a.

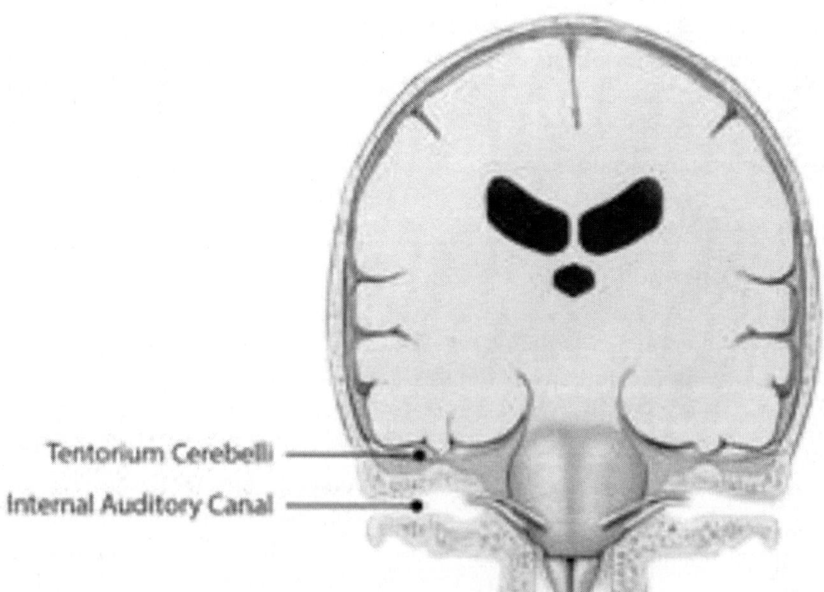


Figure 1b.

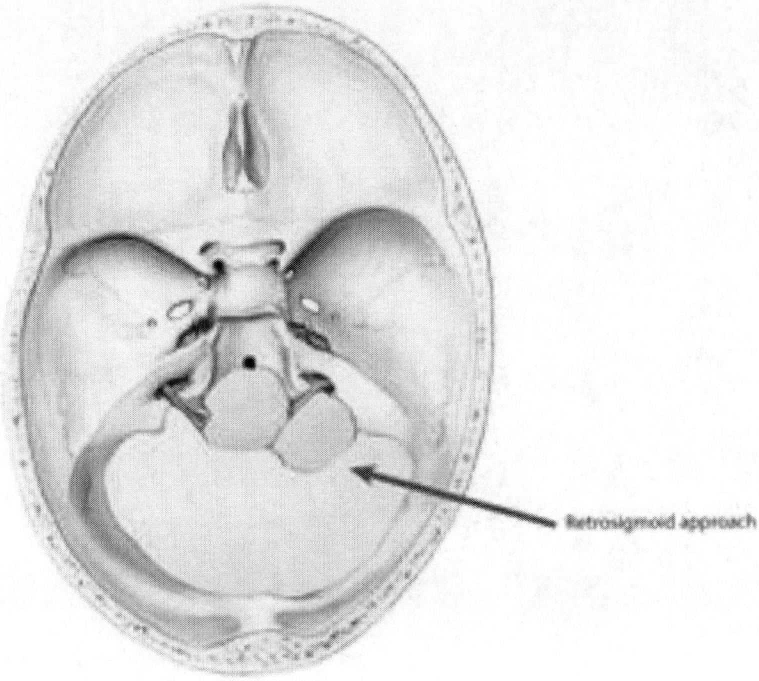


Figure 1c.

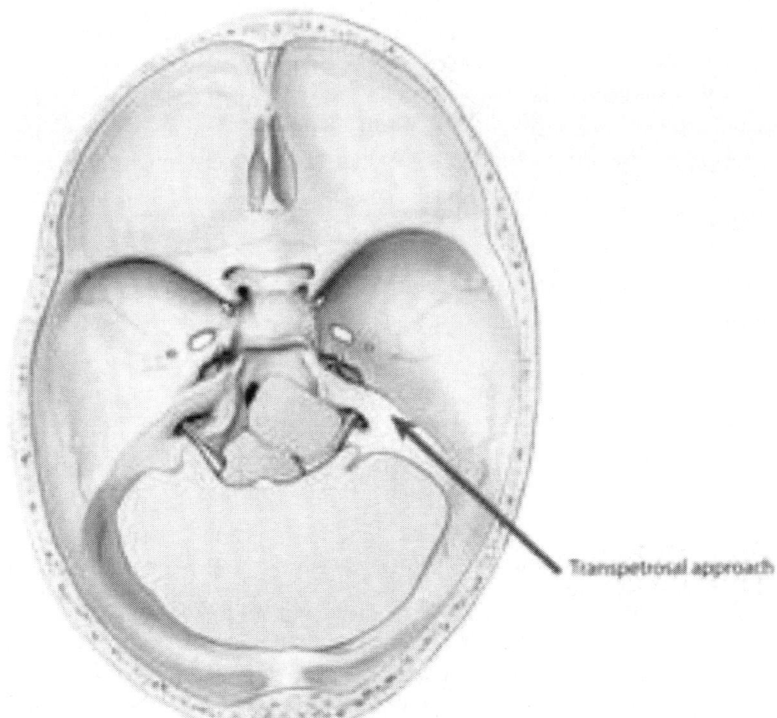


Figure 1d.

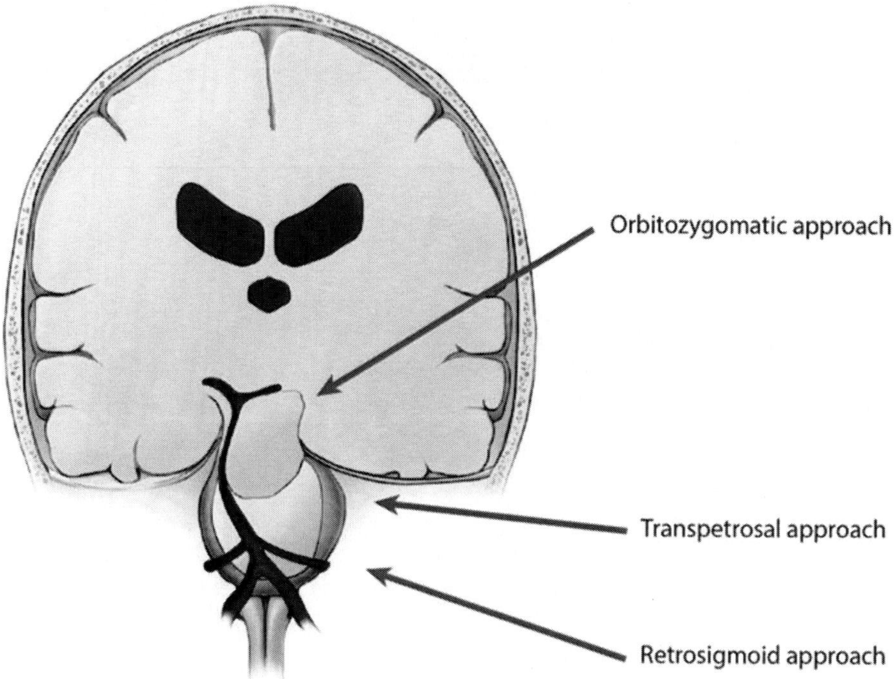


Figure 1e.

Illustration by Jennifer Kerbo ©2013.

Figure 1. The internal acoustic canal (IAC) and tentorium are landmarks that divide the middle and posterior cranial fossae, as shown in axial (A) and coronal (B) views. A retrosigmoid approach (C) is adequate for tumors located predominantly lateral to the IAC. Transpetrosal approaches (D) may be used to approach tumors with significant presence medial to the IAC. Tumors involving the middle and posterior cranial fossae are best approached in combination (E), such as through a transpetrous combined approach or through the use of two separate craniotomies (i.e., retrosigmoid plus orbitozygomatic approaches).

A burr hole is positioned over the thinnest part of the occipital bone covering the cerebellar hemisphere, and the craniotomy is extended superiorly and laterally to the transverse-sigmoid junction for maximum exposure of the CPA [29]. At our institution, we elect to use three-dimensional stereotactic navigation to aid in bony removal and improve accurate exposure. The dura is opened and the arachnoid membranes of the lateral cisterns carefully dissected to allow the release of cerebrospinal fluid and decompression of the cistern. After identification of the tumor, internal debulking is performed with ultrasonic aspiration and bipolar electrocaudery. The lateral margins are defined with sharp microsurgical dissection. Demarcation of all critical cranial nerves and neurovascular structures is always attempted. Following resection, a watertight closure of the dura should be attempted, with dural substitutes used for reinforcement. Opened mastoid air cells can be sealed using fibrin glue or large pieces of bone wax to avoid delayed cerebrospinal fluid leaks. Lumbar drainage is often used for large CPA masses at our institution and is determined on a case-by-case basis [29]. Meningiomas arising from the dura, superior to the fifth cranial nerve, are difficult to resect safely near the edge of the tentorium.

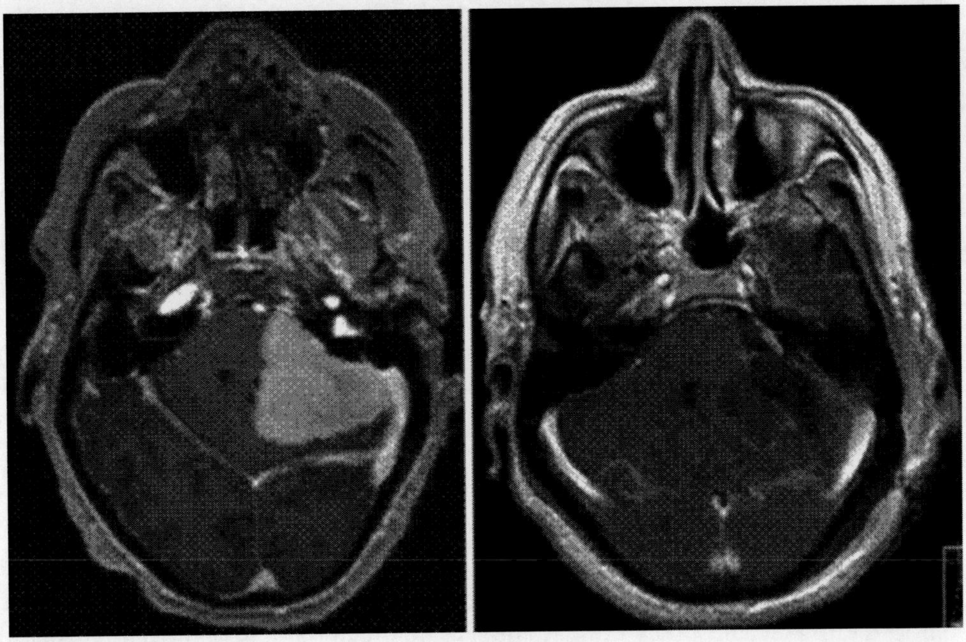

Figure 2. 75-year-old woman presented with gait difficulty and headache. Imaging revealed a petrous meningioma lateral to the internal acoustic canal with enlargement on serial imaging. An expanded retrosigmoid approach was used and gross total resection was achieved. Three dimensional stereotaxis and BAER monitoring were used intraoperatively to enhance safe resection. Preoperative axial T1-weighted MRI with gadolinium contrast injection demonstrates the homogeneously enhancing petrous meningioma (left). Postoperative axial T1-weighted MRI with gadolinium contrast confirms gross total resection of the tumor (right).

We prefer to perform a combined approach incorporating a transpetrosal or subtemporal approach to improve safe resection of these lesions.

## Transpetrosal Approaches

Transpetrosal approaches are more suitable for meningiomas positioned anterior to the IAC. They provide better exposure of ventral neurovasculature structures and posteriorly displaced cranial nerves that would otherwise be in the way if a retrosigmoid approach were used. Additionally, they require less retraction of the brain [6, 14]. However, these approaches involve complex anatomy and pose greater risk to the intrapetrosal otoneurological structures, limiting their use [6].

We work closely at our institution with otolaryngologists to minimize the risk to these structures. The anterior transpetrosal approach is best suited for smaller petroclival meningiomas medial to the IAC, without significant extension into the posterior fossa [16]. This approach allows for the adequate exposure of tumors infiltrating the posterior cavernous sinus. It may be used alone for tumors extending across the midline or in combination with a posterior petrosal approach [21]. Larger tumors extending into the posterior fossa and those lateral to the IAC both necessitate the use of the posterior petrosal approach or a combined approach. An anterior approach will not allow enough exposure for safe resection [16, 21].

## Anterior Transpetrosal (Kawase) Approach

In 1975, Bochenek and Kukwa [30] described an extended middle fossa approach to the IAC and CPA. Kawase and colleagues later modified this approach in the 1980s to gain access to the vertebrobasilar junction and the petroclival region [22]. Variations to the Kawase approach have since been widely employed. The anterior transpetrosal approach is commonly used to expose the floor of the middle cranial fossa, the petrous bone apex, and the petroclival region [8, 21, 22]. The surgical field provided by Kawase's approach is bound anteriorly by the mandibular nerve, posteriorly by the IAC, laterally by the greater superficial petrosal nerve, and medially by the petrous ridge. Exposure of the ventral pons may extend from approximately the fifth cranial nerve to the emergence of the sixth nerve. This will expose both nerves ipsilaterally and reveal cranial nerve VI on the contralateral side, in the distal part of its cisternal passage. The ipsilateral acoustic-facial bundle may also be exposed at its cisternal passage origin. This approach allows for good exposure of the upper clivus and improved visualization of the clival region across the midline. It may also expose a section of the basilar artery, as well as the segment of AICA extending from its origin to as far as the ventral aspect of its loop [16, 22]. The anterior petrosal approach allows for excellent surgical freedom to the trigeminal porous [16]. Additional transtentorial extension can broaden the access provided beyond the fifth cranial nerve and upper pontile sulcus [22]. However, this approach yields limited access to the lower cerebellomedullary angle and the lower cranial nerves [22]. Performance of a subtemporal craniotomy, with an anterior petrosectomy of the petrous apex anteromedial to the intrapetrous carotid, facilitates access to the brainstem anterior to the cranial nerves while also preserving the cochlea and hearing function [8, 22].

## Posterior Transpetrosal Approach

The posterior transpetrosal approach provides a lateral operative corridor to the region extending from the trigeminal impression to the jugular tubercle in the upper to middle clivus [8, 16]. It provides exposure to lesions deep within the posterior cranial fossa and lateral to, or below, the IAC. The posterior transpetrosal approach is considered the approach of choice for larger petroclival tumors. Resection of the petrous bone allows for an increased exposure of the lateral aspect of the brainstem and petroclival groove. This provides greater access to the petroclival region with minimal temporal lobe retraction. However, the posterior petrosal approach may provide insufficient exposure in patients with a high jugular bulb or with tumors that cross the midline of the clivus [21].

Several of the complications of this approach are associated with the mobilization and manipulation of the sigmoid sinus or with the sectioning of the tentorium. Certain patients are at a higher risk of venous drainage disruption with the use of the posterior transpetrosal approach. Patients with a dominant or single sigmoid sinus ipsilateral to the lesion, patients with transverse sinuses that do not connect to the torcular herophili, or those with venous drainage through the tentorium are included. These patients must be identified preoperatively and alternative approaches should be considered [21].

Though multiple variations of this approach have been described, all remain as extensions of the basic mastoidectomy. There are essentially three main variants of the posterior transpetrosal approach, each differentiated by the extent of petrous bone resection involved: retrolabyrinthine, translabyrinthine, and transcochlear [16, 31-37]. Aggressive bony removal provides greater anatomical exposure and increases the surgical freedom, yet this comes at the expense of a greater risk of complication [16].

Al-Mefty and colleagues [20] described the use of the retrolabyrinthine approach for petroclival access in 1988 (Figure 3). The retrolabyrinthine approach involves the least amount of petrous bone resections and is selected in cases mandating the preservation of seventh and eighth cranial nerve functions and where the anterior exposure to the brainstem is not required. This approach does not disturb the labyrinth or skeletonize the facial nerve, thus preserving hearing and facial nerve function. Although the retrolabyrinthine approach is the safest method in terms of cranial nerve morbidity, it does not provide adequate access to the central clival depression [16]. However, additional bony exposure can be obtained through the removal of one or two semicircular canals, possibly resulting in the slight preservation of hearing. The translabyrinthine approach was developed by Morrison and King [35] in the 1970s. It consisted of drilling the mastoid and labyrinth and cutting the tentorium to gain exposure to the CPA (Figure 4). The approach was modified to include a posterior fossa craniotomy by Hakuba and colleagues [38] in the 1980s. This variation may be utilized in patients with little to no hearing function, as the labyrinth and hearing are sacrificed to gain greater exposure.

All three semicircular canals are removed, and the lateral segment of the IAC is completely skeletonized. This thereby increases access to the anterolateral brainstem and inferior clivus [21]. The transcochlear approach provides the greatest degree of exposure to the petroclival region and to the anterior surface of the brainstem, yet is rarely used given its associated complications.

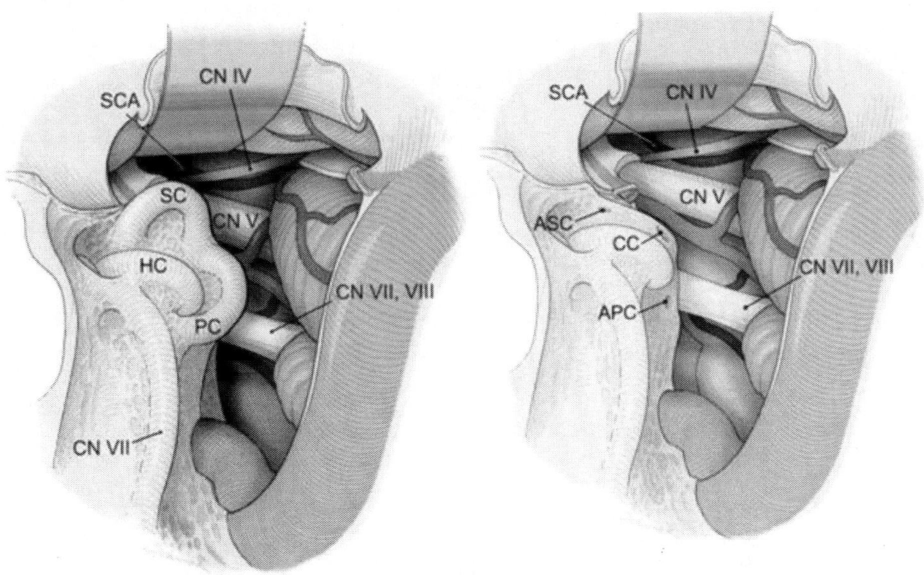


Reproduced with permission from Journal of Neurosurgery Publishing Group. Courtesy of Barrow Neurological Institute.

Figure 3. Exposure achieved using a standard retrolabyrinthine approach (left) and exposure gained with addition of the transcrusal approach (right). APC = ampulla of posterior canal; ASC = ampulla of superior canal; CC =crus commune; CN = cranial nerve; HC = horizontal canal; PC = posterior canal; SC = superior canal; SCA = superior cerebellar artery.

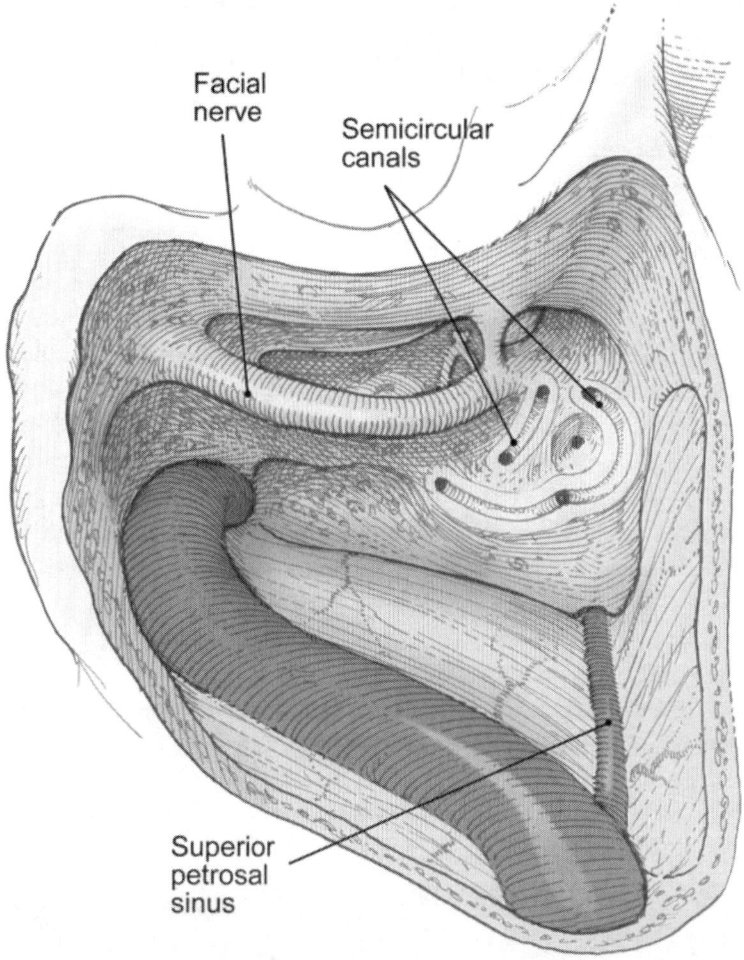




Figure 4. Translabyrinthine approach with progressive drilling of the temporal bone reveals the three semicircular canals. Anterior to cranial nerve VII, the middle ear is entered through the facial recess.

It was initially employed by House and colleagues [33] in the 1970s to allow for greater exposure of the CPA [21]. This approach sacrifices hearing and may jeopardize facial nerve function. It is exclusively considered in cases where hearing is absent and facial weakness evident. The transcochlear approach consists of the resection of the cochlea and division of the greater superficial petrosal nerve. The transotic variant involves exposure of the facial nerve *in situ* and the occlusion of the auditory canal [16, 33, 37, 39].

## Combined Transpetrosal Approach

The combined transpetrosal approach consists of performing both, anterior and posterior transpetrosal approaches, to further increase exposure across the posterior and middle cranial fossae (Figure 5) [16, 22]. The approach was first described by Hakuba and colleagues [38] and combined the preauricular and postauricular transpetrous approaches.

These involved the resection of the labyrinth and endolymphatic sac and preservation of the cochlea and ossicles in an attempt to preserve hearing function. However, seven of the eight patients in this study experienced hearing loss [29]. Sekhar and colleagues [10] employed partial resection of the labyrinth, which increased temporal exposure and preserved serviceable hearing in 80% of the patients who underwent surgery [21].

Combined approaches generally consist of a temporal craniotomy in combination with the removal of the petrous bone to a variable degree.

Lateral or anterolateral approaches used alone are inadequate for large tumors in the petroclival region that extend into the CPA [22]. In some cases, a combined approach may preserve hearing function with the utilization of a partial labyrinthectomy and partial apicetomy [10, 16, 40, 41]. A transcrural variant has been described that reportedly increases access to the central clival depression, with overall reduced risk of cranial nerve morbidity [16, 28, 40, 41]. However, some researchers maintain that the performance of the petrous apicectomy made possible through this approach is responsible for the significant improvement in exposure rather than the partial labyrinthectomy [10, 42]. The partial labyrinthectomy has been found to achieve little when used alone in cadaveric models in comparison with a retrolabyrinthine approach [16, 43, 44]. Moreover, the partial labyrinthectomy may also risk hearing function. Therefore, some authors have used the combined petrosal approach, by incorporating the retrolabyrinthine approach and the anterior transpetrosal approach, to resect the petrous apex and maximize petroclival exposure [45].

These authors recommend employing the combined transpetrosal approach for patients with large petroclival tumors where hearing and facial nerve function are to be preserved. In our practice, we have found this approach to be advantageous, though time-intensive. However, performing the cranial work prior to initiating temporal bone drilling significantly decreases the time necessary to achieve adequate exposure, allowing us to utilize this strategy routinely [16].

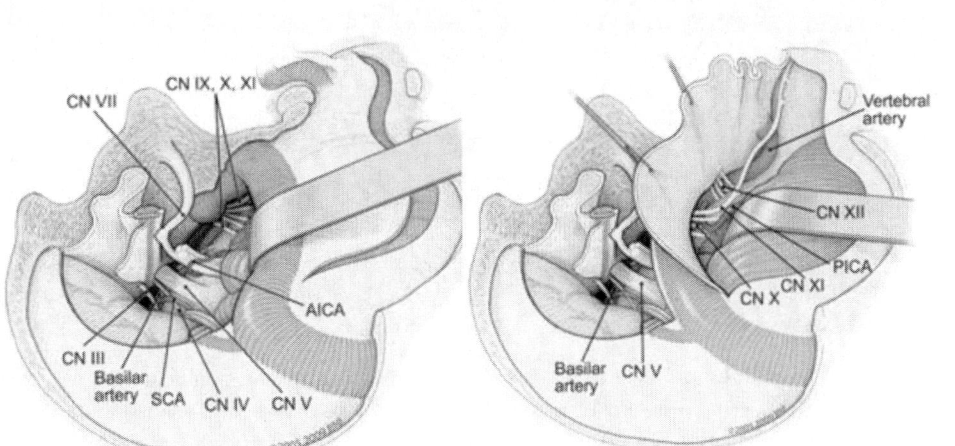


Reproduced with permission from Barrow Neurological Institute.

Figure 5. Posterior fossa exposures obtained through the use of a combined approach with retraction of the sigmoid sinus posteriorly (left) or anteriorly (right). AICA = anterior inferior cerebellar artery; CN = cranial nerve; PICA = posterior inferior cerebellar artery; SCA = superior cerebellar artery.

This combined methodology allows the tumor to be approached through the petrous bone, both anteriorly and posteriorly to the labyrinth and middle ear structures [21].

It provides a level of exposure comparable to that imparted by the transcochlear approaches, yet is without the risks associated with these techniques since the intrapetrosal neuro-otologic structures remain largely undisturbed [22]. It allows access to large tumors in the posterior fossa below the IAC through a posterior exposure, while exposing the midline clivus, contralateral side, anterior cavernous sinus, petrous apex, Meckel's cave, and ventral brainstem via an anterior approach. Better visualization of the basilar artery and perforating vessels accompanies ventral brainstem exposure and allows for safer avenues of resection (Figures 6 and 7) [21].

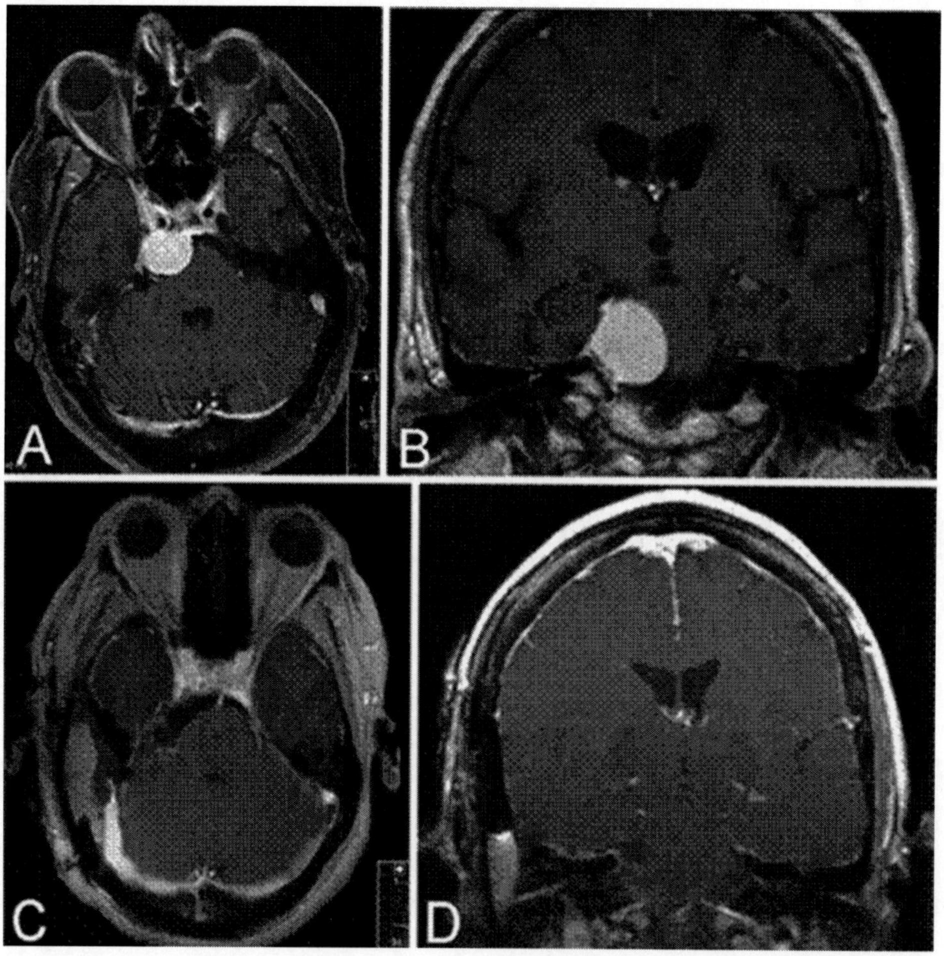


Figure 6. 50-year-old woman presented with diplopia and headaches and was found to have cranial nerve IV neuropathy on exam. Imaging revealed a large petroclival meningioma medial to the internal acoustic canal with supratentorial extension. A combined transpetrosal approach was used with an anterior petrosectomy and posterior labyrinthectomy, and near total resection (Simpson Grade III) was achieved. Preoperative axial (A) and preoperative coronal (B) T1-weighted MRI with gadolinium contrast reveals a homogeneously enhancing petroclival meningioma. Postoperative axial (C) and postoperative coronal (D) T1-weighted MRI with gadolinium contrast demonstrated near total resection of the petroclival lesion.

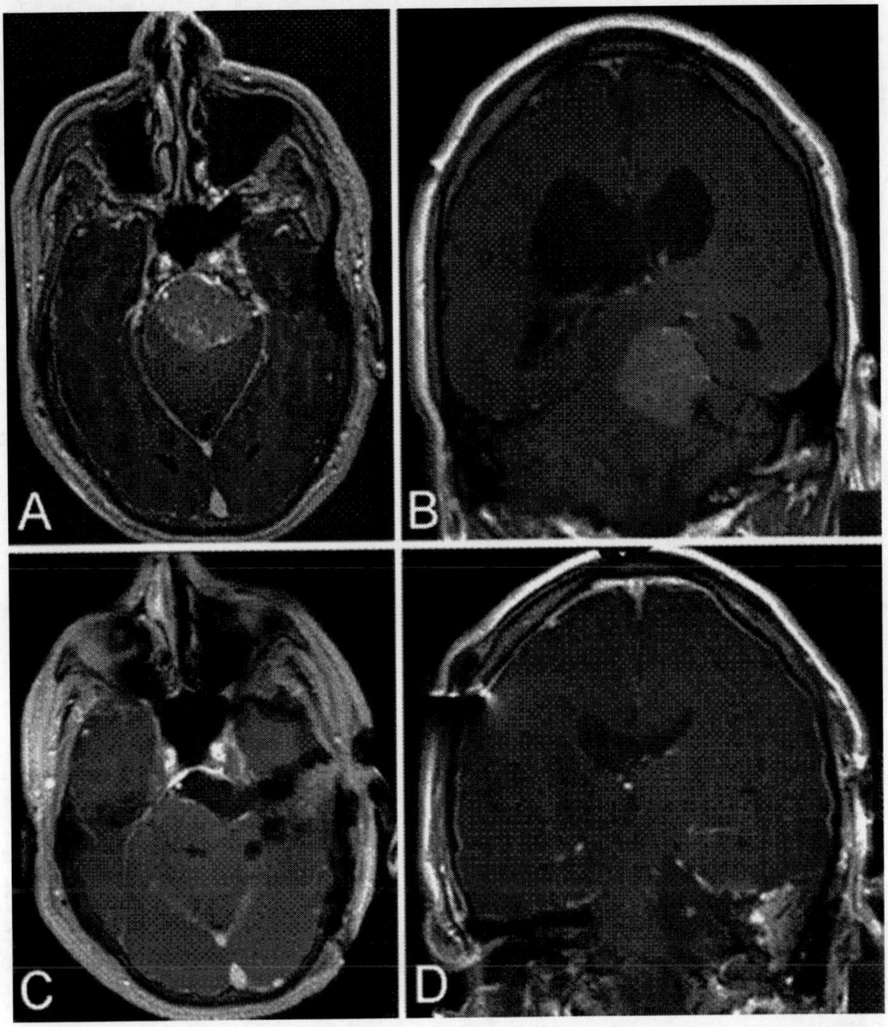


Figure 7. 48-year-old man presented with progressive gait difficulty and weakness with dysphagia. On exam, he was found to have left-sided hemiparesis, severe ataxia, hearing loss, and cranial nerve IV and VI involvement. Imaging studies revealed a large posterior petrous meningioma with extension into the middle cranial fossa and severe brainstem compression with associated hydrocephalus. The patient underwent a large combined transpetrosal approach with achievement of gross total resection. Preoperative axial (A) and preoperative coronal (B) T1-weighted MRI with gadolinium contrast shows enhancement of a petrous meningioma. Postoperative axial (C) and coronal (D) T1-weighted MRI with gadolinium contrast confirms gross total resection.

## Intraoperative Monitoring

Intraoperative neurophysiologic monitoring is used to help guide tumor dissection to protect the cranial nerves and minimize neurologic morbidity during surgical manipulation. The modalities generally employed include somatosensory evoked potential, motor evoked potentials, brain stem auditory evoked potentials, electroencephalography, and cranial nerve monitoring, most commonly of cranial nerves V and VII [8, 19].

## Discussion

Petrous meningiomas constitute a heterogeneous group of tumors with complex anatomical localizations and surgical management [3]. The management of these lesions has evolved over the past few decades as surgical technique, technology, and philosophy have progressed.

In determining management options, neurosurgeons must take into account the composite risk of surgical resection on a case-by-case basis. Age of presentation, tumor progression, clinical signs and symptoms of brainstem compression, cranial neuropathies, and co-morbidities must all be considered when offering a surgical strategy to a patient [8].

### Natural History

Few studies have examined the natural progression of these tumors. Van Havenbergh and colleagues [46] observed the petroclival tumors of 21 patients for 4 years or more, during which 76% of tumors demonstrated growth and 63% of patients experienced neurologic deterioration.

The progressive nature of these tumors was demonstrated by cranial nerve involvement. 50% of patients who presented asymptomatically developed cranial nerve deficits and 20% of patients who were initially symptomatic developed additional deficits [46]. Van Havenbergh's study observed an overall growth rate of 0.81 mm/yr in diameter and 0.81 $cm^3$/yr in volume.

When non-growing tumors were excluded, the rate was of 1.16 mm/yr in diameter and 1.10 $cm^3$/yr in volume. Greater growth was seen in small- and medium-sized tumors, though this observation lacked statistical significance [46]. Jung and colleagues [47] examined the growth rates of postoperative residual tumors following subtotal resection. They identified growth rates of 0.37 cm/yr in diameter and 4.94 cm3/yr in volume, with lower rates of growth in older patients.

The discrepant rates observed in the previous two studies discussed may suggest that remnants have greater rates of growth or that they may be reflective of the comparison between different tumor subtypes [46, 47]. The lower growth rates associated with advanced age in the study by Jung and colleagues, was not observed in Van Havenbergh's study. However, Starke and colleagues reported greater tumor progression in patients more than 65-years-old following STR [46-48].

Complete surgical resection is considered to be curative with minimal recurrence on long-term follow-up, as this is outcome is the ultimate objective in treatment. Though STR has been associated with recurrence, functional outcome and quality of life must be taken into account and often take precedence over achieving total resection for complex lesions. In cases involving complex anterior petrosal and petroclival lesions, where aggressive surgery is associated with significant complications including cranial nerve deficits, many surgeons elect to leave remnants and preserve a good functional outcome [13, 14]. STR has been shown to provide adequate tumor control and preservation of neurologic function [24, 49-55]. The use of adjuvant therapies has further promoted this shift in away from total resection and towards safe resection strategies [24, 48].

# Resection Principles and Options

## True Petrous Meningiomas

Anterior petrous meningiomas tend to become symptomatic earlier and be smaller upon discovery; however, resection is more challenging, and rates of GTR vary between 18% and 75%. Although generally larger at the time of operation, posterior petrous meningiomas are associated with GTR rates between 86% and 100% and with better postoperative functional outcomes [3, 6, 7, 9, 19, 24, 26, 56]. Table 1 demonstrates the rates of GTR and mortality in a series of studies addressing petrous meningioma surgical management.

Mortality rates associated with the resection of petrous meningiomas are shown to vary from 0% to approximately 9%.

Recurrence rates in resected posterior petrous-based meningiomas are reported to be between 3.2% and 23%, usually occurring in less than 10% of cases [9]. Though recurrence is generally associated with STR, it may follow GTR as well. Bassiouni and colleagues [9] reported achieving a GTR rate of 84.3% in 51 patients with meningiomas of the posterior petrous bone. Two recurrences were observed, both occurring in patients who underwent GTR. One of the recurrences was associated with atypical histology. In another study, five recurrent tumors were reported of which three were observed in GTR cases [9].

**Table 1. Literature reports of surgical outcomes in petrous meningiomas**

| Authors and year | Number of patients | Mortality (%) | GTR (%) |
|---|---|---|---|
| Liu et al. 2003 [3] | 21 | 0 | Total: 86 |
| Roche et al. 2003 [6] | 57 | 8.8 | PPM: 86<br>APM: 18<br>Total: 39 |
| Bassiouni et al. 2004 [9] | 51 | 0 | Total: 84.3 |
| Wu et al. 2005 [19] | 82 | 0 | PPM: 100<br>APM: 75 |
| Deveze et al. 2007 [25] | 43 | 0 | Total: 79.1 |
| Sade and Lee 2008 [12] | 58 | Not reported | PPM: 97<br>APM: 58<br>Total: 84 |
| Qu et al. 2009 [26] | 42 | 0 | Total: 90 |
| Peyre et al. 2012 [24] | 53 | Not reported | Total: 72 |

APM = anterior petrous meningioma; GTR = gross total resection; PPM = posterior petrous meningioma.

In our practice, we attempt to achieve GTR of petrous meningiomas when possible and reserve STR for cases involving debilitated patients, poor brainstem interface, or advanced tumors with extensive adhesion to and encasement of neurovascular structures. We generally employ the retrosigmoid approach for petrous meningiomas. However, we often prefer to utilize a combined transpetrosal approach for tumors arising medial to the IAC in cases involving both the posterior and middle cranial fossae. Care is taken to preserve hearing if function is intact, unless greater exposure is required.

## Petroclival Meningiomas

Rates of GTR reported for petroclival lesions in available studies range from 20% to 85%, and the mortality rates associated with surgical treatment of these tumors vary between 0% and 10% (Table 2) [8, 14, 16]. Al-Mefty and colleagues [14] performed a retrospective analysis of 64 petroclival meningioma cases and reported a GTR rate of 64% with a 9.8% recurrence rate following GTR. STR was associated with a 43% recurrence rate and this difference in rate of recurrence was statistically significant ($p = 0.00348$). More aggressive resection was not found to be associated with greater morbidity, as the vast majority of new or worsening postoperative cranial nerve deficits resolved [14].

**Table 2. Literature reports of surgical outcomes in petroclival meningiomas**

| Authors and year | Number of patients | Mortality (%) | CN deficits (%) | GTR (%) |
|---|---|---|---|---|
| Al-Mefty et al. 1988 [20] | 13 | 0 | 31 | 85 |
| Sammi et al. 1989 [63] | 24 | 0 | 70 | 71 |
| Spetzler et al. 1992 [64] | 18 | 0 | 39 | 78 |
| Bricolo et al. 1992 [4] | 33 | 9 | 76 | 79 |
| Couldwell et al. 1996 [17] | 109 | 3.7 | 33 | 69 |
| Roberti et al. 2001 [65] | 110 | 0.9 | 47 | 45 |
| Little et al. 2005 [58] | 137 | 0.7 | 22.6 | 40 |
| Park et al. 2006 [66] | 49 | 2 | 28.6 | 20 |
| Bambakidis et al. 2007 [8] | 46 | 0 | 30 | 43 |
| Natarajan et al. 2007 [59] | 150 | 0 | 20.3 | 32 |
| Seifert et al. 2010 [67] | 93 | 0 | 31 | 37 |
| Nanda et al. 2011 [60] | 50 | 0 | 32 | 28 |
| Al-Mefty et al. 2014 [14] | 64 | 1.56 | 89 | 64? |

GTR = gross total resection.

The traditional suboccipital and pterional approaches have been widely employed in the treatment of petroclival tumors, however, the use of transpetrosal approaches has become increasingly common [14]. With time and experience, we have largely replaced the aggressive combined transpetrosal approach with a conventional retrosigmoid approach in the treatment of petroclival meningiomas at our institution. This applies particularly to tumors extending lateral to the IAC or those without significant supratentorial presence [8, 16, 57]. We return to the combined transpetrosal approaches in cases involving larger tumors [10, 11, 16, 45, 58, 59].

It is important to remember that many factors that prevent GTR are independent of the surgical approach selected, the skill, or experience of the surgical team. These factors have been well described and include brainstem pial invasion, neurovascular structure encasement and firm tumor consistency [17, 58-60]. Cavernous sinus invasion has also been identified as a factor, although a recent study by Al-Mefty and colleagues [14] reported that extension into the cavernous sinus was not found to adversely affect the extent of resection achieved [16].

Factors such as tumor location relative to the IAC, involvement of one or both cranial fossae, and preoperative hearing function are important considerations in managing these lesions. We have developed a treatment algorithm for petroclival meningiomas at our institution based on these considerations (Figure 8).

## Stereotactic Radiosurgery

The use of radiosurgical treatment has increased over the past decade. It may be used as primary therapy or as an adjuvant to surgical resection in cases involving STR or complicated recurrent growth [24, 48].

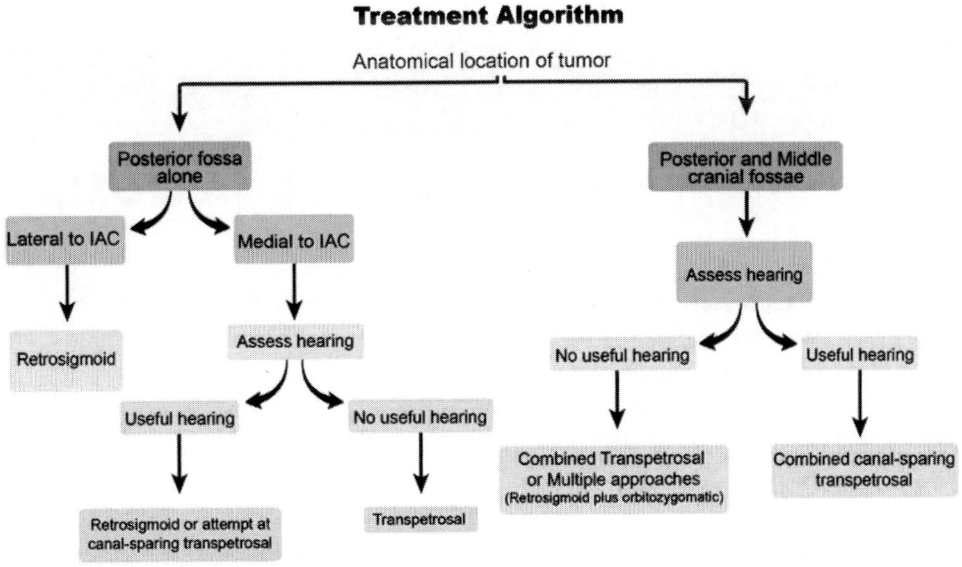


Illustration by Jennifer Kerbo ©2013.

Figure 8. Algorithm illustrates important considerations in determining surgical approaches for the treatment of petroclival tumors. IAC = internal acoustic canal.

Starke and colleagues [48] performed a retrospective review of 152 patients with posterior fossa meningiomas treated with Gamma Knife radiosurgery (GKRS) following surgical resection or as initial management.

They performed follow-ups for 2 years minimum and an overall median of 7 years. It was concluded that GKRS provides adequate control of posterior fossa meningiomas and is associated with low rates of neurological deficits. The study reported stable or decreased tumor volume in 87% of patients in addition to stable or improved neurological function in 91% at the last follow-up visit. There was radiographic progression-free survival rates of 98%, 96%, and 78% at 3, 5, and 10 years, respectively. Starke and colleagues found that tumor progression was associated with ages greater than 65-years-old and with decreased dosages to the tumor margin. They also found that meningiomas that attach at the clivus or petrous bone are associated with the development of new or worsening neurological deficit following GKRS [48].

However, many of the studies that assert good control with STR and GKRS have consisted of relatively short follow-up periods. Mathiesen and colleagues [61] examined the long-term outcome associated with STR and radiation to find that 75% of tumors recurred. This suggested the treatment strategy to delay rather than preclude recurrence. They further reported a 56% radiation-induced complication rate. Moreover, these progressing tumors are difficult to treat because resection has extremely high complication rates following initial treatment, given resultant scarring and radiation vasculopathy [13, 14, 61]. However, it has also been shown that achieving a Simpson grade I and II resection with total removal of the tumor, dura, and underlying bone does not necessarily correlate with lower recurrence rates in skull base meningiomas [24, 62]. Using more clearly defined tumor populations and better follow-up merits further study of this treatment.

We do not perform stereotactic surgery (SRS) as a routine for every case involving STR at our institution. The use of SRS in our practice is individualized and dependent on such factors such as the patient's age and the residual tumor's volume, location, and pathological characteristics. We continue to follow the patient clinically and radiologically following resection and reassess SRS initiation.

## CONCLUSION

The fundamental objective of petrous meningioma treatment is the preservation or improvement of neurological function. The indications for surgical management of petrous meningiomas include documented growth or the development of neurological symptoms [16]. Smaller, asymptomatic meningiomas that do not demonstrate brain edema, show little to no growth on serial imaging, or are highly calcified may be followed conservatively [27]. Stereotactic radiosurgery should always be discussed as an option but should be avoided as a first line therapy if surgery can be offered.

Surgical treatment in this region requires an aggressive but prudent approach, with the objective of limiting neurologic morbidity while maximizing tumor exposure, resection, and safety. The anatomical relationships of the tumor, particularly to the IAC and its superior and inferior extension, are useful in surgical planning. If sensorineural hearing loss is already present, a transpetrosal approach may be recommended for cases in which it would otherwise be avoided if hearing preservation were desired. The choice of exposure must further account for the ability and experience of the surgical team.

Complete tumor removal is remains to be the only permanent treatment considered for these lesions and is the goal of surgery. However, it may not always be possible to achieve this level of resection safely. Removal may be limited by tumor size, consistency, involvement of surrounding neurovascular structures, adhesion to the brainstem, or extension into the cavernous sinus. In these cases, STR is reasonable, and radiosurgery may be added for residual tumor. Radiosurgery as the primary method of treatment is employed for patients who are not candidates for surgery due to advanced age and operative risks, as well as in complicated cases of recurrence [14, 16, 48].

## References

[1] Nakamura M., Roser F., Mirzai S., Matthies C., Vorkapic P., Samii M. Meningiomas of the internal auditory canal. *Neurosurgery,* 2004; 55(1):119-27.

[2] Al-Mefty O. Operative Atlas of Meningiomas. Philadelphia: Lippincott-Raven. 1998.

[3] Liu J. K., Gottfried O. N., Couldwell W. T. Surgical management of posterior petrous meningiomas. *Neurosurgical focus,* 2003; 14(6):e7.

[4] Bricolo A. P., Turazzi S., Talacchi A., Cristofori L. Microsurgical removal of petroclival meningiomas: a report of 33 patients. *Neurosurgery,* 1992; 31(5):813-28.

[5] Desgeorges M., Sterkers O., Poncet J. L., Rey A., Sterkers J. M. [Surgery for meningioma of the posterior skull base. 135 cases. Choice of approach and results]. *Neuro-Chirurgie*, 1995; 41(4):265-90.

[6] Roche P. H., Pellet W., Fuentes S., Thomassin J. M., Regis J. Gamma knife radiosurgical management of petroclival meningiomas results and indications. *Acta Neurochir.*, (Wien). 2003; 145(10):883-8.

[7] Sade B., Lee J. H. Petrous Meningiomas II: Ventral, Posterior and Superior Subtypes. In: Lee J. H., editors. Meningiomas: Diagnosis, Treatment, and Outcome. London: Springer Science and Business Media; 2008. 443-447.

[8] Bambakidis N. C., Kakarla U. K., Kim L. J., Nakaji P., Porter R. W., Daspit C. P., et al. Evolution of surgical approaches in the treatment of petroclival meningiomas: a retrospective review. *Neurosurgery,* 2007; 61(5 Suppl. 2):202-9.

[9] Bassiouni H., Hunold A., Asgari S., Stolke D. Meningiomas of the posterior petrous bone: functional outcome after microsurgery. *Journal of neurosurgery,* 2004; 100(6):1014-24.

[10] Sekhar L. N., Schessel D. A., Bucur S. D., Raso J. L., Wright D. C. Partial labyrinthectomy petrous apicectomy approach to neoplastic and vascular lesions of the petroclival area. *Neurosurgery,* 1999; 44(3):537-50.

[11] Sekhar L. N., Wright D. C., Richardson R., Monacci W. Petroclival and foramen magnum meningiomas: surgical approaches and pitfalls. *Journal of neuro-oncology,* 1996; 29(3):249-59.

[12] Sade B., Lee J. H. Ventral petrous meningiomas: unique tumors. *Surgical neurology,* 2009; 72(1):61-4.

[13] Pamir M. N., Black P. M., Fahlbusch R. Overview of Petroclival Meningiomas. In: Pamir M. N., Black P. M., Fahlbusch R., editors. Meningiomas: A Comprehensive Text. Philadelphia, PA: Saunders/ Elsevier, 2010. 477-486.

[14] Al-Mefty R., Dunn I. F., Pravdenkova S., Abolfotoh M., Al-Mefty O. True petroclival meningiomas: results of surgical management. *Journal of Neurosurgery*, 2014; 120(1):40-51.

[15] Chen L. F., Yu X. G., Bu B., Xu B. N., Zhou D. B. The retrosigmoid approach to petroclival meningioma surgery. *J. Clin. Neurosci.,* 2011; 18(12):1656-61.

[16] Xu F., Karampelas I., Megerian C. A., Selman W. R., Bambakidis N. C. Petroclival meningiomas: an update on surgical approaches, decision making, and treatment results. *Neurosurgical focus,* 2013; 35(6):E11.

[17] Couldwell W. T., Fukushima T., Giannotta S. L., Weiss M. H. Petroclival meningiomas: surgical experience in 109 cases. *J. Neurosurg.,* 1996; 84(1):20-8.

[18] Yasargil M. G., Mortara R. W., Curcic M. Meningiomas of Basal Posterior Cranial Fossa. In: Krayenbuld H., editor. Advances and Technical Standards in Neurosurgery. Vienna: Springer-Verlag; 1980. 3-118.

[19] Wu Z. B., Yu C. J., Guan S. S. Posterior petrous meningiomas: 82 cases. *J. Neurosurg.*, 2005; 102(2):284-9.

[20] Al-Mefty O., Fox J. L., Smith R. R. Petrosal approach for petroclival meningiomas. *Neurosurgery,* 1988; 22(3):510-7.

[21] Ware M. L., Pravdenkova S., Erkmen K. Al-Mefty O. Petroclival and Upper Clival Meningiomas I: An Overview of Surgical Approaches. In: Lee J. H., editors. Meningiomas: Diagnosis, Treatment, and Outcome. London: Springer Science and Business Media; 2008. 403-414.

[22] Fournier H. D., Mercier P., Roche P. H. Surgical anatomy of the petrous apex and petroclival region. *Advances and technical standards in neurosurgery,* 2007; 32:91-146.

[23] Brackmann D. E., Crawford, J. V., Green J. D. Cerebellopontine Angle Tumors. In: Bailey B. J., Johnson J. T., Newlands S. D., editors. Head and Neck Surgery—Otolaryngology. 4th ed. Philadelphia, PA: Lippincott Williams and Wilkins; 2006.

[24] Peyre M., Bozorg-Grayeli A., Rey A., Sterkers O., Kalamarides M. Posterior petrous bone meningiomas: surgical experience in 53 patients and literature review. *Neurosurgical review*, 2012; 35(1):53-66.

[25] Deveze A., Franco-Vidal V., Liguoro D., Guerin J., Darrouzet V. Transpetrosal approaches for meningiomas of the posterior aspect of the petrous bone Results in 43 consecutive patients. *Clinical neurology and neurosurgery,* 2007; 109(7):578-88.

[26] Qu F. J., Zhou X. D., Wang X. L., Li F., Lu X. D., Liu Y. G., Zhong Y. H., Yang H. A., Ni S. L. The Classification of Posterior Petrous Meningiomas and Its Clinical Significance. *Journal of International Medical Research,* 2009; 37:949.

[27] Millesi M., Kueß M., Widhalm G., Knosp E. Current Surgical Strategies in the Treatment of Intracranial Meningiomas. *European Association of NeuroOncology Magazine,* 2013; 3(3):112-7.

[28] Sheth S., Branstetter B. Ft., Escott E. J. Appearance of normal cranial nerves on steady-state free precession MR images. *Radiographics : a review publication of the Radiological Society of North America, Inc.,* 2009; 29(4):1045-55.

[29] Mehdorn H. M., Buhl R. M. Petrous Meningiomas I: An Overview. In: Lee J. H., editors. Meningiomas: Diagnosis, Treatment, and Outcome. London: Springer Science and Business Media; 2008. 433-441.
[30] Bochenek Z., Kukwa A. An extended approach through the middle cranial fossa to the internal auditory meatus and the cerebello-pontine angle. *Acta oto-laryngologica*, 1975; 80(5-6):410-4.
[31] Bambakidis N. C., Gonzalez L. F., Amin-Hanjani S., Deshmukh V. R., Porter R. W., Daspit P. C., et al. Combined skull base approaches to the posterior fossa. Technical note. *Neurosurgical focus*, 2005; 19(2):E8.
[32] House W. F. Transtemporal Bone Microsurgical Removal of Acoustic Neuromas. Evolution of Transtemporal Bone Removal of Acoustic Tumors. *Arch. Otolaryngol.*, 1964; 80:731-42.
[33] House W. F., Hitselberger W. E. The transcochlear approach to the skull base. *Arch. Otolaryngol.*, 1976; 102(6):334-42.
[34] King T. T. Combined translabyrinthine-transtentorial approach to acoustic nerve tumours. *Proc. R Soc. Med.*, 1970; 63(8):780-2.
[35] Morrison A. W., King T. T. Experiences with a translabyrinthine-transtentorial approach to the cerebellopontine angle. Technical note. *J. Neurosurg.*, 1973; 38(3): 382-90.
[36] Siwanuwatn R., Deshmukh P., Figueiredo E. G., Crawford N. R., Spetzler R. F., Preul M. C. Quantitative analysis of the working area and angle of attack for the retrosigmoid, combined petrosal, and transcochlear approaches to the petroclival region. *Journal of neurosurgery*, 2006; 104(1):137-42.
[37] Tummala R. P., Coscarella E., Morcos J. J. Transpetrosal approaches to the posterior fossa. *Neurosurgical focus*, 2005; 19(2):E6.
[38] Hakuba A., Nishimura S., Jang B. J. A combined retroauricular and preauricular transpetrosal-transtentorial approach to clivus meningiomas. *Surgical neurology*, 1988; 30(2):108-16.
[39] Jenkins H. A., Fisch U. The transotic approach to resection of difficult acoustic tumors of the cerebellopontine angle. *Am. J. Otol.*, 1980; 2(2): 70-6.
[40] Horgan M. A., Anderson G. J., Kellogg J. X., Schwartz M. S., Spektor S., McMenomey S. O., et al. Classification and quantification of the petrosal approach to the petroclival region. *J. Neurosurg.*, 2000; 93(1): 108-12.
[41] Horgan M. A., Delashaw J. B., Schwartz M. S., Kellogg J. X., Spektor S., McMenomey S. O. Transcrusal approach to the petroclival region with hearing preservation. Technical note and illustrative cases. *J. Neurosurg.*, 2001; 94(4):660-6.
[42] Chanda A., Nanda A. Partial labyrinthectomy petrous apicectomy approach to the petroclival region: an anatomic and technical study. *Neurosurgery*, 2002; 51(1):147-59.
[43] Miller C. G., van Loveren H. R., Keller J. T., Pensak M., el-Kalliny M., Tew J. M., Jr. Transpetrosal approach: surgical anatomy and technique. *Neurosurgery*, 1993; 33(3):461-9.
[44] Ramina R., Neto M. C., Fernandes Y. B., Silva E. B., Mattei T. A., Aguiar P. H. Surgical removal of small petroclival meningiomas. *Acta. Neurochir.*, (Wien). 2008; 150(5):431-8.
[45] Cho C. W., Al-Mefty O. Combined petrosal approach to petroclival meningiomas. *Neurosurgery*, 2002; 51(3):708-16.

[46] Van Havenbergh T., Carvalho G., Tatagiba M., Plets C., Samii M. Natural history of petroclival meningiomas. *Neurosurgery,* 2003; 52(1): 55-62.

[47] Jung H. W., Yoo H., Paek S. H., Choi K. S. Long-term outcome and growth rate of subtotally resected petroclival meningiomas: experience with 38 cases. *Neurosurgery,* 2000; 46(3):567-74.

[48] Starke R. M., Nguyen J. H., Rainey J., Williams B. J., Sherman J. H., Savage J., et al. Gamma Knife surgery of meningiomas located in the posterior fossa: factors predictive of outcome and remission. *J. Neurosurg.*, 2011; 114(5):1399-409.

[49] Davidson L., Fishback D., Russin J. J., Weiss M. H., Yu C., Pagnini P. G., et al. Postoperative Gamma Knife surgery for benign meningiomas of the cranial base. *Neurosurgical focus*, 2007; 23(4):E6.

[50] Kreil W., Luggin J., Fuchs I., Weigl V., Eustacchio S., Papaefthymiou G. Long term experience of gamma knife radiosurgery for benign skull base meningiomas. *J. Neurol. Neurosurg. Psychiatry*, 2005; 76(10): 1425-30.

[51] Milker-Zabel S., Zabel-du Bois A., Huber P., Schlegel W., Debus J. Intensity-modulated radiotherapy for complex-shaped meningioma of the skull base: long-term experience of a single institution. *Int. J. Radiat. Oncol. Biol. Phys.*, 2007; 68(3):858-63.

[52] Nicolato A., Foroni R., Pellegrino M., Ferraresi P., Alessandrini F., Gerosa M., et al. Gamma knife radiosurgery in meningiomas of the posterior fossa. Experience with 62 treated lesions. *Minim. Invasive Neurosurg.,* 2001; 44(4):211-7.

[53] Starke R. M., Williams B. J., Hiles C., Nguyen J. H., Elsharkawy M. Y., Sheehan J. P. Gamma knife surgery for skull base meningiomas. *Journal of neurosurgery,* 2012; 116(3):588-97.

[54] Yamakami I., Higuchi Y., Horiguchi K., Saeki N. Treatment policy for petroclival meningioma based on tumor size: aiming radical removal in small tumors for obtaining cure without morbidity. *Neurosurgical review*, 2011; 34(3):327-34; discussion 34-5.

[55] Zachenhofer I., Wolfsberger S., Aichholzer M., Bertalanffy A., Roessler K., Kitz K., et al. Gamma-knife radiosurgery for cranial base meningiomas: experience of tumor control, clinical course, and morbidity in a follow-up of more than 8 years. *Neurosurgery,* 2006; 58(1):28-36; discussion 28-36.

[56] Schaller B., Merlo A., Gratzl O., Probst R. Premeatal and retromeatal cerebellopontine angle meningioma. Two distinct clinical entities. *Acta. Neurochirurgica,* 1999; 141(5):465-71.

[57] Samii M., Gerganov V., Giordano M., Samii A. Two step approach for surgical removal of petroclival meningiomas with large supratentorial extension. *Neurosurgical review*, 2010; 34(2):173-9.

[58] Little K. M., Friedman A. H., Sampson J. H., Wanibuchi M., Fukushima T. Surgical management of petroclival meningiomas: defining resection goals based on risk of neurological morbidity and tumor recurrence rates in 137 patients. *Neurosurgery,* 2005; 56(3):546-59; discussion -59.

[59] Natarajan S. K., Sekhar L. N., Schessel D., Morita A. Petroclival meningiomas: multimodality treatment and outcomes at long-term follow-up. *Neurosurgery,* 2007; 60(6):965-79; discussion 79-81.

[60] Nanda A., Javalkar V., Banerjee A. D. Petroclival meningiomas: study on outcomes, complications and recurrence rates. *J. Neurosurg.,* 2011; 114(5):1268-77.

[61] Mathiesen T., Kihlstrom L., Karlsson B., Lindquist C. Potential complications following radiotherapy for meningiomas. *Surgical neurology,* 2003; 60(3):193-8; discussion 9-200.

[62] Sughrue M. E., Kane A. J., Shangari G., Rutkowski M. J., McDermott M. W., Berger M. S., et al. The relevance of Simpson Grade I and II resection in modern neurosurgical treatment of World Health Organization Grade I meningiomas. *Journal of neurosurgery,* 2010; 113(5):1029-35.

[63] Samii M., Ammirati M., Mahran A., Bini W., Sepehrnia A. Surgery of petroclival meningiomas: report of 24 cases. *Neurosurgery,* 1989; 24(1): 12-7.

[64] Spetzler R. F., Daspit C. P., Pappas C. T. The combined supra- and infratentorial approach for lesions of the petrous and clival regions: experience with 46 cases. *Journal of neurosurgery*, 1992; 76(4):588-99.

[65] Roberti F., Sekhar L. N., Kalavakonda C., Wright D. C. Posterior fossa meningiomas: surgical experience in 161 cases. *Surgical neurology,* 2001; 56(1):8-20; discussion -1.

[66] Park C. K., Jung H. W., Kim J. E., Paek S. H., Kim D. G. The selection of the optimal therapeutic strategy for petroclival meningiomas. *Surgical neurology,* 2006; 66(2):160-5; discussion 5-6.

[67] Seifert V. Clinical management of petroclival meningiomas and the eternal quest for preservation of quality of life: personal experiences over a period of 20 years. *Acta neurochirurgica*, 2010; 152(7):1099-116.

In: Current Management of Central Nervous System … ISBN: 978-1-63483-856-6
Editors: Steven D. Chang and Anand Veeravagu 

*Chapter 8*

# Surgical Management of Cerebellopontine Angle Meningiomas

***Yiping Li, MD, Kutluay Uluc, MD and Mustafa K. Baskaya*, MD***
Department of Neurological Surgery, University of Wisconsin Medical School, Madison, Wisconsin, US

## Abstract

Cerebellopontine angle (CPA) meningiomas comprise about one percent of all intracranial meningiomas; however, they are the second most common tumor found within the CPA, after vestibular schwannomas. CPA meningiomas commonly present with unilateral hearing loss, tinnitus, ataxia, and diminished facial sensation. Although there is a role for stereotactic radiosurgery, surgery remains the treatment of choice for CPA meningiomas. A detailed understanding of CPA surgical anatomy and operative approaches is critical in preventing severe neurosurgical morbidity.

## Introduction

Nearly ten percent of all intracranial tumors originate in the cerebellopontine angle (CPA) [1]. CPA meningiomas are an uncommon subgroup of meningiomas that arise from the cells lining the arachnoid villae bordering the posterolateral pons, anterolateral cerebellum, and the internal acoustic canal (IAC).

These tumors are defined as being centered superior to the jugular foramen and inferior to the trigeminal nerve along the petrosal edge.

* Corresponding author: Mustafa K. Baskaya, MD. Department of Neurological Surgery, University of Wisconsin Medical School, K4/828 CSC, 600 Highland Avenue, Madison, Wisconsin 53792-0001, US. Tel: (608) 262-7303, fax: (608) 263-1728, e-mail: m.baskaya@neurosurgery.wisc.edu.

Meningiomas in the CPA account for up to 15% of all tumors found at this location with vestibular schwannomas (VSs) being the most common, constituting about 80% of all CPA masses [2]. In the pediatric population, meningiomas account for only 6% of all tumors found within the CPA but remain the second most common lesion after VSs [3]. Other less common tumors arising from the CPA include epidermoid cysts, arachnoid cysts, endolymphatic sac tumors, and metastasis.

Differentiating between VSs and meningiomas at the CPA is often difficult, but critical. Published results suggest that up to 25% of CPA meningiomas are mistaken for VSs [1]. VSs arise from one of the vestibular nerves and frequently present with unilateral hearing loss, tinnitus, and vertigo [2]. CPA meningiomas may arise from the superior anterior edge of the IAC, petrous bone over the CPA cistern, or petrous tentorial junction [4]. Although meningiomas in the CPA arise from a different location than VSs, because of the close proximity of various cranial nerves, their foramina, and associated neurovascular structures within the CPA, meningiomas in this location present most commonly with unilateral hearing loss, tinnitus, headache and vertigo [4]. In CPA meningiomas, however, the facial nerve is affected much earlier in the clinical course while hearing loss occurs later. Trigeminal neuralgia is also much more common as a result of an expanding CPA meningioma, rather than a VS, which often does not involve the trigeminal nerve until the tumor has grown to larger sizes [5]. Other symptoms common to both VSs and CPA meningiomas include dizziness, vertigo, and diminished sensation. Rarely, these tumors may also present with hydrocephalus, brainstem compression, and/or lower cranial nerve dysfunction [6].

Radiographically, the differences between VSs and meningiomas are more apparent. CPA meningiomas are often more broad based in appearance, rest along the petrous bone, present with a dural tail, and are associated with calcifications and adjacent hyperostosis [7]. VSs, on the other hand, are more likely to undergo cystic degeneration, widen the IAC, and have a globoid appearance [7]. Although VSs and meningiomas at the CPA present with similar symptoms and may share imaging features, these tumor types have distinct treatment and prognostic considerations.

The literature suggests that CPA meningiomas may have a higher incidence of recurrence compared with similar-sized VSs; however, from a prognostic standpoint they have increased rates of hearing preservation and trend towards reduced rates of post-operative facial nerve weakness [8]. Systematic reviews of outcomes for VSs found an estimated 8-25% of patients suffer from post-operative facial nerve palsy, and as low as 5% of patients maintain serviceable hearing despite undergoing hearing preservation surgery [9, 10].

CPA meningiomas, in contrast, have very low rates of post-operative facial palsy and hearing loss [8]. One potential explanation for this trend is that VSs often involve the IAC, causing significant compression of the facial and vestibulocochlear nerve, while only a small subset of CPA meningiomas arise from or spread to the IAC [11]. The close proximity of neural and vascular structures in and adjacent to the IAC makes surgical resection and preservation of cranial nerves more challenging. VSs most commonly arise from the superior vestibular nerve and compress the facial nerve anteriorly within the IAC, thus smaller VSs may present with more severe cranial nerve deficits compared to equal-sized meningiomas, which often arise from the petrous dura anterior and superior to the IAC [2].

CPA meningiomas involving the IAC present as a clinically distinct subgroup of CPA meningiomas. These tumors are more likely to be symptomatic on presentation, have higher recurrence rates, and be misdiagnosed as VSs [11].

Historically, meningiomas were only discovered when they became large and symptomatic; however, as technology has improved, so has early and often incidental detection of meningiomas. The natural history of asymptomatic meningiomas of <2.5 cm in diameter usually does not progress to cause symptoms [12]. Small meningiomas are therefore often followed with serial imaging and monitored for symptom progression. Meningiomas in the CPA, however, are more prone to result in symptom progression due to the close proximity of neurovascular structures within the CPA [12]. Small meningiomas at this location often compress eloquent neural structures and require surgical intervention. The indications for surgery include CPA meningiomas that cause mass effect and subsequent symptoms, tumors that are rapidly expanding on serial imaging, or for atypical appearing lesions that require a tissue diagnosis [8, 11].

## Surgical Anatomy

CPA tumors have traditionally been regarded as challenging surgical cases. As meningiomas in this location enlarge, they may envelop cranial nerves and cerebellar arteries, distort the brainstem, or even erode through the temporal bone. Understanding the key structures within this space and their relationships to certain landmarks allows for safe surgical management. The CPA is defined as a space between the middle cerebellar peduncle, the medial edge of the petrous temporal bone, and the superior and inferior limbs of the cerebellopontine fissure (CPF) (Figure 1), which is formed by the petrosal surface of the cerebellum as it bends around the pons. It is at this critical juncture where cranial nerves IV through XI may be accessible. The cranial nerves within the CPA may be divided into a superior, middle, and inferior complex, each with its own intricate anatomy and close association with the brainstem and vascular structures. The superior complex contains the trochlear and trigeminal nerves. These nerves traverse close to the upper limb of the CPF and are invariably associated with the superior cerebellar artery (SCA), superior petrosal venous complex and the superior petrosal edge of the cerebellum at the level of the pontomesencephalic junction as they travel towards the petrous apex [13, 14]. The most common operations involving the upper complex include exposure of the posterior root of the trigeminal nerve in cases of trigeminal neuralgia secondary to vascular compression or for petrous apex lesions; however, CPA tumors frequently extend towards the trigeminal nerve, thus familiarity with this region is of vital importance (Figure 2). As dissection of the CPA projects superiorly along the pontine and cerebellar surfaces, the posterior root of the trigeminal nerve may be exposed. By following the trigeminal nerve along its course, it can be observed traveling anteriorly and laterally from the pons towards the petrous apex. As the nerve reaches the petrous apex, it exits the posterior fossa and enters the middle fossa through Meckel's cave. Meckel's cave marks the posterolateral aspect of the cavernous sinus. It is a cerebrospinal fluid (CSF) - containing arachnoid pouch that protrudes from the petrous apex and houses the trigeminal nerve ganglion. At this location a smaller motor root of the trigeminal nerve may be identified and separated from the larger sensory root; however, anastomoses between the motor and sensory roots are commonly found. A myriad of bridging petrosal veins may frequently be seen either blocking access, adherent to, or intimately intertwined between the roots of the trigeminal nerve as it travels towards Meckel's cave.

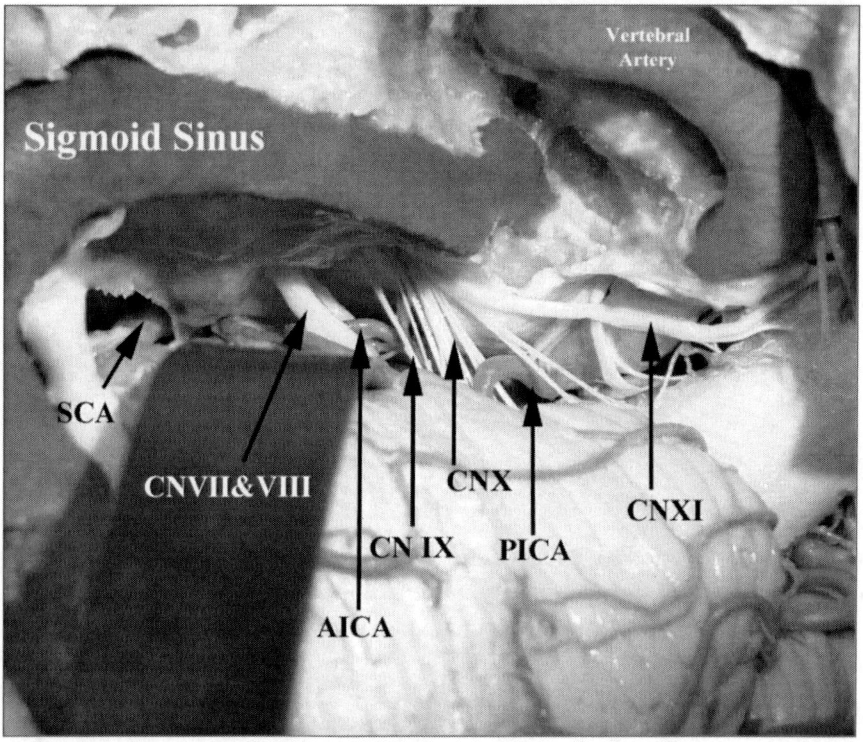


SCA: Superior cerebellar artery, CN VII and VIII: Facial and Vestibulocochlear nerve complex, AICA: Anterior inferior cerebellar artery, CNIX: Glossopharyngeal Nerve, CNX: Vagus nerve, PICA: Posterior inferior cerebellar artery, CNXI: Accessory Nerve.

Figure 1. Cadaveric dissection showing the CPA and cerebello-medullary cisterns and neurovascular structures.

Most of these veins make up the petrosal venous complex and drain into the superior petrosal vein [14]. Unexpected bleeding while operating within the superior complex may be due to tearing of these petrosal veins, although arterial bleeding via the SCA may also be encountered. The middle complex contains the abducens, facial, and vestibulocochlear nerves. These nerves traverse from the pontomedullary junction towards the IAC and are closely intertwined with the anterior inferior cerebellar artery (AICA) [15, 16]. Bordering these nerves are the pons and middle cerebellar peduncle. The most common operations involving the middle complex includes removal of acoustic neuromas, meningiomas, epidermoids, and for relief of hemifacial spasm secondary to facial nerve compression by the AICA or the vertebrobasilar system.

The majority of CPA meningiomas will involve the middle complex of the CPA but large tumors may extend to the superior or inferior complexes as well (Figure 2). Within the middle complex, the flocculus is typically encountered first and can be identified posterior and superior to the choroid plexus.

The flocculus will often be just posterior to the vestibulocochlear and facial nerves as they exit from the brainstem. This structure commonly blocks the visualization of the vestibulocochlear and facial nerves at this junction. Care must be taken when mobilizing the flocculus to avoid injury to the vestibulocochlear nerve as the nerve may be closely adherent or attached.

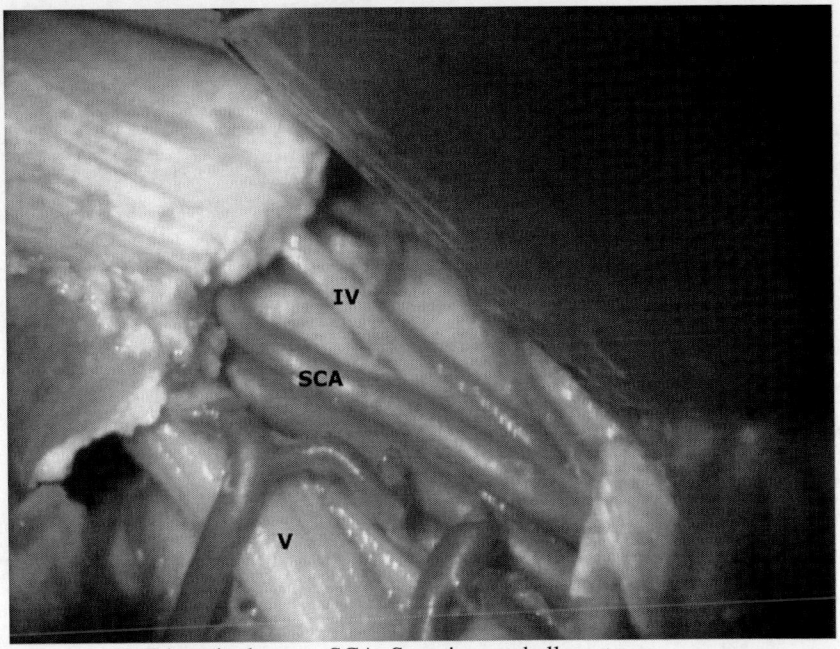


IV: Trochlear nerve, V: Trigeminal nerve, SCA: Superior cerebellar artery.

Figure 2. Exposure of the CPA in cadaveric dissection.

The vestibulocochlear nerve is typically located just posterior to the facial nerve within the cerebellopontine cistern. The AICA also arises at the pontine level and travels within this cistern and courses in close relationship to the vestibulocochlear and facial nerves as they travel towards the IAC. The subarcuate and labyrinthine arteries are branches off of the AICA that provide vascular supply to the dura of the petrous temporal bone and IAC [15, 16].

These vascular branches may also intertwine between the vestibulocochlear and facial nerve bundles within the middle complex. The AICA may also form a loop, which extends into the IAC in up to 54% of cases [15].

Both the vestibulocochlear and facial nerves can be traced towards their exit into the IAC where the facial nerve maintains an anterior relationship with the vestibulocochlear nerve. Within the cisternal segment a component of the facial nerve, which is often hidden between the vestibulocochlear and facial nerves, known as the nervus intermedius (NI) may be found. The NI arises from the facial nerve and joins the vestibulocochlear nerve within the meatal segment of the vestibulocochlear and facial nerve complex [17]. This nerve may also be found freely within the CPA cistern as it travels from the motor root of the facial nerve towards the acoustic nerve. The NI contains sensory and parasympathetic fibers of the facial nerve responsible for sensation of the external auditory meatus, taste in the anterior two thirds of the tongue, and innervation of the salivary glands [17, 18]. Injury to the NI during surgery can lead to geniculate neuralgia [18]. Being aware of its course and avoiding unnecessary disruption of the nerve is the best preventative measure. Within the IAC, the facial and vestibulocochlear nerve complex is divided into four major compartments. In the distal segment of the meatus, two bony bridges separate the vestibulocochlear nervous complex into the facial, cochlear, and inferior and superior vestibular nerves.

These bony bridges within the IAC separate the nerves in a fairly constant relationship to each other, which aids in their identification and division [19]. The lateral portion of the meatus is divided horizontally into a superior and inferior division by a bony ridge called the transverse crest. This structure partitions the facial and superior vestibular nerves superiorly and the cochlear and inferior vestibular nerves inferiorly [19]. Within the superior compartment, another bony ridge separates the facial nerve anteriorly from the superior vestibular nerve posteriorly. This vertically oriented bony ridge was described by Dr. William House and is known as "Bill's Bar" [20]. The inferior compartment contains the cochlear nerve anteriorly and inferior vestibular nerve posteriorly. The inferior compartment does not have a bony ridge complementary to Bill's Bar; nevertheless, the lateral meatus can be subdivided into four sections, each containing their respective nerves.

The inferior complex contains the glossopharyngeal, vagus, and spinal accessory nerves. These nerves traverse along the lower limb of the CPF towards the jugular foramen while bordering the medulla, inferior cerebellar peduncle, and suboccipital surface of the cerebellum. The posterior inferior cerebellar artery (PICA) passes in close relationship to these nerves as it makes a caudal loop to supply the suboccipital surface of the cerebellum [21] (Figure 1).

The most common operations involving the inferior complex includes large CPA tumors and glossopharyngeal neuralgia secondary to compression by the PICA or vertebral artery.

Within the inferior complex, the glossopharyngeal nerve is distinguished from the vagus nerve by its more superior orientation within the cerebellomedullary cistern (CMC). The glossopharyngeal nerve may also be traced towards its exit within the anterior compartment of the jugular foramen.

The anterior compartment is known as the pars nervosa and contains the glossopharyngeal nerve and venous return from the inferior petrosal sinus. The vagus nerve lies inferior to the glossopharyngeal nerve and exits within the posterior compartment of the jugular foramen. This compartment is known as the pars vascularis and contains the vagus nerve, spinal accessory nerve, and the jugular bulb.

The spinal accessory nerve may be easily distinguished from both the glossopharyngeal and vagus nerves because it is the only cranial nerve that descends below the foramen magnum and has a superior trajectory as it ascends to exit through the pars vascularis of the jugular foramen. After inspecting the cranial nerves within the inferior complex, the PICA should be identified; it commonly passes between the rootlets of the glossopharyngeal, vagus, and spinal accessory nerves [21]. Careful dissection of the arachnoid within the CMC should be performed to avoid damage to these nerves and the PICA.

## Surgical Management of CPA Meningiomas

### Preoperative Considerations

For meningiomas, the decision on when to operate is just as important as the operative approach. The surgical management of CPA meningiomas takes into account that many meningiomas at this location are incidentally found and most will remain asymptomatic throughout a patient's lifetime.

For asymptomatic incidentally found meningiomas observed over a three-year period, two thirds will show no evidence of growth, while only one third will increase over this period [22]. Meningiomas with calcifications are more likely to remain dormant or grow at a slower rate. Thus, the indications for treating CPA meningiomas are lesions that produce symptoms or demonstrate sustained growth on serial radiographs.

Once the decision of surgical resection has been established, pre-operative audiometric studies, facial nerve testing, radiographic, and/or angiographic evaluations may be performed to assess serviceable hearing and facial nerve function, and for any anatomical variations that may affect the surgical approach. Moreover, CPA meningiomas may be divided into tumors that occur anterior to, posterior to, or within the IAC, or mixed. Most CPA meningiomas primarily arise from and reside within the middle neurovascular complex. However, as these tumors enlarge, they may extend superiorly or inferiorly towards the upper or lower neurovascular complexes [11].

In cases of large extensive tumors, hydrocephalus must also be assessed pre-operatively. When hydrocephalus is present, an external ventricular drain or lumbar drain may be placed to improve relaxation of the cerebellum and improve surgical access. A ventricular shunt may also be placed two weeks prior to the operation; however, this practice has fallen out of recent favor as this adds an additional procedure and length of hospitalization.

Additional considerations during the planning of a CPA meningioma operation include intra-operative monitoring of facial and vestibulocochlear nerve function. Intra-operative neuro-monitoring is of vital importance for the preservation of these cranial nerves as it facilitates early identification and avoidance of injury [23, 24]. Although pre-operative radiographs allow the surgeon to determine and assess the location of various cranial nerves in relation to the CPA meningioma, these adjuncts may alert the surgeon when to take more caution, while also allowing the surgeon to be more aggressive during certain stages of the surgical resection. This provides the greatest chance of complete surgical resection with the least chance of surgical morbidity. The optimal surgical approach is chosen based on the patient's pre-operative cranial nerve function, the goals of surgery, and the individual anatomy and co-morbid conditions.

## Surgical Approach

In general, there are three main surgical approaches to CPA meningiomas, each with respective advantages and disadvantages. The three most commonly used approaches include the retrosigmoid approach, translabyrinthine approach, and combined transpetrosal approach for extensive meningiomas. Since the latter is rare, we will focus mainly on retrosigmoid and translabyrinthine approaches. General principles of meningioma surgery include early interruption of the blood supply to the tumor (which is often provided through the dural attachment), internal decompression, dissection of the tumor capsule and coagulating arachnoid attachments or vascular pedicles, infolding the tumor into the area of decompression, and removal of appended dura and overlying bone, if applicable [29].

Most CPA meningiomas arise from the dura along the petrous temporal bone, but may also arise from the dura of the tentorium or incisura [4]. Early identification and interruption of the blood supply will soften the tumor and aide in internal decompression. Internal decompression is accomplished by coagulating and sharply incising the tumor capsule.

The contents within the tumor capsule are then removed using a combination of ultrasonic aspiration, sharp dissection, and electro cautery. Upon completion of internal decompression, the borders of the tumor capsule are again inspected and dissected free from surrounding neural and vascular structures while infolding the tumor capsule. The tumor capsule may be coagulated to shrink the mass and ensure hemostasis. Once the tumor is dissected away, it may be removed piecemeal or en bloc and any dural attachments or overlying bone drilled and removed.

## Retrosigmoid

The retrosigmoid approach is the most familiar one and most preferred by neurosurgeons. It is frequently referred to as the "work horse" approach to the posterior fossa. This approach provides the best chance of hearing preservation and also has a reasonable chance of facial nerve preservation. The disadvantages of the retrosigmoid approach are in its angle and course, which increases the difficulty for removing tumors extending deep into the IAC and dealing with lateral cerebellum. In order to reach laterally projecting IAC tumors, there is a high operative risk of injuring the vestibule, endolymphatic sac, or posterior semicircular canal. Additionally, this method has a higher likelihood of causing iatrogenic CSF leaks and facial nerve dysfunction in comparison to the other approaches [25-27].

Access to the CPA is most commonly obtained by performing a retrosigmoid craniotomy. The patient is usually positioned in the supine position with a shoulder roll and the head is turned away from the side of exposure (Figure 3 A). This approach is generally accomplished by making a skin incision through the scalp exposing the cranium that is overlying the junction of the transverse and sigmoid sinuses. The skin incision may be linear or curved as long as there is adequate exposure of the transverse sigmoid junction, which is usually about three finger breaths behind the external auditory canal (Figure 3 B). The junction of the transverse and sigmoid sinuses may be approximated using a variety of surgical landmarks.

Traditionally the asterion has been regarded as a bony landmark that approximates the location of the transverse sigmoid junction. The asterion is a craniometric point on the skull that is formed by the intersection of lamboid, parieto-mastoid, and occipito-mastoid sutures. In most adults, the asterion is 4 centimeters posterior and 12 millimeters superior to the external auditory meatus [28]. Despite its historical importance, the asterion is no longer commonly used as a landmark for the transverse sigmoid junction because it has been found to be highly variable between individuals and frequently inaccurate (Figure 4 A-C).

The authors propose estimating the transverse sigmoid junction by making a point 4 centimeters in females and 4.5 centimeters in males posteriorly along a line drawn connecting the root of the zygoma and the inion. The mastoid tip is used to estimate the inferior-most extent of the sigmoid sinus. This surface point is also marked and used to guide the scalp incision and craniotomy. In the authors' experience, combining the utilization of these surface landmarks with estimates by neuro-navigation has proven to be extremely accurate for finding the transverse sigmoid junction [29].

Once the transverse sigmoid junction has been estimated and marked, the periosteum over the proposed craniotomy site is harvested. The periosteum is elevated and preserved in saline and often used as a dural graft during closure (Figure 5 A-C). After harvesting the periosteum, a small cranial opening is performed using a perforator or match stick drill.

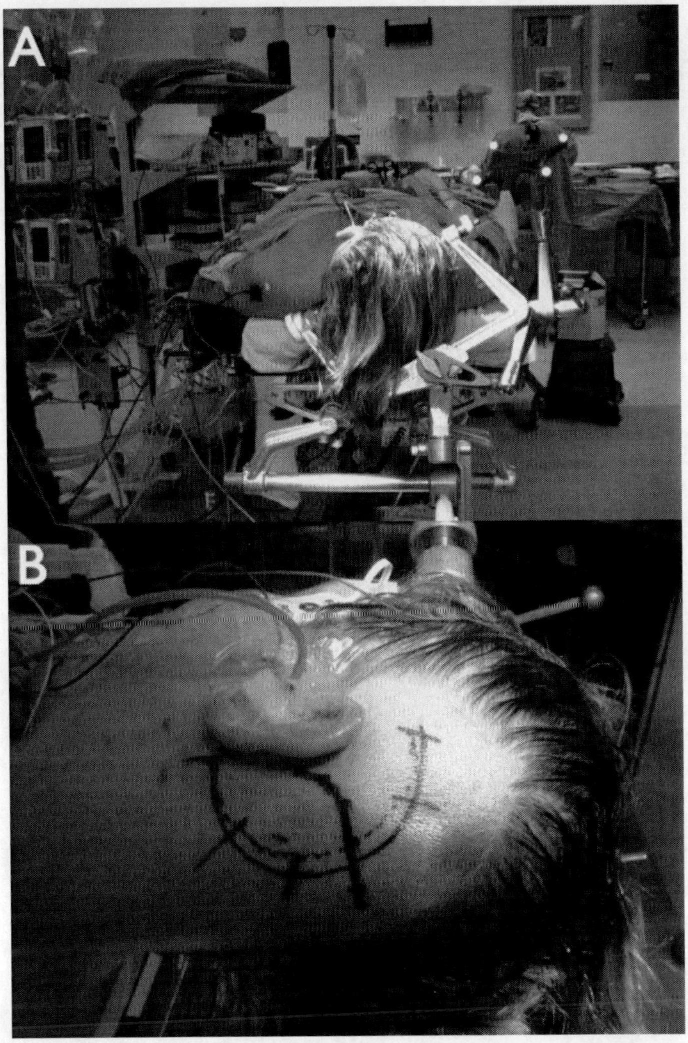


Figure 3. Photograph shows supine position and head turning 60-70° to contralateral side (A). Photograph shows C-shaped post-auricular incision and surface mapping of transverse and sigmoid sinuses (B).

A retrosigmoid craniotomy flap is turned and elevated with extreme caution to avoid injury to transverse and sigmoid sinuses (Figure 6 A-C). The mastoid bone overlying the sigmoid sinus junction is then drilled off to expose a small part of the sigmoid sinus and transverse-sigmoid sinus junction (Figure 6 D). This will facilitate wider exposure and minimize retraction on the lateral cerebellum. To prevent CSF leak, the bony edges are sealed with bone wax. This craniotomy is centered just behind the upper half of the sigmoid sinus and below the distal end of the transverse sinus, exposing the transverse sigmoid junction at the superior lateral edge of the craniotomy (Figure 5 A-D).

By performing the craniotomy at this location, the dura may be opened in a T shape allowing the transverse and sigmoid sinuses to be reflected against the edge of the craniotomy. Reflecting the dural opening in this manner optimizes exposure of the CPA. This is typically performed using 4-0 neurilon stitches to tent the dura against the craniotomy edge (Figure 7 A-B).

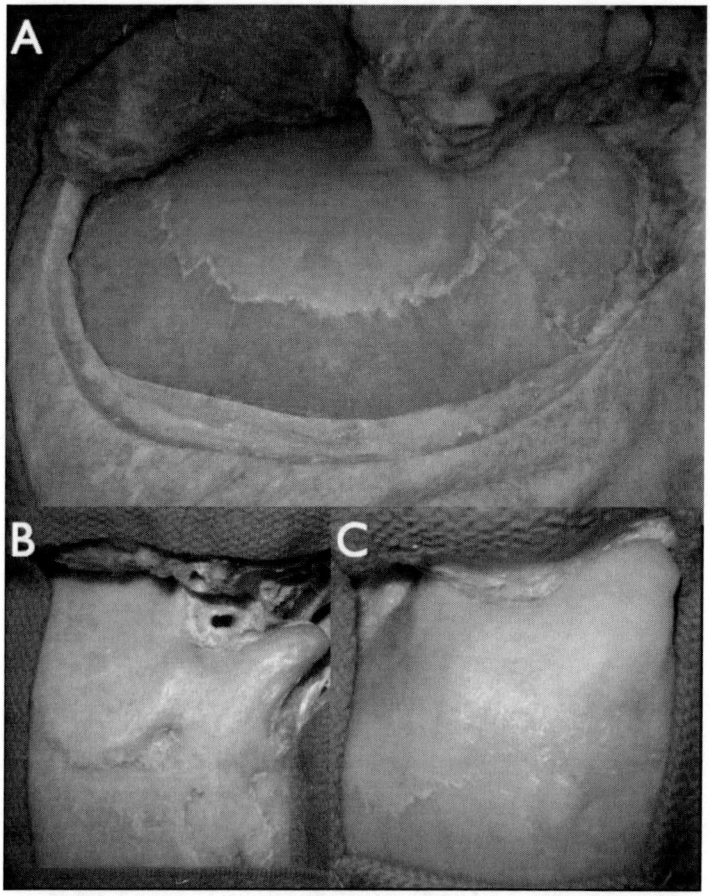


Figure 4. A-C. Cadaveric dissections performed in 3 different cadaveric heads demonstrate unidentifiable asterion.

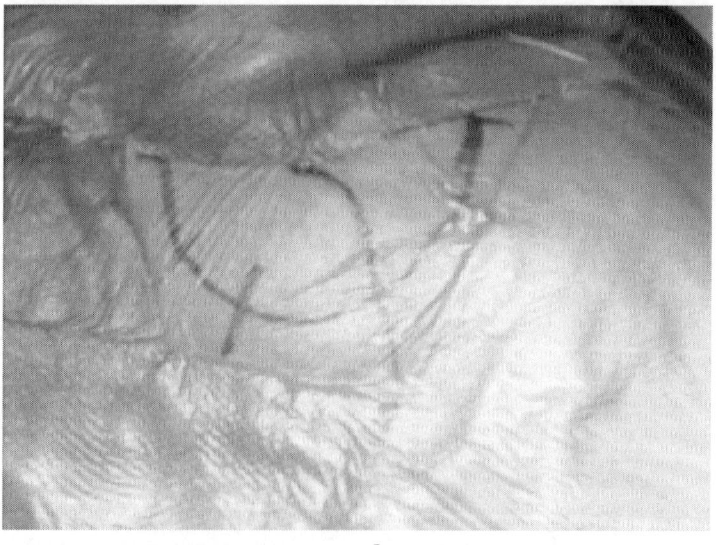

a

Figure 5. (Continued)

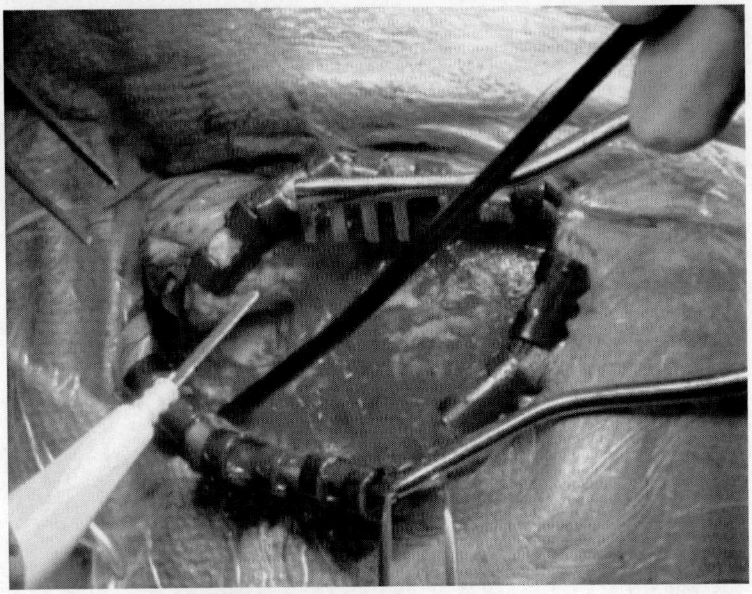

b

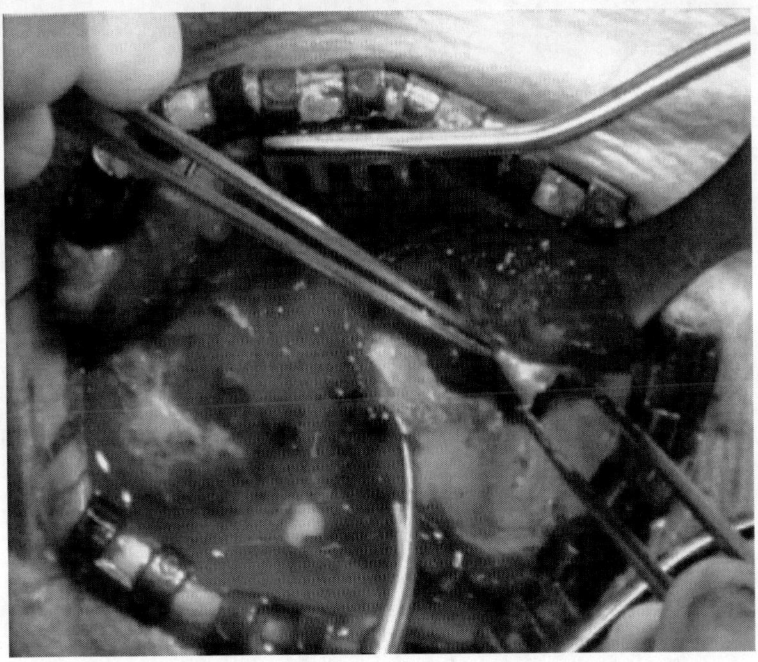

c

Figure 5. Photograph shows skin incision (A), reflection of the skin flap (B), harvesting the periosteum (C).

With the dura opened and retracted, the posterior fossa contents may be accessed by directing the dissection anteriorly and laterally. Upon initial opening of the dura just inferior and medially to the transverse sigmoid junction, the posterior fossa contents will often appear full. The posterior fossa contents are relaxed by opening the arachnoid within the CMC (Figure 7 A). By opening this space, the CSF may be removed and retraction on the cerebellum will be minimized during surgery.

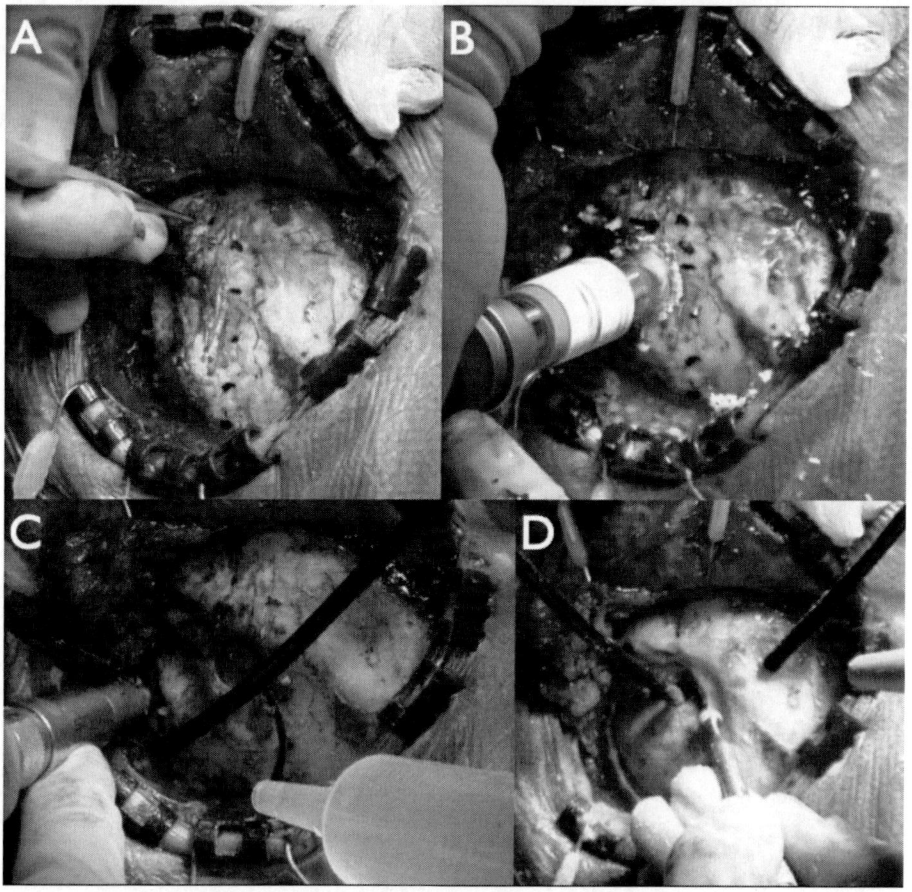


Figure 6. Photograph show marking craniotomy (A), placement of the burr hole exactly under junction of transverse-sigmoid sinuses (B), turning the bone flap (C), and drilling off the overlying bone to expose transverse-sigmoid sinus junction (D).

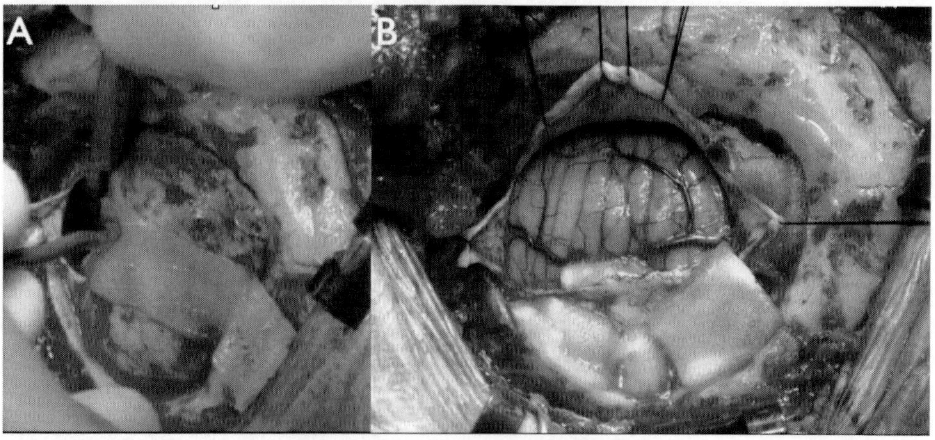


Figure 7. Photograph shows small opening of the dura inferiorly for CSF drainage from the lateral cerebello-medullary cistern (A) and reflection of the dura (B).

A lumbar or ventricular drain may also be placed pre-operatively to achieve CSF drainage and cerebellum relaxation (Figure 7 A-B).

As the cerebellum relaxes with the escape of CSF, the operating microscope should be introduced. The operating microscope should be guided to provide an intradural exposure that reveals the posterior edge of the temporal bone laterally and petrosal cerebellar surface medially. With the operating microscope in place, a patty should be placed on the lateral margin of the cerebellum for protection and to aid in retraction. Gentle retraction may be placed upon the cerebellum using a suction device or bipolar electrocautery. We usually do not place self-retaining retractors. With gentle retraction upon the cerebellum in a medial direction, the contents of the CPA may be visualized.

Careful dissection of the arachnoid membranes should be performed using both blunt and sharp dissectors to ensure that any local retraction or movement does not injure the surrounding neural or vascular structures. The petrosal vein should be preserved. As one continues the dissection anterolaterally, the arachnoid behind the glossopharyngeal and vagus nerves are often dissected open first.

Once access to this region has been established, a few key landmarks should be identified. First inspect for a small tuft of choroid plexus that travels out of the lateral recess and is typically seen protruding from the foramen of Luschka. Next, the choroid plexus is followed superiorly to identify the flocculus. The flocculus is identified because it serves as an important landmark for determining the posterior border of the vestibulocochlear and facial nerve entry zones.

Upon completion of the case, all bony edges are plugged with bone wax and a water-tight dural closure is performed. Harvested pericranium may aid in dural closure. All of these maneuvers are implemented to prevent CSF leak. The cranial flap is then re-attached and the scalp is approximated in multiple layers.

## Translabyrinthine

The translabyrinthine approach is often preferred by neuro-otologists and is a more useful method for tumors with a significant intracanalicular component and no serviceable hearing. Often, neurosurgeons and neuro-otologists work in tandem to tackle CPA meningiomas best addressed by the translabyrinthine approach, although this may be institutionally dependent.

The translabyrinthine approach has many advantages because the surgical exposure allows early identification of the facial nerve, thus, providing higher rates of facial nerve preservation, less risk to the cerebellum and the lower neurovascular complex, as well as providing adequate access to tumor extending or arising in the meatal and labyrinthine segments of the IAC (Figure 8). The disadvantage of the translabyrinthine approach is that hearing is sacrificed. In patients without serviceable hearing, this is acceptable (Figure 9 A-B and 10 A-B). Another limitation is the restricted exposure of the inferior compartment. The amount of bony drilling required in a translabyrinthine approach is also a potential disadvantage as it can result in higher rates of CSF leak and post-operative infection due to increased operative time [25, 30].

In order to perform a translabyrinthine approach the patient is positioned supine with the head turned contralateral to the side of the lesion. A C-shaped incision is planned behind the ear to expose the mastoid tip, sigmoid sinus, and transverse-sigmoid junction. The abdomen or lateral thigh should be prepped in case a fat graft or tensor fascia lata graft is needed to assist with closure.

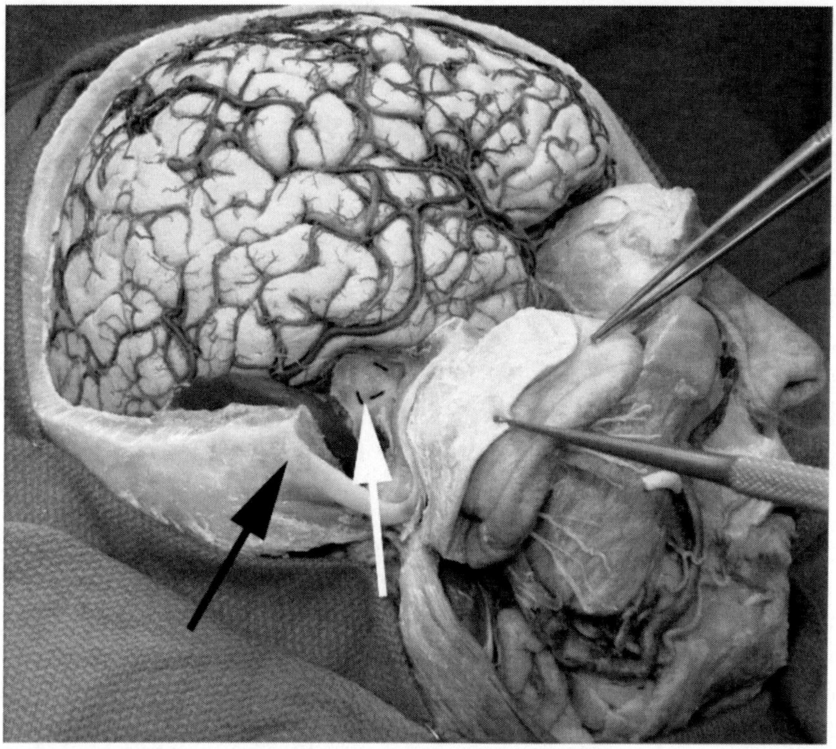

Figure 8. Cadaveric dissection demonstrates two different angles of exposure in retrosigmoid (black arrow) and translabyrinthine approach (white arrow).

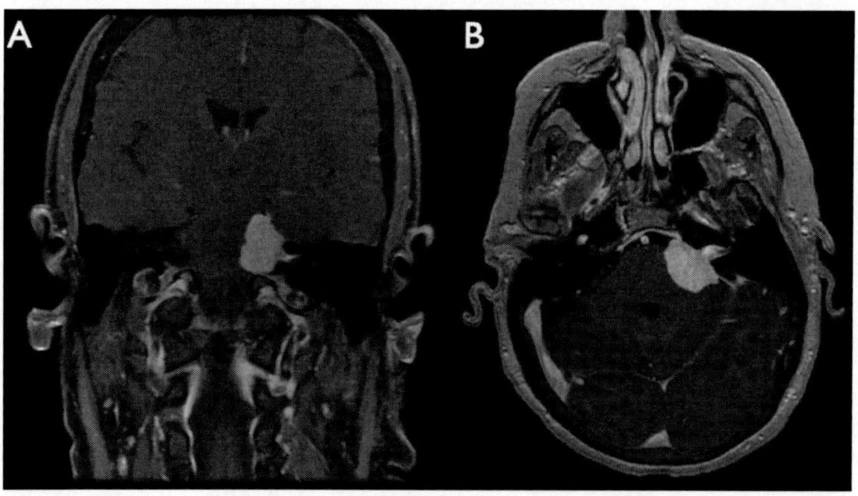


Figure 9. Preoperative post-contrast coronal T1 MRI (A) and axial MRI (B) show CPA meningioma with extension into the IAC.

After making the incision and dividing the skin and muscle, the periosteum is initially left intact then carefully elevated and harvested as an additional layer for protection against CSF leakage at the time of closure. Emissary veins, when encountered, are waxed. Dissection limits of the exposure are carried towards the mastoid tip inferiorly, 2 cm behind the sigmoid sinus posteriorly, and the spine of Henle anteriorly.

Once this is accomplished, mastoid drilling may begin. At our institution, a standard mastoidectomy begins with skeletonization of the tegmen, sigmoid sinus, and posterior border of the external auditory canal. The mastoid antrum is entered and the incus and lateral semicircular canal is identified. A diamond drill is used to remove the tegmen, exposing middle fossa dura. The presigmoid dura is also exposed in this manner (the endolymphatic duct may be transected during this process). Next a rongeur is used to remove the petrous ridge over the superior petrosal sinus heading medially. As drilling continues, the vertical segment of the facial nerve may be identified within the proximal mastoid.

The nerve is identified and traced towards the stylomastoid foramen. A thin shell of bone is left covering the nerve within the fallopian canal. The labyrinthectomy begins by drilling the lateral semicircular canal and then the posterior semicircular canal. The vestibule is exposed and the lateral semicircular canal is removed. The subarcuate artery will often be encountered in the foramen of the superior semicircular canal. The sigmoid sinus can now be followed towards the jugular bulb.

After identifying the jugular bulb, the dura of the IAC is exposed. Troughs are created superior and inferior to the IAC. The goal is to expose the IAC 270° around its circumference. Presence of a high-riding jugular bulb may limit the surgical exposure because it restricts the trough that will be drilled below the IAC. The superior trough is limited by the middle fossa dura. After exposing and opening the dura of the IAC, the superior vestibular and facial nerves are identified superior to the falciform crest and removal of the tumor may commence.

## Special Considerations

For CPA meningiomas extending towards or arising within the IAC, a retrosigmoid approach may be utilized to preserve facial and vestibulocochlear nerve function.

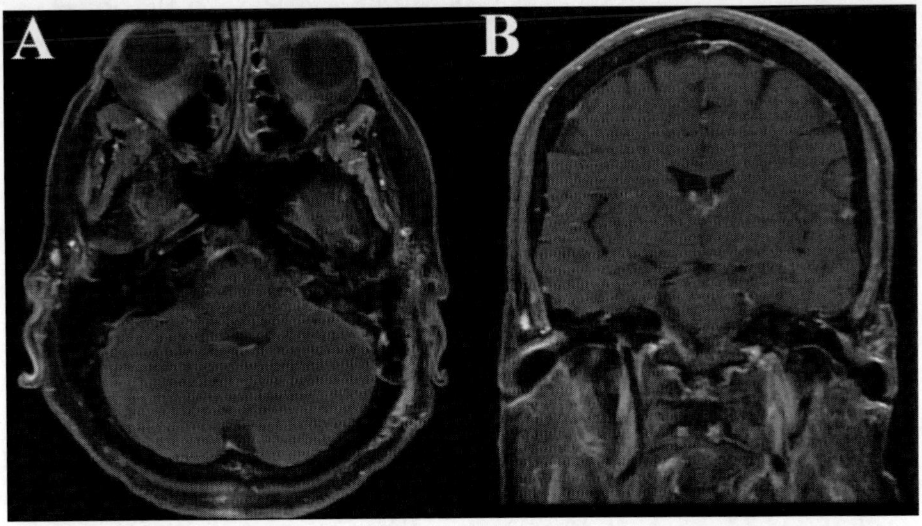


Figure 10. Postoperative postcontrast coronal T1 MRI (A) and axial T1 MRI (B) after a translabyrinthine approach with fat grafting show no residual or recurrent meningioma at 3 years.

In these cases, after removal of the extracanalicular portion of the tumor via a retrosigmoid approach, the dura over the IAC is often incised sharply and the IAC is drilled open taking care to preserve the endolymphatic sac, posterior semicircular canal, and bony labyrinth (Figure 11 A-C and 12 A-B).

Accessing the IAC via the retrosigmoid approach is often limited by these boundaries. Although there are no exact landmarks, the maximal lateral extent of temporal bone drilling should be limited to the transverse crest or about 1 cm deep within the internal auditory canal [31]. Larger CPA meningiomas, on the other hand, may arise near the IAC but extend towards Meckel's cave or the jugular foramen. Large CPA meningiomas extending towards Meckel's cave are often mistaken for but must be differentiated from petroclival meningiomas, which stem from the superior clivus or petrous apex.

Petroclival meningiomas present a separate clinical entity because they encase different neurovascular structures and the surgical approach differs from CPA meningiomas. Radiographically, petroclival meningiomas can be distinguished from CPA meningiomas arising medial to the trigeminal nerve and frequently involve the medial cranial nerves and/or the basilar artery (Figure 13 A-D and 14 A-C).

Large petroclival meningiomas are more extensive tumors than CPA meningiomas and may require combined transpetrosal approaches.

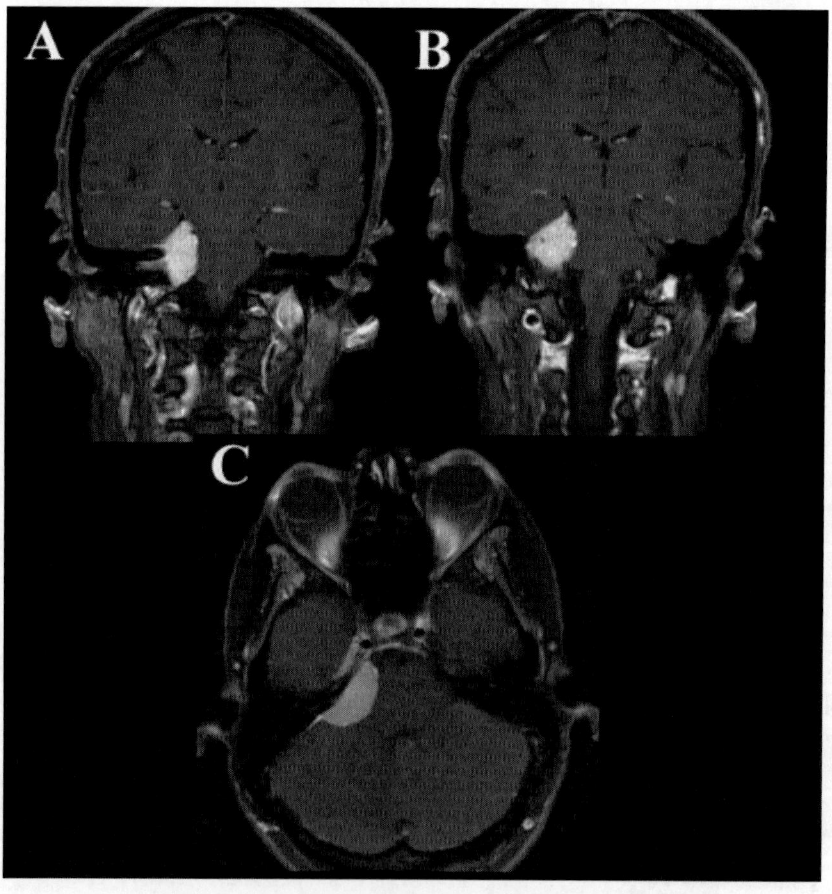


Figure 11. Preoperative postcontrast coronal T1 MRIs (A and B) and axial T1 MRI (C) show a CPA meningioma with superior extension into the tentorium and involvement of the IAC.

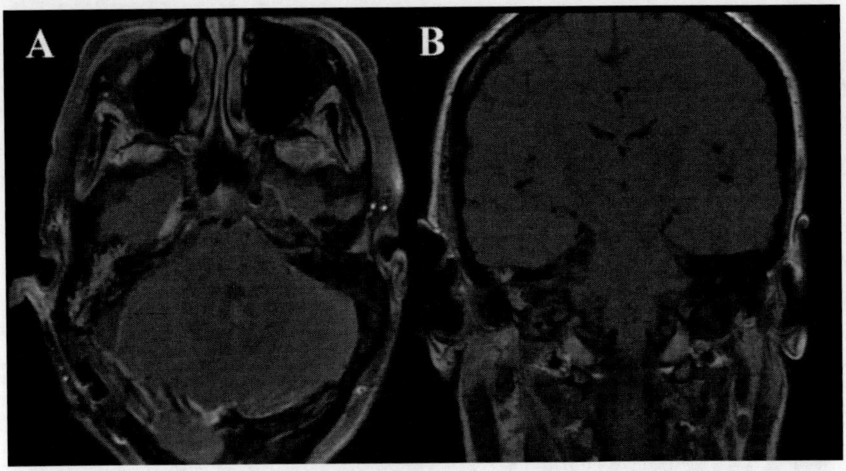


Figure 12. Postoperative postcontrast axial T1 MRI (A) and coronal T1 MRI (B) show no residual tumor after a right-sided retrosigmoid craniotomy with meatal drilling.

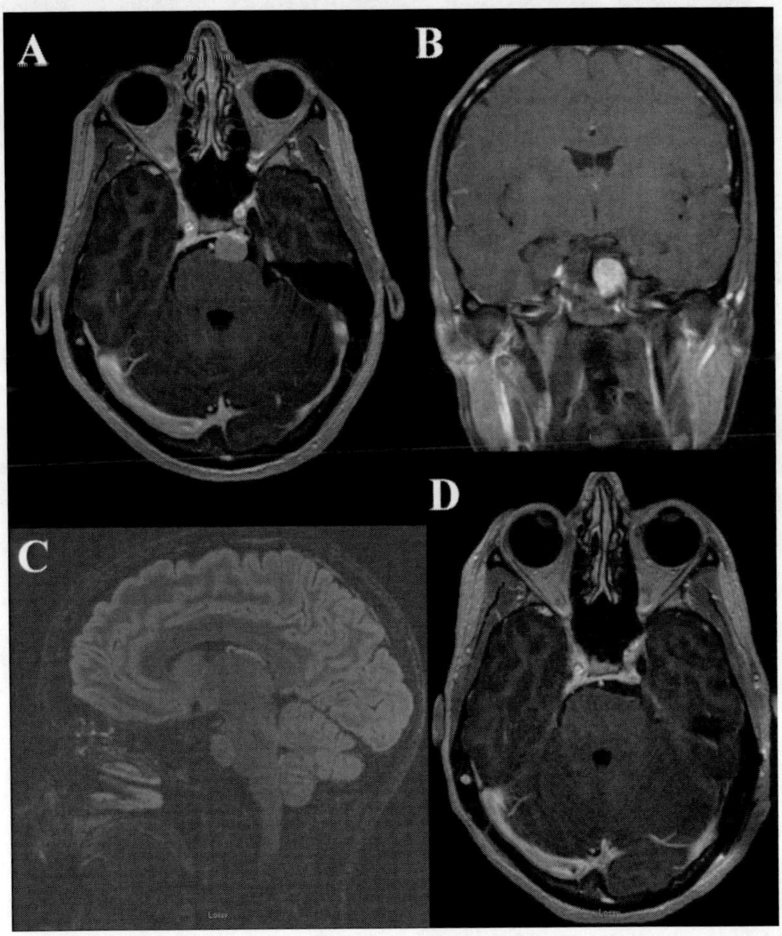


Figure 13. An axial T1 post-contrast MRI (A), coronal T1 post-contrast (B) and sagittal flair (C) show a petroclival meningioma. As seen in MRIs, this is a typical petroclival meningioma originating from the petrous-clival junction on the left, anterior to the trigeminal nerve. Postoperative axial T1 MRI shows gross total resection via a retrosigmoid craniotomy (D).

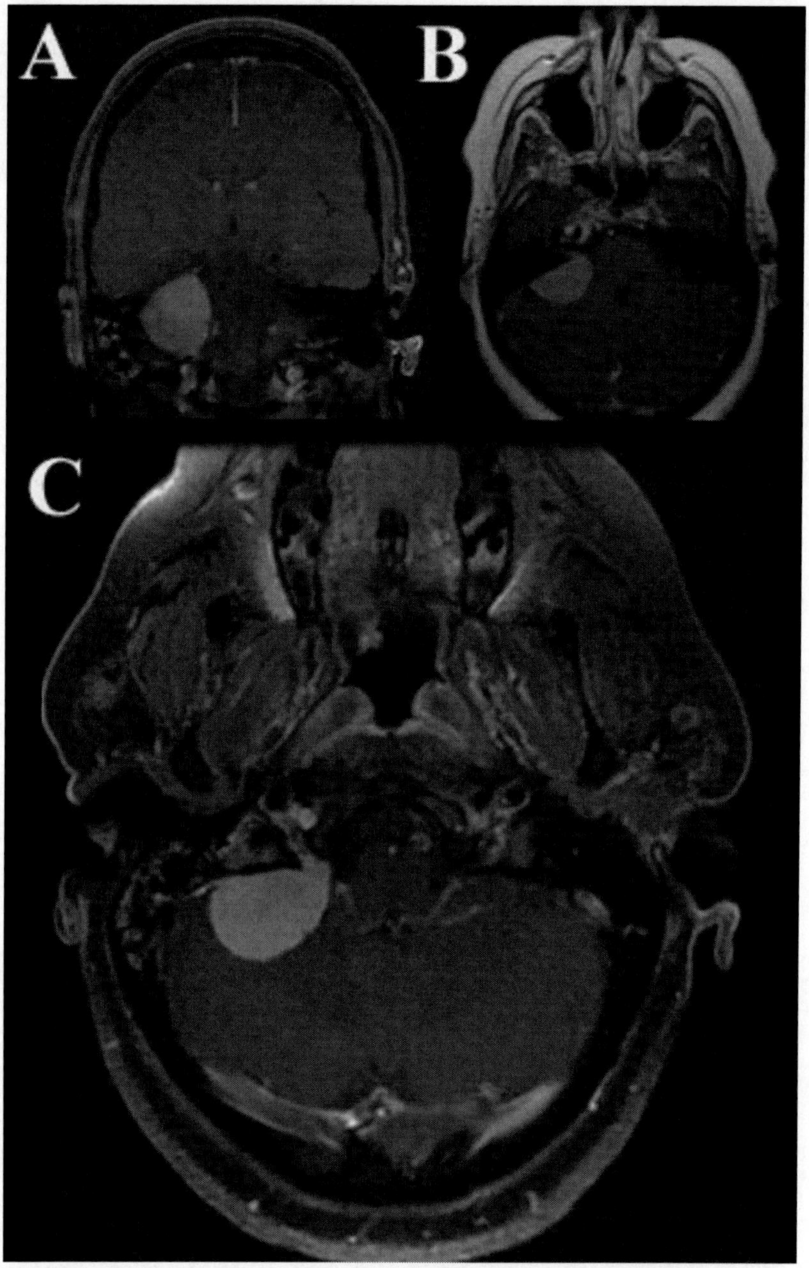


Figure 14. Preoperative postcontrast coronal T1 MRI (A), postcontrast axial T1 MRI (B and C) show a CPA meningioma with involvement of the IAC and extension into the jugular foramen.

CPA meningiomas extending towards the jugular foramen also have special considerations. CPA meningiomas involving the jugular foramen must be differentiated from lateral foramen magnum meningiomas as the latter present frequently with brainstem compression and are accessed via a far-lateral approach.

When CPA meningiomas extend inferiorly towards the jugular foramen, the skin incision and retrosigmoid craniotomy are often extended inferiorly to gain wider exposure to the lower cranial nerves and PICA (Figure 15 A-B).

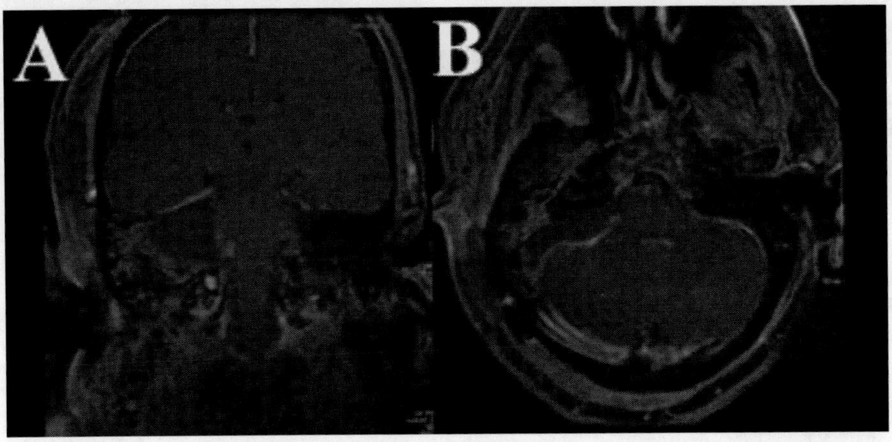


Figure 15. Postoperative coronal T1 MRI (A) and postcontrast axial T1 MRI (B) show gross total resection via retrosigmoid craniotomy extended inferiorly for jugular foramen involvement.

The normal anatomy of the CPA is often distorted with large CPA meningiomas; however, understanding consistent associations between certain structures will aid in safe surgical dissection and exposure. Upon identification of the CPA meningioma, careful initial circumferential dissection along the edges of the tumor is key for establishing the location of important neural and vascular structures. By using a nerve stimulator, the whereabouts of various cranial nerves can be established in relation to the tumor. With circumferential dissection, the base of the tumor can also be determined. These maneuvers can help reduce the rates of iatrogenic neural and vascular injury.

## Complications

Post-operative cranial nerve dysfunction must be assessed early. For patients with partial facial nerve dysfunction (House Brackmann grade III or less) in which the nerve is anatomically preserved, the partial weakness will often resolve over a period of one year.

Patients with more severe facial nerve dysfunction (House Brackmann grade IV or greater) where eye closure is impaired, natural tears and lacrilube may be used to prevent drying out the corneas, and the eye may be taped shut at night time. For patients with complete facial nerve palsy, tarsorrhaphy may also be performed to assist with eye closure [23, 24]. Unilateral vestibular nerve dysfunction is much more common post-operatively, but better tolerated.

The initial symptoms of nausea and vomiting may be distressful; however, most patients will compensate with input from the contralateral side and soon after surgery the nausea, vomiting, dizziness, and ataxia will rapidly clear [32]. In cases of large CPA meningiomas where the tumor is dissected off the brainstem, post-operative brainstem dysfunction manifesting as ataxia is often more permanent. Complications involving cranial nerves IX, X, and XII are more frequent with larger tumors extending towards the jugular foramen, and although tumors extending towards the lower neurovascular complex are less common, they are more difficult to adjust to [8]. Patients with lower cranial nerve dysfunction often require post-operative rehabilitation or tracheostomy or gastrostomy tube placement.

CSF leak and meningitis secondary to a fistula formation may manifest in the form of otorrhea, rhinorrhea, or fluid tracking down the back of the throat.

These fistulas may occur in the setting of hydrocephalus, poor wound healing, or due to injury to the apical cells, vestibule, posterior semicircular canal, peri- labyrinthine cells, or mastoid air cells [33]. The CSF subsequently leaks through a ruptured tympanic membrane into the external auditory canal, through the dura and skin, or through the nose or back of the throat via the Eustachian tube. Most CSF leaks are diagnosed within one week and are more common with lateral drilling of the internal auditory canal [33, 34].

Treatment of CSF leaks include elevating the head of bed, lumbar drain placement, surgical exploration with re-application of bone wax, pericranium or fascia lata graft application, or muscle and fat packing into the surgical bed, eustachian tumor, middle ear, and/or mastoid. CSF shunting is necessary in cases of a CSF leak secondary to hydrocephalus [33-35].

## DISCUSSION

Meningiomas arising within the CPA represent an uncommon subgroup of meningiomas due to their distinct clinical presentation, natural history, and anatomical considerations [6]. Compared to meningiomas arising from other locations, CPA meningiomas commonly compress vital neural and vascular structures enclosed within a small bony compartment. This accounts for their distinctive presentation, including hearing loss, headache, and facial numbness or pain [11]. Consequently, this also makes CPA meningiomas more likely to be symptomatic upon diagnosis and more likely to progress with conservative management [12].

A recent systematic review of untreated meningiomas suggests that over 5-year follow up most meningiomas less than 2.5 centimeters will not progress to cause symptoms [12]. However, when those tumors are broken down by location, those arising within the CPA demonstrated significantly higher rates of symptomatic progression (40%) over a 5-year period compared with the more common convexity or parafalcine meningiomas [12]. One explanation may be that the CPA contains many neural and vascular structures bordered laterally by the petrous temporal bone and medially by the brainstem, thus smaller tumors arising within this confined space are more likely to compress eloquent structures with only a modest increase in size. The principle concern for observing probable meningiomas with serial imaging is the manifestation or progression of symptoms. For CPA meningiomas, the likelihood of symptomatic progression is a realistic and probable outcome, thus, surgical intervention is the first line therapy for both symptomatic and asymptomatic CPA meningiomas [6].

When evaluating CPA meningiomas for surgical intervention, one should consider the overall tumor size, its attachment site, and whether there is involvement of the IAC, jugular foramen, and/or brainstem. Pre-operatively, the surgeon should recognize that larger CPA meningiomas (greater than 3 cm in diameter) are more likely to result in post-operative complications [6, 8]. Larger CPA meningiomas present with higher rates of brainstem compression, hydrocephalus, and jugular foramen involvement, thus, surgical resection becomes more technically challenging, requires higher rates of combined approaches, and has higher complication rates and longer operative times [6, 8, 36].

In one series, tumors larger than 3 centimeters had a nearly eight-fold increase in post-operative cranial nerve deficits (45.5% vs 5.9%) compared with smaller tumors [8]. In a separate series cranial nerve IX and X deficits were seen almost exclusively in large CPA meningiomas extending into the jugular foramen and occurred at an alarming rate of 92% [6].

CPA meningiomas can also be classified based on their sites of dural attachment. The most common presenting site was the petrous ridge followed by the tentorium, clivus, internal auditory canal, and jugular foramen, in descending order, with 71% of tumors originating from the petrous ridge [4]. The site of origin affects the direction of cranial nerve displacement and is an important consideration pre-operatively.

Most commonly, tumors arising from the petrous ridge will be anterior to the IAC (26%); however, a fairly even percentage of these tumors will also arise posterior, superior, and inferior (16%) to the IAC – again in descending order [4].

Some authors claim locating the dural origins with respect to the IAC may facilitate early tumor devascularization and avoidance of cranial nerve dysfunction; however, some studies suggest this has no effect on post-operative outcomes or complications [8, 11].

Tumor involvement of the IAC, in contrast, was found to be highly influential on post-operative outcomes [11]. CPA meningiomas may extend secondarily into the IAC or arise from within the IAC. Despite the location of tumor origin along the petrous ridge, facial nerve function and hearing preservation did not differ between CPA meningiomas arising ventral or dorsal to the IAC [11]. Facial nerve function was significantly higher in cases where there was secondary extension of the CPA meningioma into the IAC compared with those CPA meningiomas arising from within the IAC, and hearing preservation also trended towards a higher preservation rate in those tumors extending rather than arising from within the IAC [11]. The literature suggests that CPA meningiomas involve the IAC between 17 and 41% of cases [8, 11]. When this occurs, these tumors should be treated as a separate clinical entity because of the need to drill the IAC. Especially when the IAC is drilled laterally towards the labyrinth, there is a higher likelihood of injury to the facial, vestibulocochlear, or intermediate nerves. The added technical difficulties of safe IAC exposure result in higher rates of recurrence and of complications [11].

Systematic reviews of post-operative facial and vestibulocochlear nerve function after microsurgery for resection of VSs in patients with good baseline facial and hearing function suggest the overall Gardner-Robertson functional hearing preservation rate is around 52% and between 78 and 85% for House-Brackmann grade I-II facial nerve function [37-39]. In contrast, patients undergoing microsurgery for CPA meningiomas had functional hearing preservation up to 91% post-operatively and an estimated 89% chance of maintaining House-Brackmann grade I-II facial nerve function [40, 41]. In certain clinical contexts, arriving at the correct pre-operative diagnosis may affect the operative approach.

## CONCLUSION

Meningiomas of the CPA are benign lesions arising from the dura of the petrous temporal bone. These tumors are generally challenging to treat surgically; however, there are various nuances and anatomical considerations that may drastically affect surgical planning.

When one plans to operate on a CPA mass, it is important to first distinguish between CPA meningiomas and VSs. CPA meningiomas must also be carefully differentiated from petroclival and lateral foramen magnum meningiomas as these tumors are exposed via different surgical methods. The risks to hearing and facial nerve function are significantly lower in CPA meningiomas than in VSs. If a CPA meningioma is suspected, surgery is indicated and the surgeon must further investigate the tumor's dural origins, presence of involvement of the IAC and/or jugular foramen, and overall size. These tumor characteristics have significant effects on operative success, and surgical complications, thus, must be considered during the pre-operative assessment for every case.

## REFERENCES


[1] Laird, F. J., Harner, S. G., Laws, E. R. Jr, Reese, D. F. Meningiomas of the Cerebellopontine Angle. *Otolaryngol. Head Neck Surg.* 1985 Apr; 93(2): 163-7.

[2] Samii, M., Matthies, C. Management of 1000 vestibular schwannomas (acoustic neuromas): hearing function in 1000 tumor resections. *Neurosurgery* 1997 Feb; 40(2): 248-60; discussion 260-2.

[3] Holman, M. A., Schmitt, W. R., Carlson, M. L., Driscoll, C. L., Beatty, C. W., Link, M. J. Pediatric cerebellopontine angle and internal auditory canal tumors: clinical article. *J. Neurosurg. Pediatr.* 2013 Oct; 12(4): 317-24.

[4] Voss, N. F., Vrionis, F. D., Heilman, C. B., Robertson, J. H. Meningiomas of the cerebellopontine angle. *Surg. Neurol.* 2000 May; 53(5): 439-46.

[5] Samii, M., Turel, K. E., Penkert, G. Management of seventh and eighth nerve involvement by cerebellopontine angle tumors. *Clin. Neurosurg.* 1985; 32(): 242-72.

[6] Kane, A. J., Sughrue, M. E., Rutkowski, M. J., Berger, M. S., McDermott, M. W., Parsa, A. T. Clinical and surgical considerations for cerebellopontine angle meningiomas. *J. Clin. Neurosci.* 2011 Jun; 18(6): 755-9.

[7] Su, C. H., Chen, C. M., Young, Y. H. Differentiating cerebellopontine angle meningioma from schwannoma using caloric testing and vestibular-evoked myogenic potentials. *J. Neurol. Sci.* 2013 Dec. 15; 335(1-2): 155-9.

[8] Agarwal, V., Babu, R., Grier, J., Adogwa, O., Back, A., Friedman, A. H. et al. Cerebellopontine angle meningiomas: postoperative outcomes in a modern cohort. *Neurosurg. Focus* 2013 Dec; 35(6): E10.

[9] Sughrue, M. E., Yang, I., Aranda, D., Rutkowski, M. J., Fang, S., Cheung, S. W. et al. Beyond audiofacial morbidity after vestibular schwannoma surgery. *J. Neurosurg.* 2011 Feb; 114(2): 367-74.

[10] Pollock, B. E., Driscoll, C. L., Foote, R. L., Link, M. J., Gorman, D. A., Bauch, C. D. et al. Patient outcomes after vestibular schwannoma management: a prospective comparison of microsurgical resection and stereotactic radiosurgery. *Neurosurgery* 2006 Jul; 59(1): 77-85; discussion 77-85.

[11] Roser, F., Nakamura, M., Dormiani, M., Matthies, C., Vorkapic, P., Samii, M. Meningiomas of the cerebellopontine angle with extension into the internal auditory canal. *J. Neurosurg.* 2005 Jan; 102(1): 17-23.

[12] Sughrue, M. E., Rutkowski, M. J., Aranda, D., Barani, I. J., McDermott, M. W., Parsa, A. T. Treatment decision making based on the published natural history and growth rate of small meningiomas. *J. Neurosurg*. 2010 Nov; 113(5): 1036-42.

[13] Jannetta, P. J. Arterial compression of the trigeminal nerve at the pons in patients with trigeminal neuralgia. *J. Neurosurg*. 1967 Jan; 26(1): Suppl: 159-62.

[14] Hardy, D. G., Rhoton, A. L. Jr. Microsurgical relationships of the superior cerebellar artery and the trigeminal nerve. *J. Neurosurg*. 1978 Nov; 49(5): 669-78.

[15] Martin, R. G., Grant, J. L., Peace, D., Theiss, C., Rhoton, A. L. Jr. Microsurgical relationships of the anterior inferior cerebellar artery and the facial-vestibulocochlear nerve complex. *Neurosurgery* 1980 May; 6(5): 483-507.

[16] Jannetta, P. J., Abbasy, M., Maroon, J. C., Ramos, F. M., Albin, M. S. Etiology and definitive microsurgical treatment of hemifacial spasm. Operative techniques and results in 47 patients. *J. Neurosurg*. 1977 Sep; 47(3): 321-8.

[17] Rhoton, A. L. Jr, Kobayashi, S., Hollinshead, W. H. Nervus intermedius. *J. Neurosurg*. 1968 Dec; 29(6): 609-18.

[18] Tang, I. P., Freeman, S. R., Kontorinis, G., Tang, M. Y., Rutherford, S. A., King, A. T. et al. Geniculate neuralgia: a systematic review. *J. Laryngol. Otol*. 2014 May; 128(5): 394-9.

[19] Rhoton, A. L. Jr. Microsurgery of the internal acoustic meatus. *Surg. Neurol*. 1974 Sep; 2(5): 311-8.

[20] House, W. F., Belal, A. Jr. Translabyrinthine surgery: anatomy and pathology. *Am. J. Otol*. 1980 Apr; 1(4): 189-98.

[21] Lister, J. R., Rhoton, A. L. Jr, Matsushima, T., Peace, D. A. Microsurgical anatomy of the posterior inferior cerebellar artery. *J. Neurosurg*. 1982 Feb; 10(2): 170-99.

[22] Kuratsu, J., Kochi, M., Ushio, Y. Incidence and clinical features of asymptomatic meningiomas. *J. Neurosurg*. 2000 May; 92(5): 766-70.

[23] Harner, S. G., Daube, J. R., Ebersold, M. J., Beatty, C. W. Improved preservation of facial nerve function with use of electrical monitoring during removal of acoustic neuromas. *Mayo Clin. Proc*. 1987 Feb; 62(2): 92-102.

[24] Moller, A. R., Jannetta, P. J. Monitoring auditory nerve potentials during operations in the cerebellopontine angle. *Otolaryngol. Head Neck Surg*. 1984 Aug; 92(4): 434-9.

[25] Ansari, S. F., Terry, C., Cohen-Gadol, A. A. Surgery for vestibular schwannomas: a systematic review of complications by approach. *Neurosurg. Focus* 2012 Sep; 33(3): E14.

[26] Yamakami, I., Ito, S., Higuchi, Y. Retrosigmoid removal of small acoustic neuroma: curative tumor removal with preservation of function. *J. Neurosurg*. 2014 Sep; 121(3): 554-63.

[27] Rabelo de Freitas, M., Russo, A., Sequino, G., Piccirillo, E., Sanna, M. Analysis of hearing preservation and facial nerve function for patients undergoing vestibular schwannoma surgery: the middle cranial fossa approach versus the retrosigmoid approach--personal experience and literature review. *Audiol. Neurootol*. 2012; 17(2): 71-81.

[28] Day, J. D., Tschabitscher, M. Anatomic position of the asterion. *Neurosurgery* 1998 Jan; 42(1): 198-9.

[29] Cıkla, U., Kujoth, G. C., Başkaya, M. K. A stepwise illustration of the retrosigmoid approach for resection of a cerebellopontine meningioma. *Neurosurg. Focus* 2014 Jan; 36(1 Suppl.): 1.

[30] Gurgel, R. K., Dogru, S., Amdur, R. L., Monfared, A. Facial nerve outcomes after surgery for large vestibular schwannomas: do surgical approach and extent of resection matter?. *Neurosurg. Focus* 2012 Sep; 33(3):E16.

[31] Rhoton, A. L. Jr. The Cerebellopontine angle and posterior fossa cranial nerves by the retrosigmoid approach. *Neurosurgery* 2000 Sep; 47(3 Suppl.): S93-129.

[32] Glasscock, M. E. 3rd, Hays, J. W., Minor, L. B., Haynes, D. S., Carrasco, V. N. Preservation of hearing in surgery for acoustic neuromas. *J. Neurosurg.* 1993 Jun; 78 (6): 864-70.

[33] Nutik, S. L., Korol, H. W. Cerebrospinal fluid leak after acoustic neuroma surgery. *Surg. Neurol.* 1995 Jun; 43(6): 553-6;discussion 556-7.

[34] Symon, L., Pell, M. F. Cerebrospinal fluid rhinorrhea following acoustic neurinoma surgery. Technical note. *J. Neurosurg.* 1991 Jan; 74(1): 152-3.

[35] Bayazit, Y. A., Celenk, F., Duzlu, M., Goksu, N. Management of cerebrospinal fluid leak following retrosigmoid posterior cranial fossa surgery. *ORL J. Otorhinolaryngol. Relat. Spec.* 2009; 71(6): 329-33.

[36] Leonetti, J. P., Anderson, D. E., Marzo, S. J., Origitano, T. C., Schuman, R. Combined transtemporal access for large (>3 cm) meningiomas of the cerebellopontine angle. *Otolaryngol. Head Neck Surg.* 2006 Jun; 134(6): 949-52.

[37] Sughrue, M. E., Yang, I., Rutkowski, M. J., Aranda, D., Parsa, A. T. Preservation of facial nerve function after resection of vestibular schwannoma. *Br. J. Neurosurg.* 2010 Dec; 24(6): 666-71.

[38] Sughrue, M. E., Yang, I., Aranda, D., Kane, A. J., Parsa, A. T. Hearing preservation rates after microsurgical resection of vestibular schwannoma. *J. Clin. Neurosci.* 2010 Sep; 17(9): 1126-9.

[39] Yang, I., Sughrue, M. E., Han, S. J., Aranda, D., Pitts, L. H., Cheung, S. W. et al. A comprehensive analysis of hearing preservation after radiosurgery for vestibular schwannoma: clinical article. *J. Neurosurg.* 2013 Dec; 119(Suppl.): 851-9.

[40] Nakamura, M., Roser, F., Mirzai, S., Matthies, C., Vorkapic, P., Samii, M. Meningiomas of the internal auditory canal. *Neurosurgery* 2004 Jul; 55(1): 119-27; discussion 127-8.

[41] Nakamura, M., Roser, F., Dormiani, M., Matthies, C., Vorkapic, P., Samii, M. Facial and cochlear nerve function after surgery of cerebellopontine angle meningiomas. *Neurosurgery* 2005 Jul; 57(1): 77-90; discussion 77-90.

In: Current Management of Central Nervous System … ISBN: 978-1-63483-856-6
Editors: Steven D. Chang and Anand Veeravagu 

*Chapter 9*

# SURGICAL MANAGEMENT OF SPINAL MENINGIOMAS

***Richard D. Murray, MD, Sunil Kukreja, MD and Anil Nanda, MD MPH, FACS***
Department of Neurosurgery, Louisiana State University Health Science Center-Shreveport, Shreveport, Louisiana, US

## ABSTRACT

Spinal meningiomas comprise 7.5-15% of all meningiomas and often present between the fifth and seventh decade of life. Presenting symptoms and the neurologic deficits suffered by patients with these tumors are dictated by the anatomic location of the tumor. Surgical resection has been demonstrated to be a safe and effective treatment modality for spinal meningiomas. These lesions are technically challenging to the micro-neurosurgeon, with delicate vasculature and spinal nervous elements in close approximation to tumor tissue. A complete resection has the potential to be curative, with most patients having significant improvement in function. This chapter aims to discuss the epidemiology and histopathology, followed by an in depth discussion of the operative technique.

## INTRODUCTION

Spinal meningiomas are benign, slow growing tumors that arise from arachnoid cap cells and are often located in the intradural, extramedullary compartment, causing progressive extrinsic compression of the spinal neural elements [1].

Being slightly less frequent than nerve sheath tumors, they constitute the second largest group of spinal intradural tumors. The first reported case of a spinal meningioma was in 1888, when Sir Victor Horsely and Sir William Gowers described a case of a "fibromyxoma," which was successfully removed surgically [2, 3].

Later in 1938, Sir Harvey Cushing introduced the term "meningioma" for these tumors [4].

Spinal meningiomas are typically defined as meningiomas that arise within the spinal canal below the vertebral level of C2. Lesions in the region of C1/C2 and the foramen magnum are typically classified as craniovertebral junction (CVJ) and foramen magnum meningiomas respectively. They are generally low-grade, and due to their indolent course can cause significant symptoms prior to final diagnosis. Given their natural history of progressive compression of neural elements, the potential for a "cure," if completely removed, remains the cornerstone in the treatment options for these lesions. In most cases a complete surgical resection is achievable, though in certain subsets, such as densely calcified, ventral and ventrolateral tumors and en-plaque growth patterns may pose unique challenges [5].

This chapter discusses the epidemiology, histo-pathology, and imaging features, before providing an in-depth discussion of the surgical management of these lesions. Select clinical cases are presented and pearls of technique are provided.

## EPIDEMIOLOGY

The annual incidence of intradural spinal tumors ranges from three to five per million people [6]. Spinal meningiomas are less common (7.5-15% of all meningiomas) than intracranial meningiomas [7, 8]. The patients are usually between the fifth and seventh decade of their life [9]. 1.2% of patients are younger than 18 and 28.4% are older than 70 years [10]. The incidence of spinal meningioma in females is much higher than that found in men, with incidence ranging from 2.5-4.2:1 being reported [7, 11]. The female preponderance has been attributed to sex hormones and other receptors found in women. The majority of primary spinal tumors are located in the intradural extramedullary compartment and spinal meningiomas comprise around 25% of these tumors [12]. They are second in frequency, only to nerve sheath tumors, which make up about 40% of all intradual spinal cord tumors in adults [13]. Approximately 83-95% of the spinal meningiomas are intradural; however, in about 10% of cases, they can have a transdural or an extradural component. In exceptional cases, they can be found purely extradurally [14-17]. The tumors are mostly located in the thoracic spine (67-84%), followed by the cervical spine (14-27%), and lumbar spine (2-14%) [18]. However, the preference for the thoracic spine is observed only in females [19]. Younger patients have a higher rate of tumors located in the cervical spine (39%), and the majority of these tumors arise from higher cervical regions [20]. In general, the lesions arising from the thoracic spine are located dorsally within the spinal canal, whereas tumors arising from the foramen magnum and higher cervical regions are usually ventral or ventrolateral [14]. Most spinal meningiomas are WHO grade I and II. The subtypes defined for cranial meningiomas hold for spinal meningiomas, with meningothelial and psammomatous lesions most commonly identified [8, 14, 31]. Some authors have reported that psammomatous meningiomas are more common in the spine than intracranially [30, 31].

## PATHOLOGY AND HISTOPATHOLOGY

The cell of origin for spinal meningiomas, as with their intracranial counterpart, is the arachnoid cap cell.

A higher frequency of these cells is found in the root exit zones of nerves and the vascular entry zones into the spinal canal, thereby accounting for the typical lateral location of these tumors [14].

Overall, lateral tumors are more frequently observed than dorsal or ventral tumors, with a posterolateral location being the most common [14, 21, 22]. Foramen magnum and CVJ lesions have a higher incidence of lateral or ventrolateral localization, with cervical lesions being common in ventally [14, 19]. In the thoracic spine, a preponderance of dorsal and dorsolateral locations are encountered.

Though rare in comparison to other locations, in the lumbar spine, a posterior position for these tumors is more common [23].

Numerous receptors have been described in meningiomas, with progesterone being the most common. The increased occurrence in females supports the possibility of hormonal factors playing a significant role in pathogenesis [14, 24-26]. The increased tendency of spinal meningiomas to occur in the thoracic spine of post-menopausal woman may be due to increased trauma to the meninges related to osteoporotic collapse of the thoracic vertebrae [14, 27].

Most tumors have a broad attachment to the leptomeninges from which they derive their vascular supply. Typically an arachnoid plane is present between the tumor and the spinal cord, which in general remains well preserved.

It is rare, though not completely unknown, for spinal meningiomas to penetrate the pial layer overlying the spinal cord or to parasitize cord vasculature.

Macroscopically, meningiomas appear round or lobulated, with a broad base and are typically well circumscribed (Figure 1). Tumor consistency ranges from fleshy, friable and cauliflower-like to rubbery and firm. On occasion they can be densely calcified, very firm, or fibrous [28, 29]. These calcifications can range from microscopic to heavily calcified to the point of being visible on computed tomography (CT) of the spine.

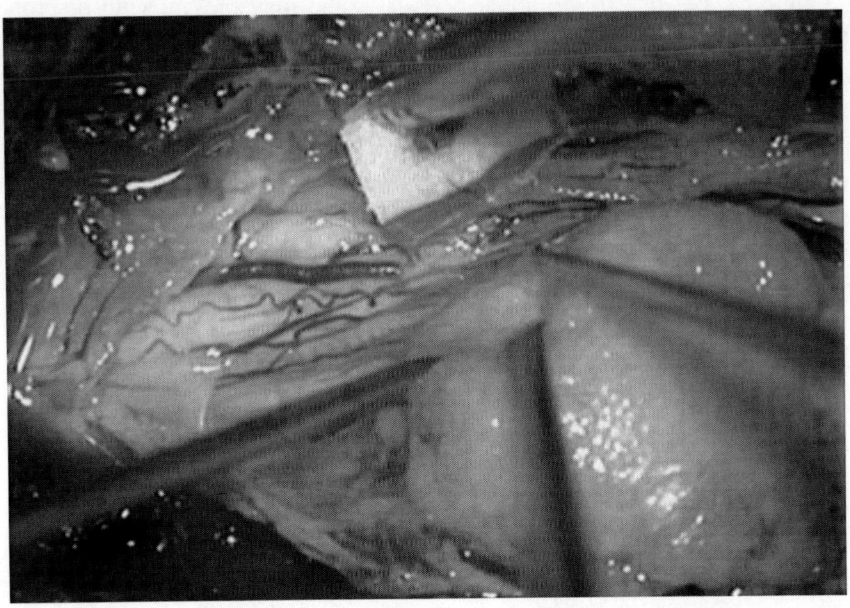

Figure 1. A meningioma adherent to the dura is being dissection away from the spinal cord using microsurgical technique.

## Clinical Presentation

Meningiomas are typically slow growing tumors allowing for various compensation mechanisms to occur. This includes displacement of cerebrospinal fluid (CSF), epidural fat and vasculature, physical displacement and compressibility of the spinal cord itself and loss of myelination prior to the loss of axons [32]. Symptoms often progress over the course of months to years, which accounts for the delay between onset of symptoms and diagnosis.

Pain is typically present for years prior to final diagnosis [7]. The duration of symptoms prior to diagnosis is in the order of 1-2 years, but can be as long as 15-20 years [19, 30, 33, 34]. The general availability of MRI has had a significant impact by reducing the average time of diagnosis by 6 months, leading to lower post-surgical disability [7, 30, 33].

The specific neurologic deficits suffered by patients with spinal meningiomas are dictated by the anatomic location of the tumor and direct compression of neural elements, though effects can also be due to vascular compromise, abnormal CSF circulation or spinal cord tethering [14]. Compression at the neural foramen may give rise to radicular pain. Dorsal root compression may give rise to sensory loss, while ventral root compression may result in weakness [14]. Direct cord compression can have variable effects, ranging from motor weakness due to anterior horn cell compromise, dorsal column fallout, or the effects of ascending and descending. Myelopathy is a relatively common finding with one study showing a 64% incidence of weakness and 32% of patients being non-ambulatory [7].

Though more common in nerve sheath tumors, spinal meningiomas may demonstrate two distinct phases of presentation. The first is due to progressive irritation of nerve roots, resulting in pain. The second stage, caused by direct spinal cord compression, is characterized by various cord syndromes, ranging from Brown-Sequard to dorsal column fallout to myelopathy [35].

The vertebral level at which these lesions arise will also have a significant effect upon the physical symptoms. Lesions in the upper cervical spine may present with disproportionate loss of dorsal column sensation in the upper limbs as compared to the lower limbs, with atrophy of the intrinsic hand muscles and variable involvement of long tracts below the level of the lesion. Thoracic lesions may cause a radiating chest pain or sensory disturbances several neurological levels below the vertebral level of the lesion. Lumbar lesions may have variable presentation depending on involvement of the lower spinal cord, conus medularis, or the cauda equina alone. Sacral lesions may involve only sympathetic nerves and as such present with sphincter disturbances only [36]. Symptoms due to vascular compromise, either via arterial compromise with distant watershed symptoms or venous congestion are also possible [7, 14]. Other rare phenomena include symptoms due to raised ICP, hydrocephalus or syringomyelia [14, 37-39]. Tethering of the spinal cord or neural elements is also a possibility, especially in the setting of a previous resection.

## Imaging Studies

In the diagnostic workup of spinal meningiomas, magnetic resonance imaging (MRI) provides the greatest amount of clinically useful information.

Other modalities that are occasionally useful include CT and CT Myelography, infrared (IR) myelography, X-ray, and ultrasound. MRI provides precise anatomic detail regarding tumor location, size and spatial relationship to adjacent structures [7, 14].

MRI with and without contrast has become the study of choice to delineate tumors of this nature. Sagittal images provide valuable information regarding the precise vertebral level involved and is helpful as a screening tool. Axial images provide information as to the exact relationship of the tumor to the cord, the degree of cord displacement, presence of a dural tail as well as the character of the tumor-cord interface [22, 29]. The presence of a CSF cleft predicts a well preserved pial plane between cord and tumor [7]. Routine imaging sequences typically include Axial, Sagittal and Coronal sequences with T1 weighted pre and post contrast images, as well as T2 weighted images [7, 14].

Typically these lesions have a broad dural attachment that enhances homogenously with contrast [40]. Similar to intracranial meningiomas, spinal meningiomas can have a dural tail [41, 42]. Occasionally, they can be of an "en-plaque" configuration [33, 43, 44].

CT provides good spatial resolution; however, it is particularly useful in assessing the degree of calcification and spinal bony anatomy. Heavily calcified tumors correspond with very firm intraoperative lesions and may predict a challenging surgical resection. When MRI is contraindicated, myelography can be added to CT and will allow for a less detailed anatomic localization. Hyperostosis is rare with spinal meningiomas, possibly due to the presence of a wide epidural space [14].

In heavily mineralized tumors, CT can be of significant utility in predicting the likelihood of a firm tumor and delineating bony relationships.

Plain radiographs have a relatively limited role to play in the age of MRI and CT. Occasionally heavily mineralized tumors may be visible on plain spine radiographs, but the anatomic definition of CT and MRI is significantly more evolved. They may play a role in determining exact vertebral level pre- and intra-operatively and in documenting the presence of anatomic variations in vertebral column configuration. The differential diagnosis based upon imaging findings would include meningiomas, schwannomas, neurofibromas and malignant nerve sheath tumors [7, 14]. Meningiomas tend to be homogenously enhancing, with a broad dural base and occasionally a dural tail.

Calcifications can manifest as a signal void on all MRI sequences and results in heterogeneous contrast uptake [7]. Meningiomas tend to be isodense to the cord on T1 and T2 sequences. Enhancement is strong and homogenous, unless significant calcification exists. It is of cardinal importance to determine the exact vertebral level at which the lesion is located. Variations in vertebral anatomy, such as an extra rib or sacralization of the lumbar vertebrae may lead to a surgical procedure targeting an incorrect level. Documenting the exact vertebral height as well as the method used to determine this (i.e., counting from lowest rib upwards, or counting from C1 downwards) is vital in ensuring intra-operative consistency in arriving at the correct level.

Pitfalls/Pearls:

1. Densely mineralized tumors can be very difficult to remove with microsurgical techniques and may require the use of ultrasonic aspirators
2. Document the vertebral level of the tumor as well as the technique used to determine this prior to surgery. Then ensure that this same technique is used to arrive at the correct level during surgery.

## SURGICAL ANATOMY

Most spinal meningiomas can be successfully managed via a dorsal midline approach. In most cases tumors either arise from a lateral or dorsal origin, or alternatively displace the cord laterally to such an extent that an adequate surgical corridor is created, a dorsal or dorsolateral approach is adequate in the large majority of cases. Cases in which the tumor origin is directly ventral and firm or fibrous are the most challenging. Factors which play a role in choosing a surgical approach includes, vascularity of the tumor and spinal cord, vertebral level and anatomical structures in relation to the vertebral column, amount of mineralization present, relationship to the spinal cord, operating distance, expected ease of reconstructing the dura in a watertight fashion and surgeon preference and experience [29].

A number of different approaches have been described and are listed in Table 1.1.

In general terms, each specific region of the spine poses unique anatomical challenges. The cervical spine has the oropharynx, esophagus and trachea, recurrent laryngeal nerve, carotid, jugular veins, and vertebral artery to consider. In the thoraco-cervical junction, the ribs come into play, with the aortic arch, thoracic duct and pleural cavities playing a role. In the thoracic spine, the ribcage, scapula and clavicle, lungs and pleural cavities and large vessels limit access, while in the thoraco-lumbar region the liver, diaphragm and vena cava are structures to consider. In the lumbo-sacral region, the vena cava and aorta with its branches, as well as the pelvic viscera all limit access to the anterior aspects of the vertebral column.

## MANAGEMENT

The final treatment algorithm depends on a number of clinical and imaging characteristics. Small asymptomatic lesions incidentally discovered in elderly patients could potentially be followed with serial imaging only.

**Table 1.1.**

| | |
|---|---|
| Cervical | Anterior and lateral retropharyngeal |
| | High Anterior cervical approach |
| | Anterolateral (Smith Robinson) |
| | Lateral Approach |
| | Midline posterior |
| Upper Thoracic | Anterior trapdoor |
| | Midline sternotomy |
| | Transthoracic |
| | Costotransversectomy |
| | Midline posterior |
| Lower Thoracic | Transthoracic |
| | Transdiaphragmatic thoracolumbar |
| | Retropleural |
| | Midline Posterior |
| Lumbar | Midline Posterior |
| | Posterolateral |
| | Retroperitoneal |

In most symptomatic patients though, surgery offers the potential of a cure in a treatable disease process. Combinations of treatment modalities are also in use, with radiosurgery being an option for small or incompletely resected lesions.

## Pre-Operative Considerations

Risks specific to this surgery are paralysis, worsening of neurologic deficits, failure to improve, incomplete resection, need for repeat surgery, CSF leak, meningitis, pain, instability and new bladder, bowel and/or sexual dysfunction.

The utility of electrophysiologic monitoring should be considered. Electromyography (EMG) can play a role in identifying individual nerve roots and monitoring root function.

Somatosensory evoked potentials (SSEP) monitor dorsal column function. Motor Tracts are monitored via motor evoked potentials (MEP).

Even though meningiomas tend to be well circumscribed, a combination of monitoring modalities can aid in surgical decision making and may provide additional information as to post-operative prognosis for improvement [14].

## Detailed Account of Surgical Management

Most spinal meningiomas are approached via a dorsal midline approach, encompassing a posterior laminectomy over one or multiple vertebral levels. This typically provides adequate working space and the shortest working distance, minimal cord manipulation and appropriate dural closure, while avoiding post-operative biomechanical instability.

In some instances, more esoteric approaches need to be considered. Individual treatment decisions are largely a matter of clinical judgment and patient preference [29].

**1.2. Table with steps of surgery**

| |
|---|
| Positioning |
| Pre-op localization of skin incision |
| Skin incision |
| Soft tissue dissection |
| Intra-op localization |
| Bony removal |
| Tumor localization with ultrasound |
| Dural opening |
| Inspection |
| Access maneuvers |
| Tumor dissection |
| Irrigation of CSF space and tumor bed |
| Dural closure |
| Soft tissue closure |
| Post-operative management |

# SURGICAL APPROACH

A dorsal approach to the spine is adequate for most spinal meningiomas. As these lesions are most commonly located posterolaterally in the thoracic spine and anterolaterally in the cervical spine, this approach is well suited for this pathology [35]. Lateral displacement of the cord by the tumor can result in an improved lateral working channel which may prove adequate to remove the tumor.

## Surgical Approach Image 1

This tumor displaces the cord laterally, thereby creating an operative corridor. Note the spinal nerve roots draped over the surface of the tumor.

## Surgical Approach Image 2

Same case as in Image 1. The working corridor created by the tumor has been utilized, debulking the center of the tumor and preserving the spinal nerve roots that cross over the surface of the tumor. A patient is typically positioned prone on the operating table, with special attention paid to ensuring the abdomen is free of compression to reduce venous pressure. For cervical lesions, the head is kept fixated in a Mayfield head clamp™, with the neck mildly flexed. Thoracic lesions can be approached with the patient positioned on gel rolls or pillows, or alternatively on a Jackson spine table™.

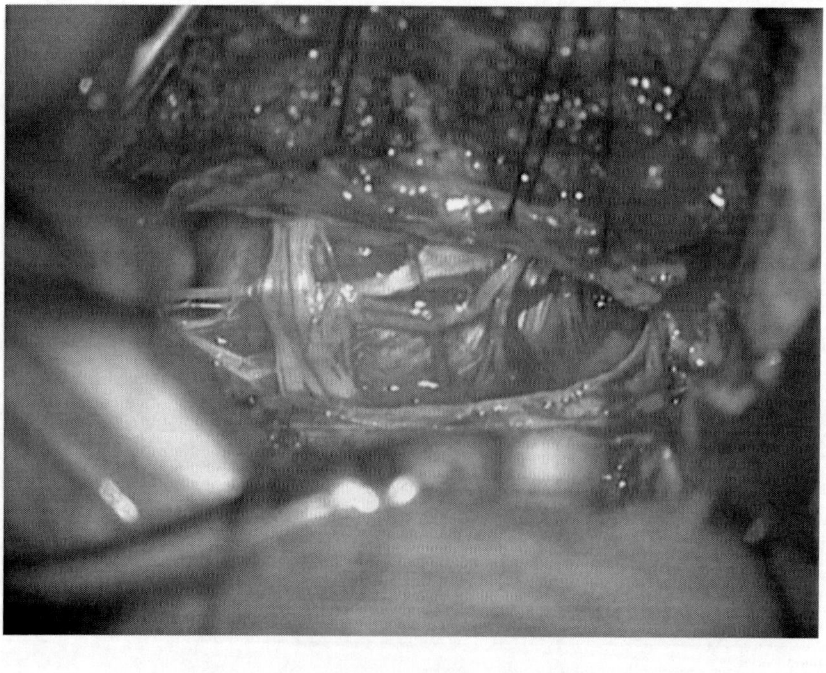

Image 1.

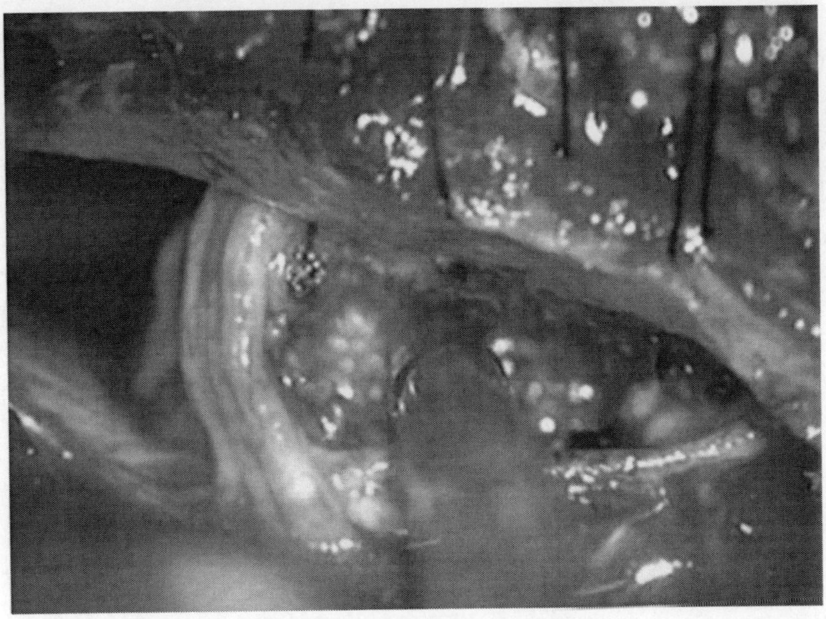

Image 2.

The approach to lumbar pathology is eased by using a Wilson frame™, which counteracts the lumbar lordosis, thereby opening the interspinous distance which facilitates surgical access. Pre-operative localization via XR is then carried out, which places the surgical incision in the correct region. In the lumbar and cervical spine, this can be done via lateral x-rays. In the thoracic region, it may be more beneficial to use anterior-posterior x-rays. It is of cardinal importance to ensure that the same counting strategy is followed to localize the tumor as was done pre-operatively with reference films.

The skin incision is typically midline, with bilateral subperiosteal exposure of the bony anatomy. The paraspinal musculature can then be retracted via self-retaining retractors or via table mounted retractor systems. Extending this incision in a superior and inferior direction may aid in achieving further soft tissue retraction laterally. If tumor extent dictates a more lateral dural incision, a paramedian skin incision may aid in achieving less muscle bulk below the retractor system and therefore a more lateral surgical reach.

Once adequate soft tissue is resected and another x-ray is taken. This is to ensure that vertebral levels remain properly identified and correlated with the correct tumor location.

An alternative strategy for localization of the intradural tumors has been successfully used at our institution on numerous occasions. An intra-operative CT scan is performed with the O-arm™, which then allows the use of intra-operative navigation with the Stealth™ system. The surgeon then accurately determines the correct level of interest, tailor the laminectomy according to intra-operative anatomy and ensure dural exposure is adequate.

Bony removal is typically done via a bilateral midline laminectomy over one or more vertebral levels, depending on the extent of the tumor. The goal of bony exposure is to visualize the complete extent of the dural attachment of the tumor, with additional rostro-caudal extent to facilitate watertight dural closure [14]. The lateral extent of and the amount of displacement of the spinal cord by the tumor determines how much bony resection may be required.

Since bony removal has to be performed in a very careful fashion in order to avoid traumatizing an already compromised spinal cord, the laminectomy is typically performed via high speed drilling to thin the laminae, followed by resection with micro ronguers [35]. Thereafter piecemeal resection of the ligamentum flavum and medial aspects of the facet joints are carried out to further facilitate exposure. Extending the bony resection laterally, to include more of the facet joints, resecting a rib head or even a pedicle may at times be required to facilitate tumor resection [35, 45]. Even though compromising biomechanical stability is typically not a concern, the possibility has to be considered and a management strategy anticipated prior to initiating a case. It may also be of benefit to resect more portions of the neighboring spinous processes, which can enlarge the surgical corridor and access.

After completion of the bony and ligamentous exposure, an intra-operative ultrasound is brought into the field and used to determine the cranio-caudal extent of the tumor and the precise relationship to the spinal cord. The goal of this step is to ensure that bony exposure is optimal and if not found to be so, that this deficit is corrected prior to opening the dura, so as to ensure that all macro-dissection and bone work is done prior to dural opening, with dural protection in place. This also aids in limiting the amount of blood and debris entering into the CSF spaces.

It has been previously described, that inspection of the dura and noting the area above which dural pulsations are visible, will demonstrate the superior extent of the tumor [14]. This is based upon a similar mechanism as that demonstrated by the Queckenstedt test [46]. This is likely to be most helpful for larger tumors, completely limiting the transmission of CSF pulsations inferior to the tumor or tumors in which the dural base covers a large area. In smaller lesions, it is unlikely to be a reliable marker of tumor extent. Another helpful aid is to visually inspect the dura, which often demonstrates a visible tumor contour. Alternatively, gentle palpation may be of use.

Once adequate bony exposure is established, meticulous hemostasis must be obtained. Failure to control epidural bleeding at this stage can generate significant bothersome epidural oozing, once the tamponade effect of the inflated thecal sac is removed, which could result in venous oozing throughout the case, obscuring anatomical detail, increasing operative time and contaminating CSF.

The durotomy is planned to encompass the entire circumferential border of the tumor and minimize spinal cord exposure [14]. The dura is then opened in a linear fashion, typically in the midline. This incision can be exaggerated to one side, depending on the location of the tumor. The need for adequate exposure to the tumor has to be balanced against the ease of achieving a watertight dural closure at the end of the case.

For ventrally located tumors, the planned dural excision should ideally encompass the full extent of the tumor with an adequate margin of 3-4 mm and include the area of the dural tail. This helps to ensure a complete resection, while also providing early control of the tumor's vascular supply, thereby limiting intra-operative bleeding. In cases of complete or suspected complete occlusion of CSF flow, entering the dura above the level of the tumor and releasing CSF slowly, ensuring that pressure shifts within the CNS is controlled.

The dura is then tacked up with small retention sutures to the edges of the opening. The arachnoid sheath is also opened along the entire length of the tumor and tacked to the edges of the dura. It has been described that tilting the patient slightly head down, may aid in limiting the amount of air and blood entering into the thecal sac. This may play a role in limiting post-operative arachnoiditis [3].

Prior to initiating the microsurgical dissection portion of the case, we find it helpful to pause at this time, re-inspect to ensure meticulous hemostasis. After the tamponade effect of the expanded thecal sac is removed, often a small amount of venous oozing can restart. Investing time at this stage pre-empts the need to retrace surgical steps at a later stage to control this venous leakage.

Inspecting the interface between the tumor and the cord is then carried out. Additional resection of dentate ligaments can be carried out, which may aid in enlarging lateral access to the cord. Using very gentle suture retraction on the dentate ligaments can help to improve the surgical corridor. Care needs to be taken in the high cervical region so as to not injure the ascending cervical portion of the accessory nerve, which runs directly ventral to the dentate ligament. In extreme cases, in the thoracic spine one or more nerve roots may need to be sectioned to gain access to ventral lesions [7, 30, 35, 45].

At times, a ventrally or ventrolaterally situated tumor displaces the cord enough to provide an adequate surgical access corridor from a dorsal approach.

Surgical debulking of the tumor is then carried out. The tools used depend on the consistency of the tumor. Soft, friable tumors can be addressed with microinstruments, bipolar and suction, whereas more firm or calcified tumors may require ultrasonic aspirator assistance. The goal of this step is to debulk the center of the tumor, which in general aids to establish a better delineation of the tumor-cord interface. The capsule of the tumor is kept intact, so as to allow countertraction during dissection of the tumor cord interface.

Typically the interface between the cord and the tumor is a well-developed plane, which once clarified can be dissected with microsurgery and separated completely from the cord. It is rare that a tumor will infiltrate the surface of the cord. Two types of interfaces have been described by Salpietro et al. [22]. A "floating interface" is characterized by a hypointense peritumoral rim seen on MRI.

This typically signifies a small well preserved CSF space between the arachnoid and the intermediate leptomeningeal layer, which makes the tumor easily dissectible off the spinal cord. In the second type, the "deep interface," no such peritumoral rim is seen on MRI and the arachnoid layer is poor or absent. In these cases the tumor is difficult to separate from the spinal cord and is adherent to structures, but is usually completely dissectible, due to a preserved pial layer. Meticulous micro-dissection of this tumor cord interface is then carried out, taking care to preserve cord vasculature.

Devascularizing the tumor is a useful strategy. This minimizes the amount of bleeding encountered, which eases the microsurgical dissection. This can be done via circumferential dural coagulation and sectioning or alternatively by locating and coagulating feeding vessels, after the vessels have been confirmed to be components of tumor vasculature.

Dorsally located tumors can typically be resected completely, along with complete excision of the dural attachment and subsequent dural reconstruction via dural graft. In other cases, for instance ventral cervical tumors, even though complete excision of the tumor can be achieved, dural resection is not practical.

In such cases, it may be prudent to resect all visible tumor and to coagulate and scrape the remaining dura. In WHO grade I meningiomas, there is not a significant difference in recurrence rates between a Simpson Grade I and II. However, in WHO grade II and III, a Simpson Grade I resection should be aimed for [23].

En-plaque meningiomas are associated with a significant amount of scarring and make dissection more difficult [14, 47].

Recurrent meningiomas also poses unique problems, being much more adherent to structures and not possessing the pial plane typically found in these lesions, they may even infiltrate the pia and be densely adherent to the spinal cord, nerve roots and surrounding structures [9, 33].

Once tumor resection is completed and meticulous hemostasis has been achieved, irrigating the resection cavity with warm saline is carried out. This irrigation helps to remove all debris and blood. Removal of the debris and blood may help to decrease the development of arachnoiditis, tethering, syrinx formation and hydrocephalus [14, 28].

Factors which play a role in achieving a complete resection include anterior location, degree of mineralization, narrow canal and recurrent or en-plaque morphologies.

The next step is to reconstruct the dura.

This can be done via a combination of running watertight sutures, coupled with dural sealant materials, dural regeneration matrixes or by patching dural gaps with dural graft. In rare cases it is not possible to reconstruct the dura in a watertight manner and partial reconstruction via dural regeneration matrixes in combination with dural sealants and temporary CSF diversion must be considered.

Since the spinal dura can be divided into an inner and an outer layer, some authors have advocated stripping the entire inner layer as circumscribed by the base of the tumor, then reconstructing the outer layer of the dura in a watertight fashion [48]. The soft-tissue is then closed in a multi-layer fashion, with the skin being closed with watertight sutures.

## Surgical Approach Image 3

Stripping the inner layer of dura on which the meningioma had previously been based.

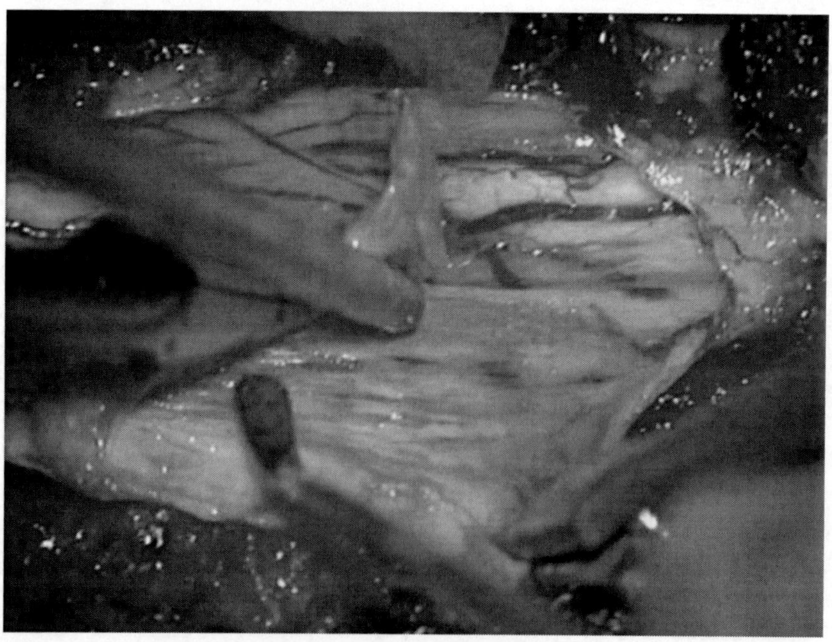

Image 3.

Pitfalls/Pearls:

1. Meticulous hemostasis early in the case is essential. This decreases the amount of time spent later in the case controlling peripheral leakage.
2. Prior to opening the dura, place ¼ x 3 inch cottonoids linearly lateral to the dural edges. This helps to control and wick away any bleeding during the rest of the case.
3. Placing small ½ x ½ cottonoids or alternatively squares of gelfoam inside the thecal sac, at the superior and inferior extent of the opening helps to limit the entry of debris and blood into the thecal sac.

## Post-Operative Management

Post-operative management is case specific and to a large extent depends on the quality of the dural reconstruction and suture line. Standard measures include limiting any action which may increase ICP, such as Valsalva maneuvers or straining. A brief period of bedrest may benefit surgical wound healing and prevent pseudomeningocele development.

## Prognosis and Recovery

Prognosis after surgical removal of spinal meningiomas is generally excellent. Various studies have reported a favorable neurological outcome after surgical removal in the range of 60-98% [8, 19, 31, 33-35].

A number of factors are associated with a worse prognosis, including pial invasion and subtotal resection, as well as advanced age, profound neurologic deficits and prolonged symptoms prior to diagnosis [23, 35, 49]. Sphincter disturbance is a particularly ominous sign [21, 35]. In general complete resection is often achieved, with some large studies reporting rates of 82-99% [8, 31, 34].

Factors which are associated with complete resection include absence of need for ventral exposure, absence of bony involvement, presence of a peritumoral hypodense rim on MRI [14, 22, 29]. Recurrence rates after complete resection range from 1.3-6.4% [19, 50, 51].

In most cases it can be expected that some degree of neurological recovery can be expected after surgery. Prognostic factors that are associated with a better outcome include younger age, complete removal of tumor, posterior or posterolateral location, location below C4 and short duration of symptoms [20, 29, 43, 45, 52, 53]. Factors which are associated with a worse outcome include pre-operative sphincter dysfunction, anterior location within the spinal canal, highly calcified tumors, recurrent and en-plaque tumors, as well as WHO grade II and III subtypes [20, 21, 35, 43, 52].

One study, utilizing the National Inpatient Sample in the US, found that 6.4% of patients suffered in hospital complications. 42% of Patients were discharged to facilities other than their home or "self-care" and that the pediatric population and advanced age had the highest rates of adverse outcomes [10]. Some patients continue to deteriorate after surgery. In these patients the factors to consider include recurrence, delayed post-operative scarring, syringomyelia or instability, and myelopathy [33, 35].

## FUTURE DIRECTIONS

The role of adjuvant radiotherapy is still unclear in cases of incomplete resection, though spinal radiosurgery offers a unique opportunity for local control. An intriguing concept has recently been reported regarding the use of intra-operative 5-ALA.

This has been well described in intracranial meningiomas, but has only recently been studied in spinal meningiomas [54, 55]. Protoporphyrin IX, which is metabolized from 5-aminolevulinic acid (5-ALA), accumulates in tumor tissue and shows fluorescence when exposed to excitation light. This may aid in identifying tumor infiltration along dural margins, which might not be visible under routine operative microscope view.

Fluorescence should be interpreted with caution, given the variable amounts of fluorescence that may be achieved between tumors and even within the same tumor.

## CONCLUSION

Surgery remains the mainstay of treatment for symptomatic spinal cord meningiomas. These lesions are well suited for surgery, with well-preserved tissue planes and residence in accessible anatomic locations.

Factors which need to be considered during surgical planning include the approach used and approach related complications, extent of surgical resection achievable with any specific approach, and ease of dural reconstruction after tumor extirpation.

## CASE STUDY 1

51-year-old male, known with a history of diabetes and hypertension, presents with a nine month history of progressive weakness in the right hand, coupled with numbness from the mid-thoracic region downwards. He reports not being able to maintain his balance when walking and has had numerous falls in recent months. Neck pain is a more recent feature of his symptoms, having started as a dull ache roughly 6 months prior to presentation.

Physical exam reveals decreased strength in C7 and T1 distribution, as well as myelopathic signs in the lower extremities.

### Case Study 1 - Image 1

T1 Sagittal post contrast image of the cervical spine demonstrating a brightly enhancing intradural extra-axial mass with a broad dural base, located anterior to the cord at the level of C7-T1.

## Case Study 1 - Image 2

T2 sagittal MRI of the cervical spine with an extra-axial intradural lesion in the lower cervical region anterior to the spinal cord.

## Case Study 1 - Image 3

T1 Axial post contrast image of the lower cervical spine which demonstrates a lesion anterolateral to the spinal cord, which fills the canal and displaces the cord postero-laterally.

***Operative Course***

This tumor displaces the cord in a postero-lateral direction, thereby creating a corridor for surgical access lateral to the cord, from a dorsal approach. Patient was placed prone on a spine table, with the head fixed in caliper traction. A dorsal midline incision was made, soft tissue dissection was carried out over the lamina, followed by a multilevel laminectomy, ensuring adequate rostro-caudal exposure of the dura and the intradural tumor.

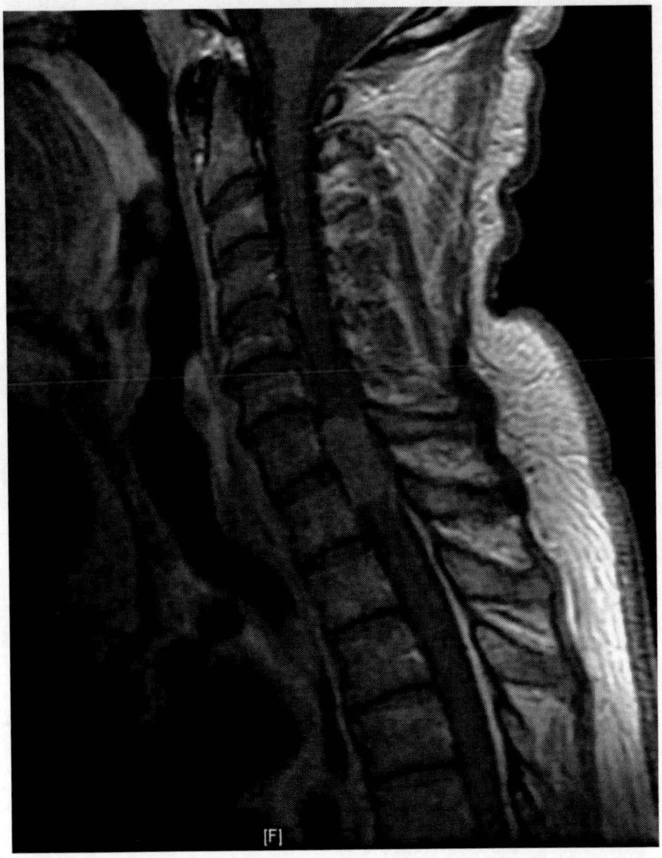


Image 1.

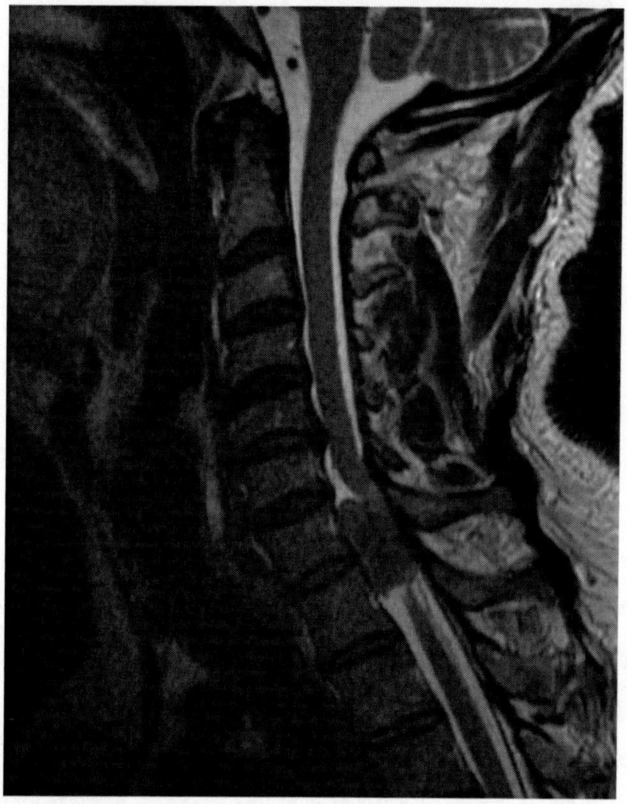

Image 2.

## Case Study 1 - Image 4

Intraoperative image demonstrating tumor lateral to cord in the superior aspect of the picture, with the spinal cord being displaced to the contralateral side.

The tumor was then approached via this corridor, with central debunking and disconnecting the tumor-dura interface. This then created enough space to dissect the tumor away from the cord.

## Case Study 1 - Image 5

Once disconnected from the dura and the cord, large portions of the tumor could be removed. Once all microscopically visible remnants of the tumor was removed, the remaining dura was coagulated and closed in a watertight fashion.

## Case Study 1 - Image 6

Post-operative MRI demonstrating complete resection of tumor, with edema of the spinal cord.

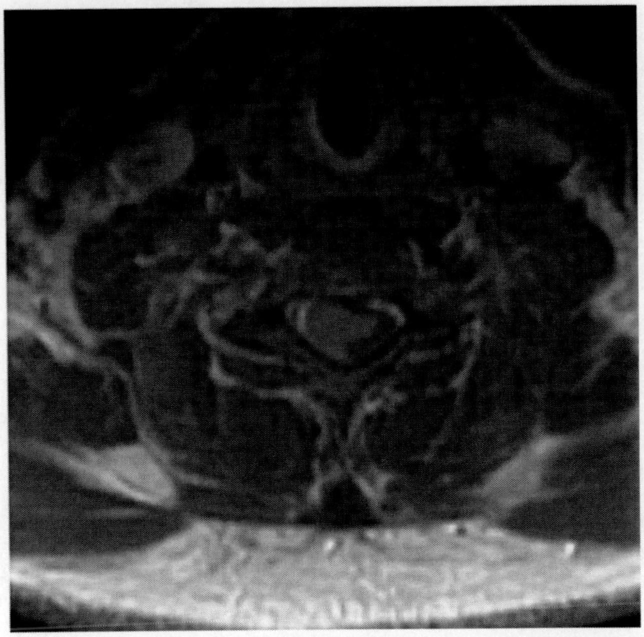

Image 3.

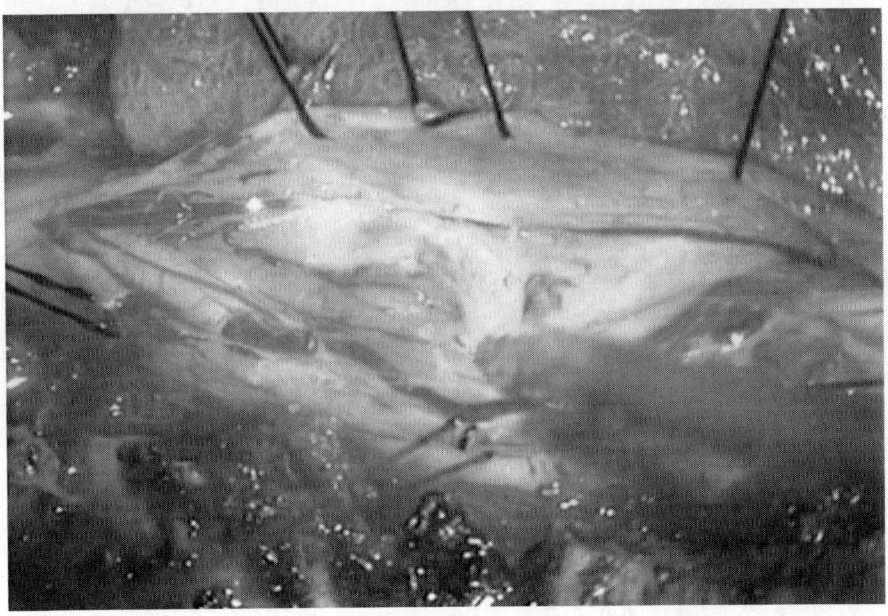

Image 4.

***Post-Operative Course***

The hospital course was uneventful and the patient was discharged to a rehabilitation facility, where he continued to make significant gains. At latest follow up, he was continuing to progressively improve in strength, balance and gait. At latest follow up, there was no sign of tumor recurrence.

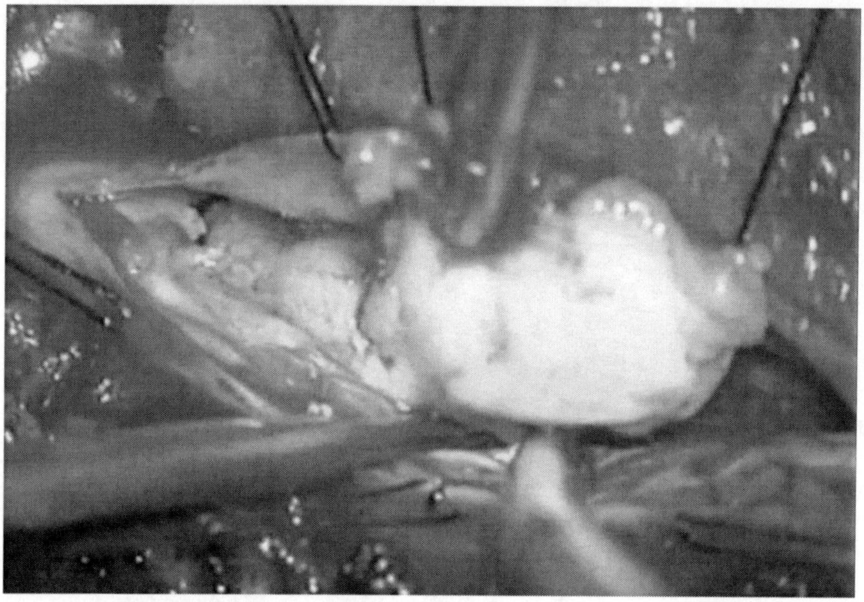

Image 5.

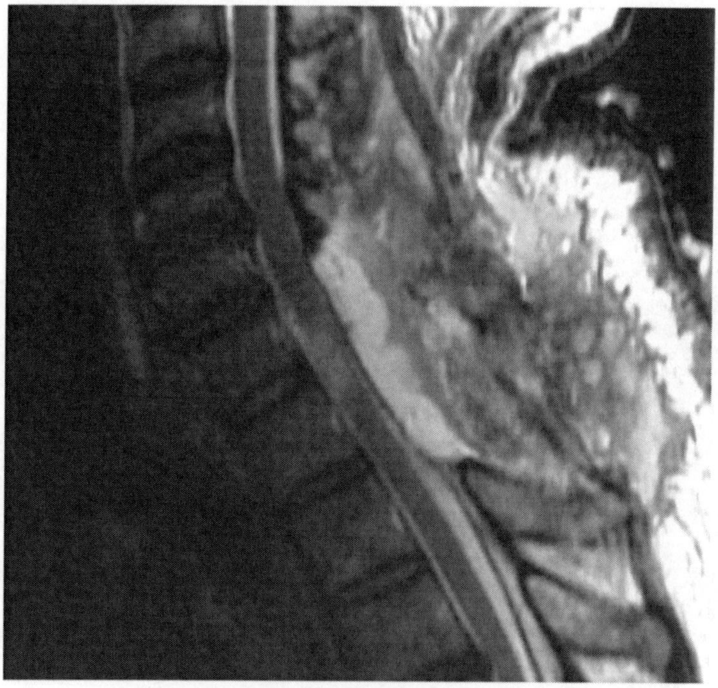

Image 6.

## Case Study 2

A female patient in her late twenties with a history of Neurofibromatosis presents with 6 months of symptoms related to worsening gait and balance.

Physical exam demonstrated intact strength in her lower extremities, with signs of frank myelopathy. Imaging studies demonstrated a densely calcified mass in her lower thoracic spine.

## Case Study 2 - Image 1

Sagittal T1 with contrast image of the thoracic spine demonstrating broad dural base and bright enhancement with contrast.

## Case Study 2 - Image 2

Axial T1 with contrast of the thoracic spine demonstrating broad dural base and bright enhancement with contrast.

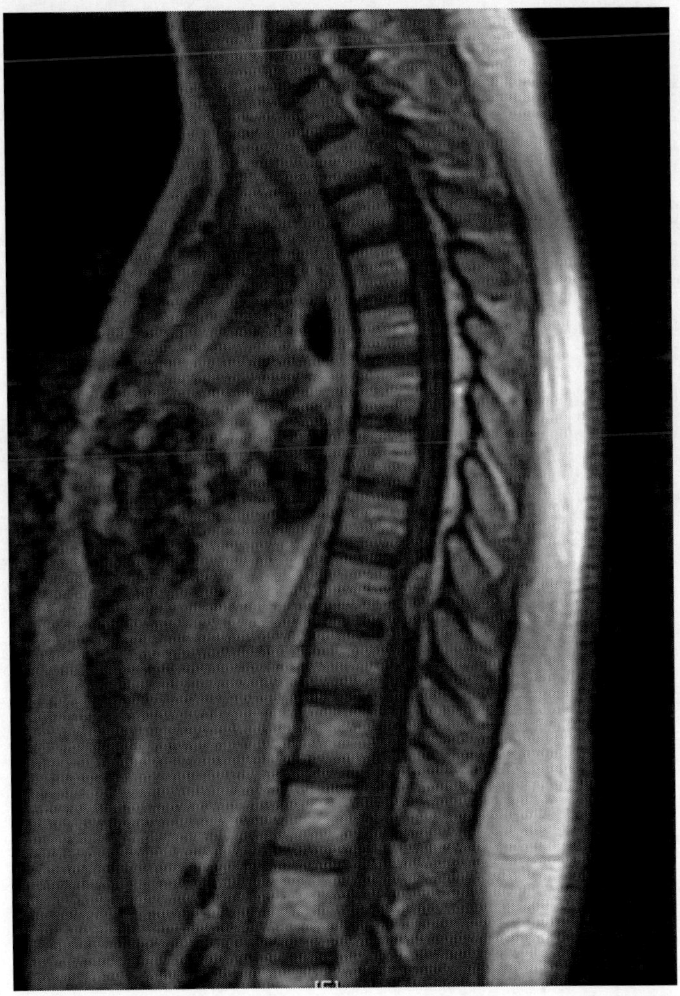

Image 1.

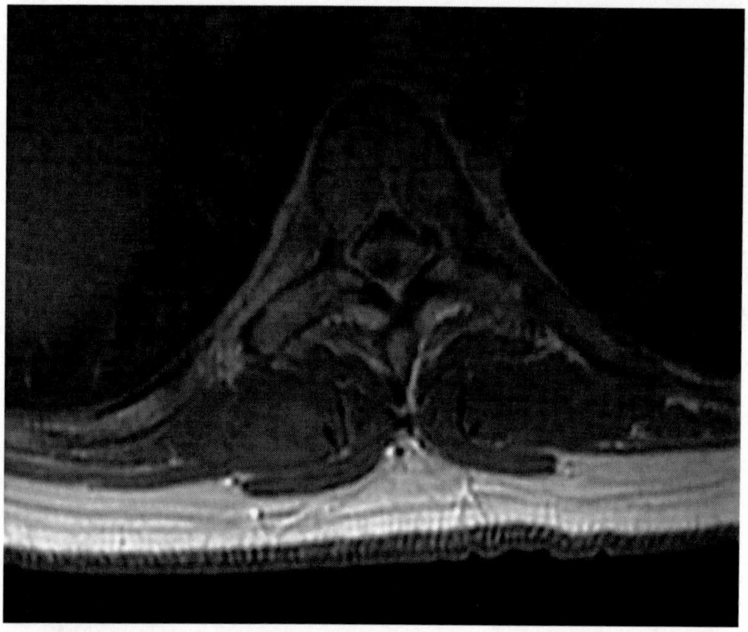

Image 2.

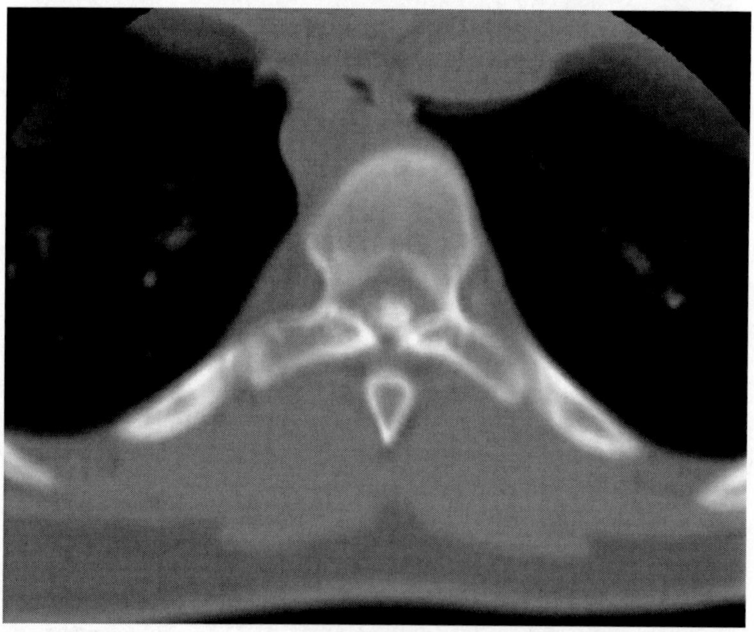

Image 3.

## Case Study 2 - Image 3

Axial CT of the thoracic spine demonstrating a densely calcified lesion posterior to spinal cord.

## Case Study 2 - Image 4

Sagittal CT of the thoracic spine with a densely calcified mass in the posterior portion of the spinal canal.

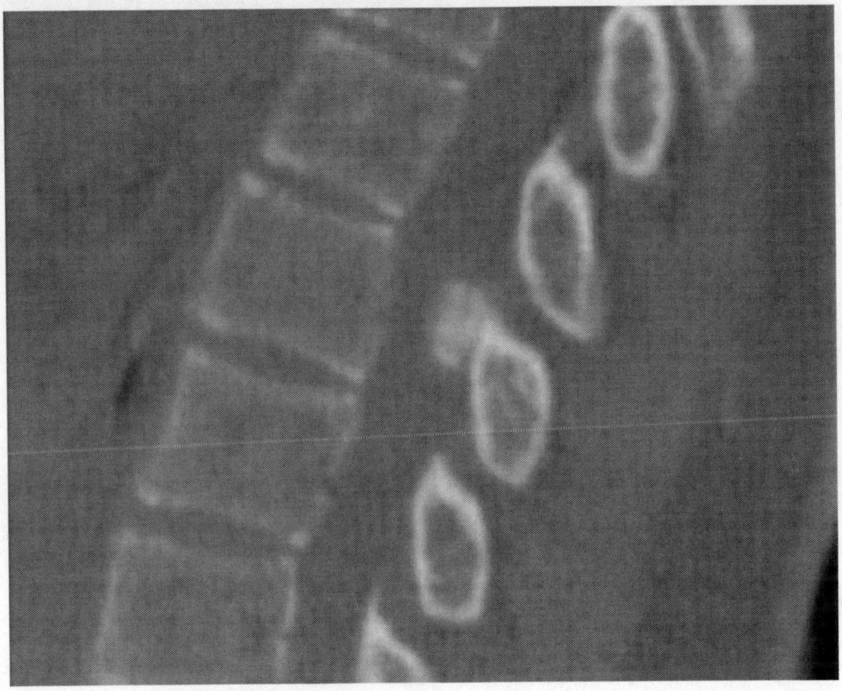

Image 4.

### *Operative Course*

This patient was placed prone on a spine table, an intra-operative CT scan of the thoracic spine was performed. Neuronavigation was then used to accurately identify the region of interest and to tailor the laminectomy as required by the tumor.

## Case Study 2 - Image 5

A densely calcified mass, posterior to the cord was dissected away from the cord.

### *Post-Operative Course*

The patient had an uncomplicated hospital course and has made significant improvements in function.

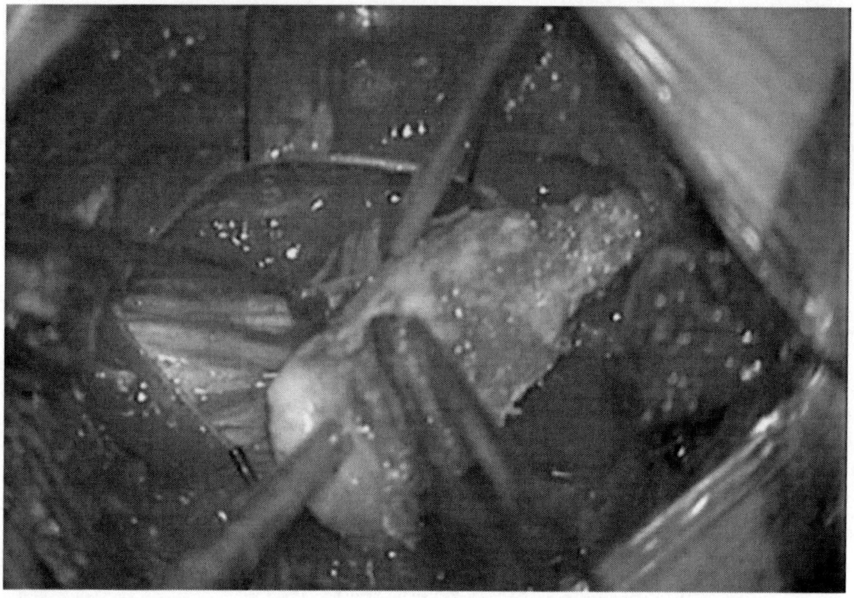

Image 5.

## REFERENCES

[1] Mawrin, C., Perry, A. Pathological classification and molecular genetics of meningiomas. *J. Neurooncol.* [Internet]. 2010 Sep. [cited 2014 Sep. 13]; 99(3):379–91. Available from: http://www.ncbi.nlm.nih.gov/pubmed/20809251.

[2] Powell, M. Sir Victor Horsley-an inspiration. *BMJ* [Internet]. 2006 Dec. 23 [cited 2014 Sep. 13]; 333(7582):1317–9. Available from: http://www.pubmedcentral.nih.gov/article render.fcgi?artid=1761176&tool=pmcentrez&rendertype=abstract.

[3] Guidetti, B. Removal of extramedullary benign spinal cord tumours. *Advances and Technical Standards in Neurosurgery*, vol. 1. 1974. pp. 173–97.

[4] Cohen-Gadol, A. A., Spencer, D. D., Krauss, W. E. The development of techniques for resection of spinal cord tumors by Harvey W. Cushing. *J. Neurosurg. Spine* [Internet]. 2005 Jan. [cited 2014 Sep. 13];2(1):92–7. Available from: http://www.ncbi.nlm.nih.gov /pubmed/15658135.

[5] Talacchi, A., Biroli, A., Soda, C., Masotto, B., Bricolo, A. Surgical management of ventral and ventrolateral foramen magnum meningiomas: report on a 64-case series and review of the literature. *Neurosurg. Rev.* [Internet]. 2012 Jul. [cited 2014 Sep. 13];35 (3):359–67; discussion 367–8. Available from: http://www.ncbi.nlm.nih.gov/pubmed/ 22430127.

[6] Helseth, A., Mørk, S. J. Primary intraspinal neoplasms in Norway, 1955 to 1986. A population-based survey of 467 patients. *J. Neurosurg.* [Internet]. 1989 Dec. [cited 2014 Sep. 13];71(6):842–5. Available from: http://www.ncbi.nlm.nih.gov/pubmed/ 2585075.

[7] Gottfried, O. N., Gluf, W., Quinones-Hinojosa, A., Kan, P., Schmidt, M. H. Spinal meningiomas: surgical management and outcome. *Neurosurg. Focus* [Internet]. 2003 Jun. 15;14(6):e2. Available from: http://www.ncbi.nlm.nih.gov/pubmed/15669787.

[8] Solero, C. L., Fornari, M., Giombini, S., Lasio, G., Oliveri, G., Cimino, C. et al. Spinal meningiomas: review of 174 operated cases. *Neurosurgery* [Internet]. 1989 Jul. [cited 2014 Jul. 25];54(1):95. Available from: http://www.ncbi.nlm.nih.gov/pubmed/2671779.

[9] Souweidane, M. M., Benjamin, V. Spinal cord meningiomas. *Neurosurg. Clin. N. Am.* [Internet]. 1994 Apr. [cited 2014 Sep. 4];5(2):283–91. Available from: http://www.ncbi.nlm.nih.gov/pubmed/8032227.

[10] Ambekar, S., Sharma, M., Kukreja, S., Nanda, A. Complications and outcomes of surgery for spinal meningioma: a Nationwide Inpatient Sample analysis from 2003 to 2010. *Clin. Neurol. Neurosurg.* [Internet]. Elsevier B.V.; 2014 Mar. [cited 2014 Aug. 14];118:65–8. Available from: http://www.ncbi.nlm.nih.gov/pubmed/24529232.

[11] Cheng, M. K. Spinal cord tumors in the People's Republic of China: a statistical review. *Neurosurgery* [Internet]. 1982 Jan. [cited 2014 Sep. 13];10(1):22–4. Available from: http://www.ncbi.nlm.nih.gov/pubmed/7057974.

[12] Abul-Kasim, K., Thurnher, M. M., McKeever, P., Sundgren, P. C. Intradural spinal tumors: current classification and MRI features. *Neuroradiology* [Internet]. 2008 Apr. [cited 2014 Sep. 13];50(4):301–14. Available from: http://www.ncbi.nlm.nih.gov/pubmed/18084751.

[13] Halliday, A. L., Sobel, R. A., Martuza, R. L. Benign spinal nerve sheath tumors: their occurrence sporadically and in neurofibromatosis types 1 and 2. *J. Neurosurg.* [Internet]. 1991 Feb. [cited 2014 Sep. 14];74(2):248–53. Available from: http://www.ncbi.nlm.nih.gov/pubmed/1846409.

[14] Tsai, E. C., Butler, J., Benzel, E. C. Chapter 57 Spinal Meningiomas. *Meningiomas: diagnosis, treatment and outcome*. 2008. pp. 529–39.

[15] Calogero, J. A., Moossy, J. Extradural spinal meningiomas. Report of four cases. *J. Neurosurg.* [Internet]. 1972 Oct. [cited 2014 Sep. 9];37(4):442–7. Available from: http://www.ncbi.nlm.nih.gov/pubmed/5070871.

[16] Gambardella, G., Toscano, S., Staropoli, C., Longo, M., D'Amico, D., Marafioti, T. et al. Epidural spinal meningioma. Role of magnetic resonance in differential diagnosis. *Acta Neurochir.* (Wien) [Internet]. 1990 Jan. [cited 2014 Sep. 10];107(1-2):70–3. Available from: http://www.ncbi.nlm.nih.gov/pubmed/2096614.

[17] Frank, B. L., Harrop, J. S., Hanna, A., Ratliff, J. Cervical extradural meningioma: case report and literature review. *J. Spinal Cord Med.* [Internet]. 2008 Jan;31(3):302–5. Available from: http://www.pubmedcentral.nih.gov/articlerender.fcgi?artid=2565566&tool=pmcentrez&rendertype=abstract.

[18] Birch, B., DK, R. Intradural extramedullary spinal lesions in EC B (ed.). *Spinal surgical techniques, complication avoidance and management*, vol. 1. 2005. pp. 948–60.

[19] Levy, W. J., Bay, J., Dohn, D. Spinal cord meningioma. *J. Neurosurg.* [Internet]. 1982 Dec;57(6):804–12. Available from: http://www.ncbi.nlm.nih.gov/pubmed/7143063.

[20] Cohen-Gadol, A. A., Zikel, O. M., Koch, C. A., Scheithauer, B. W., Krauss, W. E. Spinal meningiomas in patients younger than 50 years of age: a 21-year experience. *J. Neurosurg.* [Internet]. 2003 Apr;98(3 Suppl):258–63. Available from: http://www.ncbi.nlm.nih.gov/pubmed/12691381.

[21] Peker, S., Cerçi, A., Ozgen, S., Isik, N., Kalelioglu, M., Pamir, M. N. Spinal meningiomas: evaluation of 41 patients. *J. Neurosurg. Sci.* [Internet]. 2005 Mar. [cited 2014 Sep. 13];49(1):7–11. Available from: http://www.ncbi.nlm.nih.gov/pubmed/15990713.

[22] Salpietro, F. M., Alafaci, C., Lucerna, S., Iacopino, D. G., Tomasello, F. Do spinal meningiomas penetrate the pial layer? Correlation between magnetic resonance imaging and microsurgical findings and intracranial tumor interfaces. *Neurosurgery* [Internet]. 1997 Jul. [cited 2014 Sep. 4];41(1):254–7; discussion 257–8. Available from: http://www.ncbi.nlm.nih.gov/pubmed/9218314.

[23] Setzer, M., Vatter, H., Marquardt, G., Seifert, V., Vrionis, F. D. Management of spinal meningiomas: surgical results and a review of the literature. *Neurosurg. Focus* [Internet]. 2007 Jan. [cited 2014 Jul. 25];23(4):E14. Available from: http://www.ncbi.nlm.nih.gov/pubmed/17961038.

[24] Pravdenkova, S., Al-Mefty, O., Sawyer, J., Husain, M. Progesterone and estrogen receptors: opposing prognostic indicators in meningiomas. *J. Neurosurg.* [Internet]. 2006 Aug. [cited 2014 Sep. 13];105(2):163–73. Available from: http://www.ncbi.nlm.nih.gov/pubmed/17219818.

[25] Gruber, T., Dare, A. O., Balos, L. L., Lele, S., Fenstermaker, R. A. Multiple meningiomas arising during long-term therapy with the progesterone agonist megestrol acetate. Case report. *J. Neurosurg.* [Internet]. 2004 Feb. [cited 2014 Sep. 13];100(2):328–31. Available from: http://www.ncbi.nlm.nih.gov/pubmed/15086241.

[26] Milenković, S., Berisavac, J., Cvetković-Dozić, D., Skender-Gazibara, M., Bojović, V., Berisavac, I. Hormone receptors in benign intracranial meningiomas. *J. BUON* [Internet]. [cited 2014 Sep. 13]; 9(3):295–8. Available from: http://www.ncbi.nlm.nih.gov/pubmed/17415829.

[27] Preston-Martin, S., Monroe, K., Lee, P. J., Bernstein, L., Kelsey, J., Henderson, S. et al. Spinal meningiomas in women in Los Angeles County: investigation of an etiological hypothesis. *Cancer Epidemiol. Biomarkers Prev.* [Internet]. 1995 Jun. [cited 2014 Sep. 13];4(4):333–9. Available from: http://www.ncbi.nlm.nih.gov/pubmed/7655327.

[28] Schwartz, T., McCormick, P. Spinal Cord tumors in Adults. *Youmans Neurological Surgery*, Vol. 4. 2004. pp. 4817–34.

[29] Haque, R., Kellner, C. P., McCormick, P. C. Chapter 39 Current Surgical Techniques in the treatment of spinal meningiomas. *Al-Mefty's meningiomas*. 2011. pp. 375–82.

[30] King, A. T., Sharr, M. M., Gullan, R. W., Bartlett, J. R. Spinal meningiomas: a 20-year review. *Br. J. Neurosurg.* [Internet]. 1998 Dec; 12(6):521–6. Available from: http://www.ncbi.nlm.nih.gov/pubmed/10070460.

[31] Gezen, F., Kahraman, S., Canakci, Z., Bedük, A. Review of 36 cases of spinal cord meningioma. *Spine* (Phila Pa 1976) [Internet]. 2000 Mar. 15;25(6):727–31. Available from: http://www.ncbi.nlm.nih.gov/pubmed/10752106.

[32] Rasmussen, T. B., Kernohan, J. W., Adson, A. W. Pathologic classification, with surgical consideration, of intraspinal tumors. *Ann. Surg.* [Internet]. 1940 Apr. [cited 2014 Sep. 14];111(4):513–30. Available from: http://www.pubmedcentral.nih.gov/articlerender.fcgi?artid=1390770&tool=pmcentrez&rendertype=abstract.

[33] Klekamp, J., Samii, M. Surgical results for spinal meningiomas. *Surg. Neurol.* [Internet]. 1999 Dec. [cited 2014 Sep. 2];52(6):552–62. Available from: http://www.ncbi.nlm.nih.gov/pubmed/10660020.

[34] Roux, F. X., Nataf, F., Pinaudeau, M., Borne, G., Devaux, B., Meder, J. F. Intraspinal meningiomas: review of 54 cases with discussion of poor prognosis factors and modern therapeutic management. *Surg. Neurol.* [Internet]. 1996 Nov. [cited 2014 Jul. 25];46(5): 458–63; discussion 463–4. Available from: http://www.ncbi.nlm.nih.gov/pubmed/8874546.

[35] Ozgen, S., Konya, D. Chapter 46 Spinal Meningiomas. *Meningiomas: A comprehensive Text*. 2010. pp. 569–80.

[36] Nadkarni, T. Spinal Schwannomas and Meningiomas. *Ramamurthi and Tandon's Textbook of Neurosurgery*. Jaypee; 2012. pp. 1202–9.

[37] Wang, A. M., Haykal, H. A. Thoracic spinal meningioma associated with hydrocephalic dementia. *AJNR Am. J. Neuroradiol.* [Internet]. [cited 2014 Sep. 10];8 (2):383–4. Available from: http://www.ncbi.nlm.nih.gov/pubmed/3105299.

[38] Feldmann, E., Bromfield, E., Navia, B., Pasternak, G. W., Posner, J. B. Hydrocephalic dementia and spinal cord tumor. Report of a case and review of the literature. *Arch. Neurol.* [Internet]. 1986 Jul. [cited 2014 Sep. 10];43(7):714–8. Available from: http://www.ncbi.nlm.nih.gov/pubmed/3729751.

[39] Turner, G. A., Jayasinghe, G., Rossato, R. G. Cervical meningioma and lumbar stenosis: a case presenting as immobility. *Aust. N. Z. J. Med.* [Internet]. 1997 Aug. [cited 2014 Sep. 10];27(4):442–3. Available from: http://www.ncbi.nlm.nih.gov/pubmed/9448889.

[40] Schroth, G., Thron, A., Guhl, L., Voigt, K., Niendorf, H. P., Garces, L. R. Magnetic resonance imaging of spinal meningiomas and neurinomas. Improvement of imaging by paramagnetic contrast enhancement. *J. Neurosurg.* [Internet]. 1987 May [cited 2014 Sep. 10];66(5):695–700. Available from: http://www.ncbi.nlm.nih.gov/pubmed/3572496.

[41] Alorainy, I. A. Dural tail sign in spinal meningiomas. *Eur. J. Radiol.* [Internet]. 2006 Dec. [cited 2014 Sep. 10];60(3):387–91. Available from: http://www.ncbi.nlm.nih.gov/pubmed/16876365.

[42] Quekel, L. G., Versteege, C. W. The "dural tail sign" in MRI of spinal meningiomas. *J. Comput. Assist. Tomogr.* [Internet]. [cited 2014 Sep. 10];19(6):890–2. Available from: http://www.ncbi.nlm.nih.gov/pubmed/8537521.

[43] Messori, A., Rychlicki, F., Salvolini, U. Spinal epidural en-plaque meningioma with an unusual pattern of calcification in a 14-year-old girl: case report and review of the literature. *Neuroradiology* [Internet]. 2002 Mar. [cited 2014 Sep. 10];44(3):256–60. Available from: http://www.ncbi.nlm.nih.gov/pubmed/11942384.

[44] D'Amico, A., Napoli, M., Cirillo, M., D'Arco, F., D'Anna, G., Caranci, F. et al. Imaging of cervical extradural en-plaque meningioma. A case report. *Neuroradiol. J.* [Internet]. 2012 Nov. [cited 2014 Sep. 10];25(5): 598–603. Available from: http://www.ncbi.nlm.nih.gov/pubmed/24029096.

[45] Zozulya, Y. P., Slynko, Y. I., Al-Qashqish, I. I. Surgical treatment of ventral and ventrolateral intradural extramedullary tumors of craniovertebral and upper-cervical localization. *Asian J. Neurosurg.* [Internet]. 2010 Jul. [cited 2014 Sep. 11];5(2):35–45. Available from: http://www.pubmedcentral.nih.gov/articlerender.fcgi?artid=3201079&tool=pmcentrez&rendertype=abstract.

[46] Queckenstedt, H. Zur Diagnose der Ruckenmarkskompression. *Dtsch Z. Nervenheilkd.* 1916;(55):325–33.

[47] Caroli, E., Acqui, M., Roperto, R., Ferrante, L., D'Andrea, G. Spinal en plaque meningiomas: a contemporary experience. *Neurosurgery* [Internet]. 2004 Dec. [cited 2014 Sep. 10];55(6):1275–9; discussion 1279. Available from: http://www.ncbi.nlm.nih.gov/pubmed/15574209.

[48] Saito, T., Arizono, T., Maeda, T., Terada, K., Iwamoto, Y. A novel technique for surgical resection of spinal meningioma. *Spine* (Phila Pa 1976) [Internet]. 2001 Aug. 15 [cited 2014 Sep. 10];26(16):1805–8. Available from: http://www.ncbi.nlm.nih.gov/pubmed/11493855.

[49] Haegelen, C., Morandi, X., Riffaud, L., Amlashi, S. F. A., Leray, E., Brassier, G. Results of spinal meningioma surgery in patients with severe preoperative neurological deficits. *Eur. Spine J.* [Internet]. 2005 Jun. [cited 2014 Jul. 25];14(5):440–4. Available from: http://www.pubmedcentral.nih.gov/articlerender.fcgi?artid=3454661&tool=pmcentrez&rendertype=abstract.

[50] Mirimanoff, R. O., Dosoretz, D. E., Linggood, R. M., Ojemann, R. G., Martuza, R. L. Meningioma: analysis of recurrence and progression following neurosurgical resection. *J. Neurosurg.* [Internet]. 1985 Jan. [cited 2014 Sep. 14];62(1):18–24. Available from: http://www.ncbi.nlm.nih.gov/pubmed/3964853.

[51] Namer, I. J., Pamir, M. N., Benli, K., Saglam, S., Erbengi, A. Spinal meningiomas. *Neurochirurgia* (Stuttg.) [Internet]. 1987 Jan. [cited 2014 Sep. 14];30(1):11–5. Available from: http://www.ncbi.nlm.nih.gov/pubmed/3561635.

[52] Ciappetta, P., Domenicucci, M., Raco, A. Spinal meningiomas: prognosis and recovery factors in 22 cases with severe motor deficits. *Acta Neurol. Scand.* [Internet]. 1988 Jan. [cited 2014 Sep. 13];77(1):27–30. Available from: http://www.ncbi.nlm.nih.gov/pubmed/3354308.

[53] Schaller, B. Spinal meningioma: relationship between histological subtypes and surgical outcome? *J. Neurooncol.* [Internet]. 2005 Nov. [cited 2014 Sep. 13];75(2):157–61. Available from: http://www.ncbi.nlm.nih.gov/pubmed/16132511.

[54] Muroi, C., Fandino, J., Coluccia, D., Berkmann, S., Fathi, A.-R., Landolt, H. 5-Aminolevulinic acid fluorescence-guided surgery for spinal meningioma. *World Neurosurg.* [Internet]. Elsevier Inc; 2012 [cited 2014 Jul. 25];80(1-2):223.e1–3. Available from: http://www.ncbi.nlm.nih.gov/pubmed/23247024.

[55] Coluccia, D., Fandino, J., Fujioka, M., Cordovi, S., Muroi, C., Landolt, H. Intraoperative 5-aminolevulinic-acid-induced fluorescence in meningiomas. *Acta Neurochir.* (Wien) [Internet]. 2010 Oct. [cited 2014 Jul. 25];152(10):1711–9. Available from: http://www.ncbi.nlm.nih.gov/pubmed/20535506.

In: Current Management of Central Nervous System ... ISBN: 978-1-63483-856-6
Editors: Steven D. Chang and Anand Veeravagu 

*Chapter 10*

# SURGICAL MANAGEMENT OF FORAMEN MAGNUM MENINGIOMAS

***Tej D. Azad, BA, Owais Ahmad, MD, Ian D. Connolly, MS, Anand Veeravagu, MD, Inderpreet Bhatti, BA and Steven D. Chang, MD***

Department of Neurosurgery, Stanford University
School of Medicine, Stanford, CA, US

## ABSTRACT

Foramen magnum meningiomas (FMM) are insidious tumors that pose marked challenges to the skull base neurosurgeon. The indolent clinical course of FMM and the gradual onset of symptoms contribute to its delayed diagnosis and relatively large size at presentation. Symptoms are often produced by the compression of surrounding structures (such as the upper cervical spinal cord, lower cranial nerves, and vertebral artery) within a critically confined space. Several surgical approaches have been offered to achieve complete tumor resection. We provide an overview of key clinical considerations in the management of patients with FMM and detail important surgical approaches to these lesions.

**Keywords:** meningioma, foramen magnum, craniovertebral junction, skull base, far lateral approach

## INTRODUCTION

Meningiomas are slow growing benign tumors that originate from arachnoid cells of the craniovertebral junction (CVJ) [1]. They comprise 70% of all benign tumors and 14.3% to 19% of all primary intracranial neoplasms [2]. Foramen magnum meningiomas (FMM) comprise 1.8% to 3.2% of all meningiomas. FMM are challenging lesions to treat due to their indolent and insidious nature.

George et al. defined the location of these lesions in the foramen magnum as a meningioma occurring in the region ranging anteriorly from the inferior third of the clivus to the superior edge of the body of the C2 vertebrae, laterally from the jugular tubercle to the upper laminae of the C2 vertebrae, and posteriorly from the anterior border of the squamous occipital bone to the spinal process of the C2 vertebrae [3].

Within this region, the tumor can be further described by its location on the anterior, posterior, and lateral axes. Anterior FMM have an insertion that is on both sides of the anterior midline and displace the spinal cord posteriorly, creating a narrow corridor for surgical intervention. Lateral FMM often adhere between the midline and the dentate ligament, a white fibrous sheet spanning from the pia mater medially to the dura laterally within the spinal column. Unlike anterior FMM, lesions at this location shift the spinal cord posteriorly and laterally, yielding a wider corridor for surgical intervention. FMM can also be located ventrally to the dentate ligament and are referred to as posterior FMM. Anterolateral FMM are the most commonly observed lesion, comprising 68% to 98% of FMM.

The location in relation to the vertebral artery (VA) and size of the tumor can be used for further classification. Lesions are most commonly found inferior to the VA, however, they can occur superiorly or laterally. FMM are considered 'small' when the lesion size is less than one third of the lateral diameter of the foramen magnum. 'Medium' and 'large' classifications are reserved for tumors that are measured between one third to one half of the lateral diameter of the foramen magnum and greater than one half of the lateral diameter of the foramen magnum, respectively. Additionally, tumors can be classified according to the compartment of development: intradural, extradural, and intraextradural. Intradural tumors are most commonly observed while extradural tumors are typically more invasive with higher rates of subtotal resection (STR).

The diagnosis of FMM is challenging. Early symptoms are nonspecific due to the slow growth of these tumors. This often results in a long interval between the onset of disease related symptoms and its diagnosis.

Tumor resection is considered to be the ideal treatment as it is recommended to patients with reasonably sized tumors in the foramen magnum with limited space for further growth. There are several surgical approaches to resecting FMM, with significant consideration to their dural attachment and location of the tumor.

## Clinical Presentation

Despite the growing capabilities of magnetic resonance imaging (MRI), the mean duration of symptoms before the diagnosis of FMM is 30.8 months with a mean age at the time of diagnosis reported as 55 years [4]. FMM produce symptoms that are similar to degenerative and demyelinating diseases causing possible misdiagnosis as multiple sclerosis, cervical myelopathy, syringomyelia, or amyotrophic lateral sclerosis. Symptoms are often due to the compression of adjacent structures such as the medulla oblongata, the upper cervical spinal cord, the lower cranial nerves, or the VA. The most commonly reported early symptom is neck pain, manifesting from compression of the C2 nerve distribution. This pain may present independently or may be accompanied by occipital headaches and sensory disturbances such as cold or burning dysesthesias, astereognosis, and anesthesia.

With continued tumor progression, patients may experience spastic quadriparesis, lower cranial nerve palsies, and difficulty maintaining balance. Atrophy of the intrinsic muscles of the hand, trapezius, and sternocleidomastoid has also been noted as a later presentation [1].

## SURGICAL ANATOMY

There are several critical neuroanatomical and vascular structures within the foramen magnum. The foramen magnum itself contains the cerebellar tonsils, the inferior vermis, the fourth ventricle, the caudal aspect of the medulla, the lower cranial nerves (IX-XII), the rostral aspect of the spinal cord and the upper cervical nerves (C1 and C2). Cranial nerves IX through XI originate as rootlets along the anterior medulla, with cranial nerve XI originating midway between the anterior and posterior spinal rootlets of the spinal cord. After the spinal accessory rootlets join the $9^{th}$, $10^{th}$ and the cranial portion of the $11^{th}$ nerve, these nerves exit the skull through the jugular foramen. Cranial nerve XII exits anteriorly from the medulla in the preolivary sulcus, passing posterior to the VA on its way to the hypoglossal canal.

The critical vascular structures relevant to FMM include the VAs (V3 and V4 segments), posterior inferior cerebral arteries (PICA), the anterior and posterior spinal arteries, and the meningeal branches of the vertebral, external, and internal carotid arteries. V3, also known as the suboccipital segment, arises from the C2 transverse process and extends to the dura of the foramen magnum. It is surrounded by a periosteal sheath that invaginates into the dura, when piercing the foramen magnum lateral dura. This sheath is continuous with the outer layer of the dura. The C2 radicular artery, the posterior meningeal artery, and the posterior spinal artery are small collateral branches that arise from this segment.

The V3 segment of the VA consists of three portions: vertical, horizontal and oblique. The vertical portion lies between the transverse processes of C2 and C1, while the horizontal portion lies in the groove of the posterior arch of the atlas. The oblique portion originates from the groove and continues up to the dura mater. These relative positions can change with head rotation and during surgical positioning. In a neutral head position, the vertical and horizontal portions are perpendicular. Whereas head rotation is required for the anterolateral surgical approach, causing the vertical and horizontal segments to be stretched and consequently run in parallel.

After piercing the lateral aspect of the occipitoatlantal dura mater, V3 becomes the V4. The V4 ascends from the dura to the anterior aspect of the pontomedullary sulcus and forms the basilar artery after joining its opposing segment. At the level of the foramen magnum, the V4 is at the origin of the PICA, the anterior spinal artery, and the anterior and posterior meningeal arteries. It is important to note that there are occasional anatomical variants of the VA that are important to know and identify preoperatively:

- In 40% of patients, the size of the VA differs. One side may be dominant while the alternate side can be hypoplastic or atretic
- The V3 segment may end at the posterior inferior cerebellar or occipital artery
- The V3 segment may have an intradural course that corresponds to a VA duplication
- A pro-atlantal artery may consist of a persistent congenital anastomosis between the carotid artery and the VA

- The groove of the atlas arch can form a tunnel if the occipitoatlantal membrane is calcified or ossified

## CLASSIFICATION

Appropriate classification of FMM can be useful to conceptualize the relative benefits of the surgical approaches that will be discussed and to navigate through the critical structures that can be involved in FMM resection. FMM originate in the spine and displace the VA superiorly. Those that begin at the entrance of the VA often encase the VA and displace it away from the petrous bone, while also displacing the medulla away from the VA. FMM with cranial origins are anterior or anterolateral to the entrance of the VA and they displace the VA and medulla away from the petrous bone. This results in the VA and the medulla to be in close apposition if the origin was along the lower clivus at or above the vertebrobasilar (VB) junction. If the origin is further inferior to the clivus than the VB junction, the tumor may shift the relation between the medulla and the VA. Spinocranial FMM originate inferior to the foramen magnum and thus displace the cranial nerves to the superior aspect of the tumor, enabling safe resection from below without overt risk to the cranial nerves. Cranial FMM, which arise at the anterior lip of the foramen magnum, are medial to the jugular foramen and will shift the cranial nerves posteriorly and laterally.

## SURGICAL APPROACH

Though surgical resection has demonstrated promise for many patients with FMM, the decision to pursue an operative course of treatment must be made judiciously. Patient and tumor characteristics must be taken into account in order to arrive at the optimal management strategy for patients with FMM. There is evidence that small tumors in elderly patients who remain asymptomatic may be best managed with careful observation, rather than surgical intervention [5].

For many patients, surgical resection is the optimal management strategy. The goal of surgery for FMM is to preserve and improve neurological function by radical tumor removal, regardless of tumor size. Complete removal should be attempted during the first operation, as radical resection of a recurrent tumor is less likely to be achieved. Due to clinical and anatomic constraints, the surgeon may be forced to accept STR. In such situations when tumor fragments remain adherent to vital neurovascular structures, adjuvant radiosurgical treatment may be considered.

The choice of surgical approach remains a source of debate in the management of FMM. This is in part due to the number of surgical techniques that have been offered to achieve successful resection but also due to the challenging anatomic location of these tumors in the foramen magnum. Though many surgical approaches have been proposed, certain methods present theoretical advantages rather than clinically useful benefits. For example, the transoral-transclival removal proposed by Miller and Crockard requires dural repair that can often prove to be clinically challenging [6]. This is an exemplar of other anterior approaches, which have not received widespread acceptance.

Anterior approaches have been associated with an increased risk of cerebrospinal fluid (CSF) leakage and infection [7, 8]. Moreover, the goal of complete resection can be difficult to achieve due to inadequate exposure of the tumor's lateral margins and inadequate proximal control of the vertebral arteries [7, 8].

While the risks associated with transoral approach are considered to outweigh potential benefits, alternative ventral approaches have emerged that take advantage of advances in endoscopic technique. Endoscopic transoral approaches have been proposed for lesions of the ventral CVJ and shown to be effective [9]. However, the advent of endoscopic endonasal approaches to the CVJ has limited adoption of the endoscopic transoral approach [10]. While case series using the endoscopic endonasal approach have centered on lesions of the upper to middle clivus and suprasellar regions, the foramen magnum can also be accessed. The major benefit of this approach is the avoidance of brain retraction, which is often required in open approaches to the ventral foramen magnum [11]. The major complication of the endoscopic endonasal approach is CSF leakage, though this will likely improve with sophistication of reconstructive technique. Further studies are needed to determine the efficacy of this approach for FMM [12].

Posterior and posterolateral FMM can be safely resected through a standard midline suboccipital approach. However, controversy remains regarding the optimal management of anterior or anterolateral lesions. For these ventral lesions, the standard midline suboccipital approach can result in undue brainstem retraction, higher rates of STR, and postoperative morbidity, due to inadequate exposure [13, 14]. Outcomes following the suboccipital approach for ventral FMM are contested. Some have argued that the patients operated on through conventional suboccipital approaches have worse clinical outcomes than patients that arc operated on through the lateral transcondylar route [8, 13].

Others have presented evidence of gross total resection (GTR) and equivalent outcomes for these tumors using a suboccipital approach [15-17].

Independent of the technical variations and the degree of bone removal, modern surgical approaches to the lower clivus and anterior foramen magnum derive from the posterolateral craniotomy originally described by Roberto Heros and Bernard George [3, 18]. Selection of surgical approach should take several factors into consideration, including tumor size and location, osseous involvement, patient neurological status, and location of the tumor relative to the dura (Table 1). Here we will provide a detailed description of the suboccipital and far lateral/transcondylar approaches to FMM.

## Suboccipital

A standard midline suboccipital craniectomy in concert with an upper cervical laminectomy (C1, occasionally C2) is the preferred approach for most of the lesions that originate posterior to the dentate ligaments. Patients may be oriented in a semi-sitting position, with the head slightly flexed and secured in the Mayfield head holder or in lateral decubitus.

A vertical skin incision is initiated at the superior nuchal line and is carried down through the galea and over the occipital bone. The incision is continued down through the posterior border of the sternocleidomastoid and trapezius muscles, paravertebrally to the level of C3.

**Table 1. Factors to consider for selection of surgical approach**

| |
|---|
| Tumor size |
| Tumor location |
| Extent of osseous involvement |
| Neurological status of patient |
| Dural involvement |

The spinous process of C2 is a tactile guide to the position of the foramen magnum. It allows subperiosteal dissection of the suboccipital region to be carried along the posterior arch of C1. The paravertebral muscles are detached from the occipital squama and progressively sectioned with a scalpel. A retractor is progressively inserted in the incision, exposing the suboccipital triangle and maintaining the paravertebral muscle in the appropriate position. At this point, the posterior arch of C1 is identified and dissected free with a periosteal elevator to expose the mastoid process. The VA is unperturbed and the ipsilateral half of the arch of the atlas is then resected with the Leksell rongeur.

The suboccipital craniectomy is created unilaterally using a high-speed drill to thin the occipital bone. The occipital craniectomy, performed with a Leksell rongeur, includes the foramen magnum and extends to the posterior edge of the occipital condyle. If further exposure is needed, C2 and C3 laminectomy can be included. The decision to preserve the occipital condyle is tenuous and deserves careful consideration. Emissary veins opened during dissection should be coagulated, waxed immediately, and again at the end of the procedure. At this point, the surgical microscope should be introduced.

The spinal dura is opened longitudinally, medially from the entry of the VA. Extreme care must be taken when opening the circular sinus because the large venous plexus can make homeostasis significantly more challenging. The cisterna magna is opened to drain the CSF and the tumor is exposed under the arachnoid. The brainstem and VA should be identified. Exposure can be improved with gentle elevation of the cerebellum. If the tumor is anteriorly placed, the spinal cord may be displaced posteriorly and laterally. The spinal section of the accessory nerve and posterior rootlets of the first two cervical spinal nerves may be identified on the posterior aspect of the tumor. The dentate ligament, C1 and C2 rootlets can be sacrificed if necessary. However, the vessel traveling along the nerve root should be preserved to avoid spinal cord ischemia.

Before closure, the patient's blood pressure must be brought to a normotensive level for at least 10 to 15 minutes and the surgical field should be observed for oozing. The dura is closed with a pericranial graft or artificial dural substitute. The suture line is covered with fibrin glue. The closure of superficial planes consists of three layers of suture, with nylon stitches on the skin.

## Far Lateral/ Transcondylar

Different patient positioning strategies have been successfully applied and advocated by various authors, such as modified park bench, true lateral, supine with 45° body rotation, prone, and sitting. There are considerations for each strategy and potential risks.

For example, a sitting position for FMM resection may provide a wider view, gravity retraction of posterior fossa structures, and superior venous return, but is also associated with a higher risk of air embolism.

Commonly, patients are positioned in lateral decubitus and are three-quarter prone with the patient's head turned 20° to 30° toward the floor. The patient's head is secured to the operating table using a 3-pin Mayfield skull clamp, and all pressure points are adequately padded. Intraoperative neurophysiological monitoring is invaluable due to at-risk cranial nerves (VII–XI). Somatosensory evoked potentials and motor evoked potentials are also useful to mediate risk of iatrogenic injury during surgery.

A common incision is the "inverted hockey stick" incision, which requires an inverted U–shaped incision beginning at the level of the mastoid tip, curving superiorly to the superior nuchal line. The incision should curve posteriorly toward the inion and then inferiorly through the midline to the level of the C2. The skin flap is mobilized laterally and inferiorly following dissection down to the fascial plane of the superficial muscle layer. The superficial and intermediate musculature layers of the sternocleidomastoid are detached from their insertions and reflected laterally. Preservation of a muscular cuff along the nuchal line is an important aid in facilitating wound closure. The muscles are also disconnected in the midline from the spinous processes for exposure of the posterior arch of the atlas and the C2 lamina, as needed.

After identification of the spinous process of C2 and the posterior tubercle of C1, subperiosteal dissection is performed to identify the sulcus arteriosus and the VA. The VA is displaced superiorly to view C1, the lateral margin of the laminectomy at that level. Though rarely necessary, skeletonization of the VA can be performed and may be of use in surgery for minor lesions ventral to the CVJ or when proximal control of the extradural segment of the VA is required. If this is required, the dorsal aspect of the transverse foramen can be removed to mobilize the VA medially and caudally. Removal of the ipsilateral posterior arch of C1 with a contralateral partial hemilaminectomy is completed using a high-speed drill.

A modification at this point, designated a "lazy" far lateral approach has recently been proposed. The key nuance in this approach is the management of the VA. When the lazy far lateral approach is used, the VA is reflected laterally, encased in its periosteal sheath, and wrapped in the dura. This greatly minimizes the risk for vertebral injury while preserving a wide working space. To accomplish this step, drilling must be performed laterally, and an incision should be made medially to the location at which the VA pierces the dura. The authors report no surgical mortality or VA injuries in 44 patients who received this modified approach [19].

A posterolateral retrocondylar craniotomy is performed. This procedure includes the posterolateral rim of the foramen magnum, extending laterally to expose the medial edge of the sigmoid sinus. It is usually completed with the footplate of a high-speed drill. If partial mastoidectomy is necessary, the mastoid bone air cells must be meticulously obliterated with a bone wax-bone dust mixture to prevent postoperative CSF leak and infection. The lateral edge of the foramen magnum is drilled away, continuing into the condylar fossa and to the condyle. Venous bleeding should be expected at the condylar canal, containing the condylar emissary vein. This important landmark is a useful marker for the posterior aspect of the occipital condyle. Any bleeding that occurs can be controlled with bone wax obliteration and drilling may continue directly along this channel through the bone wax.

Drilling of the occipital condyle is a contested technical advantage among surgeons employing the far lateral approach.

Proponents advocate that it provides a more direct approach to the anterior clivus and anterolateral lesions, increasing the visibility from a standard posterolateral retrocondylar craniotomy by 16° [20].

It must be noted that these measurements were achieved using cadaveric studies that did not account for space-occupying lesions that expand the surgical corridor.

As a technical aside, an important concept for surgical management of foramen magnum lesions is the definition of the surgical corridor. The corridor involves the space between the lateral margin of the CVJ and the medial aspect of the occipital condyle. This corridor is often enlarged by a space-occupying lesion that displaces the brainstem, such as FMM. It can also be expanded manually by bone removal and drilling. Most tumors have created a surgical corridor that is wide enough for safe resection without extensive condyle drilling, once symptomatic. Nanda et al. affirmed that the resectability of an FMM is influenced by the nature, location, and extension of the tumor and not by the extent of bone removal [20]. However, the authors noted that occipital condyle drilling is necessary to treat anteriorly located lesions without sufficient lateral extension in addition to large meningiomas associated with VA encasement or bone invasion.

If drilling of the condyle is determined to be necessary, it begins with removal of the cortical bone from its posteromedial aspect. Cancellous bone is found and drilled until the posterior wall of the hypoglossal canal is encountered, which represents the anterior limit of the condyle drilling and the second layer of cortical bone. The intracranial opening of the hypoglossal canal is usually located just above the occipital condyle, at the junction of its middle and posterior thirds.

It extends anterolaterally with the extracranial foramen located at the junction of the anterior and middle thirds of the condyle. In the cases where it is indicated, drilling of the posterior third of the occipital condyle provides access to the majority of anterior or anterolateral FMM without overt sacrifice of craniovertebral stability.

A C-shaped incision is fashioned in the dura, extending medially from the transverse-sigmoid junction, paramedian to the occipital sinus, and caudally at the midline. The amount of cervical dural opening is dictated by the portion of the tumor that extends below the craniocervical junction. The dura is reflected laterally and held in place with nylon sutures. If further lateral mobilization of the VA is necessary for adequate exposure, the dural opening can be modified and centered on the dural ring involving this artery. A large cuff is left surrounding the VA sheath to aid in watertight closure at the end of the resection. The posterior meningeal artery arising from the horizontal suboccipital VA can be coagulated and divided for better exposure. This also represents the initial step of tumor devascularization.

After the dura is opened, lateral FMM are usually immediately visible and their dural attachment is directly accessible. However, anterior or anterolateral FMM may be completely or partially hidden by the neural elements. The primary step following the dural opening is to identify and open the surgical corridor [21]. The VA is identified by following the course of the V3 segment where it pierces the dura mater. As previously described, the rostral dentate ligament lies at the level of the foramen magnum and is a consistent indicator of that transitional point. The upper 2 or 3 dentate ligaments may be sectioned to reduce traction on the spinal cord during dissection. The first cervical nerve root may be divided to mobilize the upper cervical cord with negligible clinical consequences. Every effort should be made for early detachment of the tumor from its dural insertion and consequently from its vascular supply.

This maneuver makes tumor resection through the small corridor between the cranial nerves and brainstem easier. Henceforth, the microdissection should be guided by the relationship between the tumor and the VA. Foramen magnum meningiomas that arise below the VA push the lower cranial nerves superiorly and posteriorly. The resection should begin at the inferior pole of the lesion.

After the capsule is opened, internal debulking can be achieved with suction technique, $CO_2$ laser, or ultrasonic aspirator, depending on the surgeon's preference and tumor consistency. The predictability of the path of the lower cranial nerves can be lost in FMM that arise above the VA. It may be valuable to identify their distal segment just proximal to the jugular foramen and dissect them free from the tumor in such cases.

Some FMM will demonstrate an invasive pattern of growth, resulting in the encasement of the VA. In these cases, preoperative evaluation of the intracranial course of the VA and the PICA is necessary. An arachnoidal plane at the tumor-vascular interface can often be elicited, though a small tumor ring may need to be abandoned around the intracranial VA. Once the tumor has been removed, the dural base must be inspected, scraped free of residual tumor debris and thoroughly coagulated.

After the tumor is removed and hemostasis is achieved, the dura is closed. Tenting sutures are transected and the dural flap is reflected back from lateral to medial. Watertight suturing should be pursued. If not possible, dural substitutes may be employed. The occipital bone fragment is then replaced. The ends of the oblique muscles are rejoined, and the semispinalis and splenius capitis muscles are sutured in layers. Afterwards, watertight sutures are applied to the aponeurosis, the subcutaneous tissue is sutured, and the skin is closed with sutures or staples.

### Stereotactic Radiosurgery

Stereotactic radiosurgery (SRS) has been shown to be a safe management strategy for small, minimally symptomatic FMM [22]. A recent multi-institutional study of SRS for posterior fossa meningiomas included 18 patients with FMM. The authors reported that meningiomas in clival, petrous, or cerebellopontine angle locations, compared with petroclival, tentorial, and foramen magnum location, were predictive of neurological decline after radiosurgery (OR 1.95). Further study of SRS for FMM will be valuable, but early evidence supports safe use of SRS in properly selected patients [23].

## Complications

The most frequent surgical complications associated with far lateral exposure for resection of FMM are lower cranial nerve deficits, particularly cranial nerves IX through XII [24]. Talacchi et al., in a recently published series of 64 patients with ventral and ventrolateral FMM, reported a high incidence of cranial nerve IX–X and XII dysfunctions postoperatively (44% and 33%, respectively) [24]. At their final outcome assessment, however, 66% of the cranial nerve deficits improved completely and all but 2 patients had returned to normal productive life.

Sekhar et al. demonstrated that tumor size was the most important single variable associated with early postoperative worsening in the surgical management of meningiomas of the petroclivus and foramen magnum. They identified tumor size and pial invasion as factors associated with sustained neurological deficits [25].

Craniovertebral instability is a rare outcome, but is directly related to the extent of occipital condyle resection. Removal of $\geq$50% of the condyle has been shown to produce significant hypermobility at the CVJ and necessitates posterior craniovertebral fusion [26]. A CSF fistula is a relatively common complication, occurring in 16% to 20% of patients, though is often transient [27, 28]. Incidence of CSF fistula can be mediated with careful dural and wound closure as well as perioperative external lumbar drainage. Recently reported surgical series have shown a progressive decline in mortality related to the surgical treatment of FMM. Mortality rates as high as 29% in the early 1980s have been replaced by increasingly favorable outcomes. An overall perioperative mortality rate of 0% to 3% appears to be a reasonable current estimate [24, 27].

## Clinical Outcomes

Clinical outcomes following FMM resection are generally favorable. A meta-analysis by Komotar et al. of the far lateral approach found that 80.6% of patients improved following surgery and only 9% worsened [12].

Several authors have noted dramatic improvement following resection, reporting patients with severe quadriparesis before surgery who can independently perform activities of daily living and regain normal gait at early follow up [13, 24, 29]. Reports of relatively robust clinical improvement provide room for discussion given the variation in reported resection rates for FMM. Surgical series vary markedly in the reported degree of FMM resection. In 18 surgical case series of FMM, only three reported 100% GTR. Degree of GTR ranged from 67% to 100% (Table 2). Factors that limited resection included inadequate exposure, tumor adherence to local structures, VA encasement, tumor recurrence, and invasion of the pia in the absence of an observed arachnoid plane [4].

A recent critical review by Komotar et al. of nearly 150 studies with reported FMM resection rates concluded that the far lateral approach achieved GTR in 93.2% and STR in 5.4%. Markedly worse rates were reported for studies that used the extreme lateral approach; GTR in 74.7% and STR in 25.3% [12]. Studies that drew on the far lateral approach reported no recurrences, while use of the extreme lateral approach resulted in higher recurrence rates (5.6%). It should be noted that recurrence was not observed (0%) in all cases where GTR was achieved, regardless of the approach [12].

## Conclusion

Foramen magnum meningiomas are rare lesions that present marked challenges to any surgeon. Though many surgical approaches have been proposed, we provide detailed accounts of what we consider the premier approaches for both ventral and dorsal meningiomas of the foramen magnum.

**Table 2. Outcomes for surgical management of FMM**

| Study (Author, Year) | N | GTR (%) | Mortality (%) | Morbidity (%) | Mean Follow-up, months (range) | Recurrence (%) |
|---|---|---|---|---|---|---|
| Sen 1990 [30] | 6 | 67.0 | 17.0 | 66.0 | - | - |
| Kratimenos 1993 [31] | 15 | 85.7 | 13.3 | 0.0 | - | - |
| Akalan 1994 [32] | 16 | 82.4 | 0.0 | - | 51.6 (6-84) | - |
| Bertalanffy 1996 [33] | 19 | 100.0 | 0.0 | 0.0 | 60.0 | - |
| George 1997 [14] | 31 | 96.8 | 9.7 | 0.0 | 57.6 (12-120) | 0.0 |
| Pirotte 1998 [34] | 6 | 100.0 | 16.0 | 16.0 | - | - |
| Salas 1999 [35] | 51 | 69.0 | 1.4 | 2.9 | 18.2 (1-50) | - |
| Arnautovic 2000 [36] | 18 | 67.0 | 0.0 | 5.6 | 40.0 (0 - 80) | 5.6 |
| Roberti 2001 [37] | 21 | 76.0 | 9.5 | 21.5 | 19.0 (0.2-63.6) | - |
| Goel 2001 [17] | 17 | 82.4 | 0.0 | 5.9 | 43.0 | - |
| Nanda 2002 [20] | 10 | 100.0 | 0.0 | 0.0 | - | - |
| Pamir 2004 [28] | 19 | 94.7 | 0.0 | 4.5 | 40.0 (2-120) | 0.0 |
| Bassiouni 2006 [13] | 25 | 96.0 | 4.0 | 8.0 | 73.2 (12-168) | 0.0 |
| Borba 2009 [29] | 15 | 80.0 | 0.0 | 13.3 | 23.6 (6-56) | 6.7 |
| Kandenwein 2009 [15] | 16 | 87.5 | 6.0 | 31.0 | 43.5 (24-119) | 0.0 |
| Wu 2009 [27] | 114 | 86.0 | 1.8 | - | 90.3 (1-180) | 0.9 |
| Pirotte 2010 [5] | 22 | 73.0 | 4.5 | 27.3 | 88.0 (24-168) | - |
| Talachhi 2012 [24] | 64 | 81.0 | 0.0 | - | 88.0 | 0.0 |

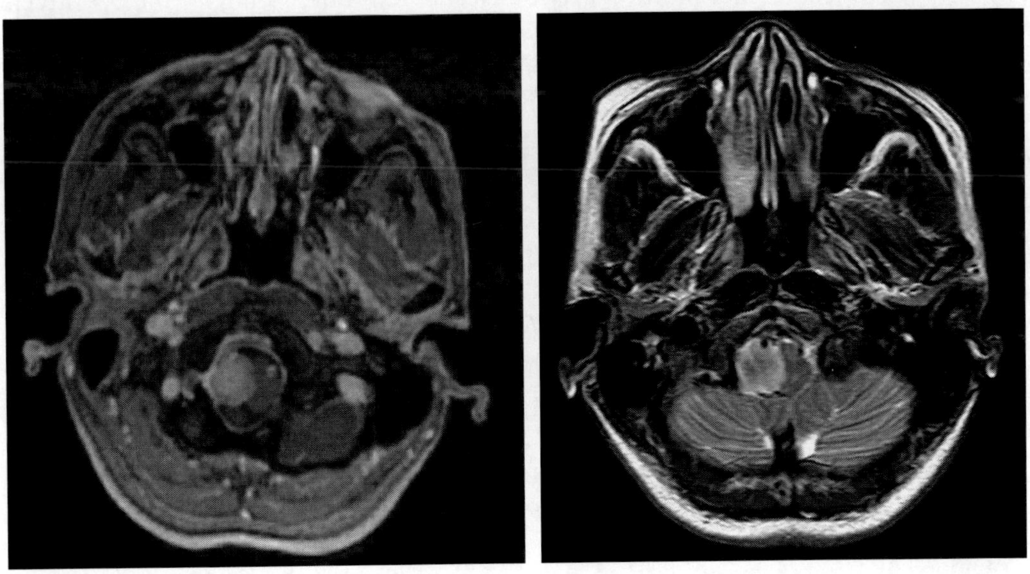

Figure 1. Pre-operative MRI demonstrating 1.7 × 1.5 cm FMM; T1 with contrast (left) and T2 (right).

The suboccipital approach for ventral FMM, far lateral approach for dorsal lesions, and other surgical approaches have respective benefits and shortcomings. Specific clinical and anatomic factors, as well as surgeon experience, should be carefully weighed to determine the optimal surgical management.

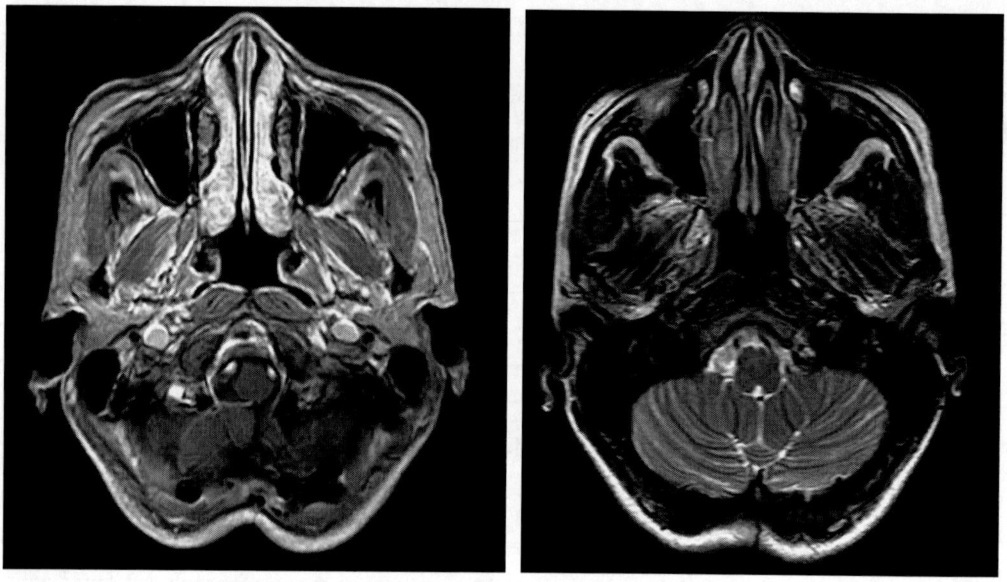

Figure 2. Post-operative MRI demonstrating GTR; T1 with contrast (left) and T2 (right).

## Illustrative Case

A 48-year-old female presented with a 10- to 15-year history of headaches. She ultimately underwent a series of MRIs that revealed an FMM measuring 1.7 times × 1.5 cm (Figure 1). Patient underwent surgical resection of this tumor and GTR was achieved. The patient suffered no perioperative complications and was neurologically intact. Postoperative MRIs confirmed complete resection of the tumor (Figure 2).

## References


[1] Boulton, M. R., Cusimano, M. D. Foramen magnum meningiomas: concepts, classifications, and nuances. *Neurosurgical focus*. 2003;14(6):e10.

[2] Wara, W. M., Sheline, G. E., Newman, H., Townsend, J. J., Boldrey, E. B. Radiation therapy of meningiomas. *The American journal of roentgenology, radium therapy, and nuclear medicine*. 1975;123(3):453-8.

[3] George, B., Dematons, C., Cophignon, J. Lateral approach to the anterior portion of the foramen magnum. Application to surgical removal of 14 benign tumors: technical note. *Surgical neurology*. 1988;29(6):484-90.

[4] Flores, B. C., Boudreaux, B. P., Klinger, D. R., Mickey, B. E., Barnett, S. L. The far-lateral approach for foramen magnum meningiomas. *Neurosurgical focus*. 2013;35(6): E12.

[5] Pirotte, B. J., Brotchi, J., DeWitte, O. Management of anterolateral foramen magnum meningiomas: surgical vs conservative decision making. *Neurosurgery*. 2010;67(3 Suppl. Operative):ons58-70; discussions.

[6] Miller, E., Crockard, H. A. Transoral transclival removal of anteriorly placed meningiomas at the foramen magnum. *Neurosurgery*. 1987;20(6):966-8.
[7] Rhoton, A. L., Jr. Meningiomas of the cerebellopontine angle and foramen magnum. *Neurosurgery clinics of North America*. 1994;5(2):349-77.
[8] Sen, C. N., Sekhar, L. N. Surgical management of anteriorly placed lesions at the craniocervical junction--an alternative approach. *Acta neurochirurgica*. 1991;108(1-2): 70-7.
[9] Yadav, Y. R., Madhariya, S. N., Parihar, V. S., Namdev, H., Bhatele, P. R. Endoscopic transoral excision of odontoid process in irreducible atlantoaxial dislocation: our experience of 34 patients. *Journal of neurological surgery Part A, Central European neurosurgery*. 2013;74(3):162-7.
[10] Dlouhy, B. J., Dahdaleh, N. S., Menezes, A. H., Md. Evolution of transoral approaches, endoscopic endonasal approaches, and reduction strategies for treatment of craniovertebral junction pathology: a treatment algorithm update. *Neurosurgical focus*. 2015;38(4):E8.
[11] Dehdashti, A. R., Ganna, A., Witterick, I., Gentili, F. Expanded endoscopic endonasal approach for anterior cranial base and suprasellar lesions: indications and limitations. *Neurosurgery*. 2009;64(4):677-87; discussion 87-9.
[12] Komotar, R. J., Zacharia, B. E., McGovern, R. A., Sisti, M. B., Bruce, J. N., D'Ambrosio, A. L. Approaches to anterior and anterolateral foramen magnum lesions: A critical review. *Journal of craniovertebral junction and spine*. 2010;1(2):86-99.
[13] Bassiouni, H., Ntoukas, V., Asgari, S., Sandalcioglu, E. I., Stolke, D., Seifert, V. Foramen magnum meningiomas: clinical outcome after microsurgical resection via a posterolateral suboccipital retrocondylar approach. *Neurosurgery*. 2006;59(6):1177-85; discussion 85-7.
[14] George, B., Lot, G., Boissonnet, H. Meningioma of the foramen magnum: a series of 40 cases. *Surgical neurology*. 1997;47(4):371-9.
[15] Kandenwein, J. A., Richter, H. P., Antoniadis, G. Foramen magnum meningiomas--experience with the posterior suboccipital approach. *British journal of neurosurgery*. 2009;23(1):33-9.
[16] Gupta, S. K., Khosla, V. K., Chhabra, R., Mukherjee, K. K. Posterior midline approach for large anterior/anterolateral foramen magnum tumours. *British journal of neurosurgery*. 2004;18(2):164-7.
[17] Goel, A., Desai, K., Muzumdar, D. Surgery on anterior foramen magnum meningiomas using a conventional posterior suboccipital approach: a report on an experience with 17 cases. *Neurosurgery*. 2001;49(1):102-6; discussion 6-7.
[18] Heros, R. C. Lateral suboccipital approach for vertebral and vertebrobasilar artery lesions. *Journal of neurosurgery*. 1986;64(4):559-62.
[19] Moscovici, S., Umansky, F., Spektor, S. "Lazy" far-lateral approach to the anterior foramen magnum and lower clivus. *Neurosurgical focus*. 2015;38(4):E14.
[20] Nanda, A., Vincent, D. A., Vannemreddy, P. S., Baskaya, M. K., Chanda, A. Far-lateral approach to intradural lesions of the foramen magnum without resection of the occipital condyle. *Journal of neurosurgery*. 2002;96(2):302-9.
[21] Bruneau, M., George, B. Foramen magnum meningiomas: detailed surgical approaches and technical aspects at Lariboisiere Hospital and review of the literature. *Neurosurgical review*. 2008;31(1):19-32; discussion 3.

[22] Zenonos, G., Kondziolka, D., Flickinger, J. C., Gardner, P., Lunsford, L. D. Gamma Knife surgery in the treatment paradigm for foramen magnum meningiomas. *Journal of neurosurgery*. 2012;117(5):864-73.

[23] Sheehan, J. P., Starke, R. M., Kano, H., Barnett, G. H., Mathieu, D., Chiang, V. et al. Gamma Knife radiosurgery for posterior fossa meningiomas: a multicenter study. *Journal of neurosurgery*. 2015:1-11.

[24] Talacchi, A., Biroli, A., Soda, C., Masotto, B., Bricolo, A. Surgical management of ventral and ventrolateral foramen magnum meningiomas: report on a 64-case series and review of the literature. *Neurosurgical review*. 2012;35(3):359-67; discussion 67-8.

[25] Sekhar, L. N., Wright, D. C., Richardson, R., Monacci, W. Petroclival and foramen magnum meningiomas: surgical approaches and pitfalls. *Journal of neuro-oncology*. 1996;29(3):249-59.

[26] Vishteh, A. G., Crawford, N. R., Melton, M. S., Spetzler, R. F., Sonntag, V. K., Dickman, C. A. Stability of the craniovertebral junction after unilateral occipital condyle resection: a biomechanical study. *Journal of neurosurgery*. 1999;90(1 Suppl.): 91-8.

[27] Wu, Z., Hao, S., Zhang, J., Zhang, L., Jia, G., Tang, J. et al. Foramen magnum meningiomas: experiences in 114 patients at a single institute over 15 years. *Surgical neurology*. 2009;72(4):376-82; discussion 82.

[28] Pamir, M. N., Kilic, T., Ozduman, K., Ture, U. Experience of a single institution treating foramen magnum meningiomas. *Journal of clinical neuroscience: official journal of the Neurosurgical Society of Australasia*. 2004;11(8):863-7.

[29] Borba, L. A., de Oliveira, J. G., Giudicissi-Filho, M., Colli, B. O. Surgical management of foramen magnum meningiomas. *Neurosurgical review*. 2009;32(1):49-58; discussion 9-60.

[30] Sen, C. N., Sekhar, L. N. An extreme lateral approach to intradural lesions of the cervical spine and foramen magnum. *Neurosurgery*. 1990;27(2):197-204.

[31] Kratimenos, G. P., Crockard, H. A. The far lateral approach for ventrally placed foramen magnum and upper cervical spine tumours. *British journal of neurosurgery*. 1993;7(2):129-40.

[32] Akalan, N., Seckin, H., Kilic, C., Ozgen, T. Benign extramedullary tumors in the foramen magnum region. *Clinical neurology and neurosurgery*. 1994;96(4):284-9.

[33] Bertalanffy, H., Gilsbach, J. M., Mayfrank, L., Klein, H. M., Kawase, T., Seeger, W. Microsurgical management of ventral and ventrolateral foramen magnum meningiomas. *Acta neurochirurgica Supplement*. 1996;65:82-5.

[34] Pirotte, B., David, P., Noterman, J., Brotchi, J. Lower clivus and foramen magnum anterolateral meningiomas: surgical strategy. *Neurological research*. 1998;20(7):577-84.

[35] Salas, E., Sekhar, L. N., Ziyal, I. M., Caputy, A. J., Wright, D. C. Variations of the extreme-lateral craniocervical approach: anatomical study and clinical analysis of 69 patients. *Journal of neurosurgery*. 1999;90(2 Suppl.):206-19.

[36] Arnautovic, K. I., Al-Mefty, O., Husain, M. Ventral foramen magnum meninigiomas. *Journal of neurosurgery*. 2000;92(1 Suppl.):71-80.

[37] Roberti, F., Sekhar, L. N., Kalavakonda, C., Wright, D. C. Posterior fossa meningiomas: surgical experience in 161 cases. *Surgical neurology*. 2001;56(1):8-20; discussion 1.

In: Current Management of Central Nervous System ... ISBN: 978-1-63483-856-6
Editors: Steven D. Chang and Anand Veeravagu 

*Chapter 11*

# SURGICAL MANAGEMENT OF CONVEXITY MENINGIOMAS

***Michael Safaee MD, Stephen T. Magill MD, PhD, and Michael W. McDermott MD***
Department of Neurological Surgery
University of California, San Francisco, US

## ABSTRACT

Convexity meningiomas are a benign neoplasm of mesenchymal origin. These tumors account for 15% of all intracranial meningiomas. Most of these tumors are discovered incidentally and patients tend to be asymptomatic at detection. Patients with small, asymptomatic tumors can be monitored with surveillance imaging and strict attention to the onset of new neurological symptoms. Additionally, patients that undergo surgical resection demonstrate favorable outcomes including robust overall survival and low rates of disease recurrence. Surgical intervention for convexity meningioma carries a low morbidity and mortality risk. In this chapter we detail the management of patients with convexity meningiomas and discuss the current literature.

## INTRODUCTION

Meningiomas account for up to 33% of primary intracranial tumors and are the most common non-glial tumors of the cranial vault [1, 2]. Convexity meningiomas refer to those that do not extend into the skull base or involve dural venous sinuses [3], with the majority located around the coronal suture and frontotemporal junction [4]. They represent between 15-20% of all meningiomas and the majority are benign, with approximately 65-80% categorized as Grade I by the 2007 WHO standards [5, 6].

## Clinical Presentation

Meningiomas, particularly Grade I lesions, possess a slow growth pattern and therefore present in a more indolent fashion. As a result they can be larger than expected at the time of diagnosis. However due to the increased use and improved quality of intracranial imaging modalities, these tumors can also be found incidentally in approximately 14-20% of cases [7, 8]. The most common presenting symptoms include headache and new onset seizure. Headaches are reported in up to half of all patients, with seizures in up to one-third [7, 8]. Seizure incidence varies by tumor location, with temporal meningiomas associated with the highest risk. Additional location-symptom associations include personality change (frontal), speech disturbances (Broca's or Wernike's areas), weakness or seizure (perirolandic), sensory deficits, hemi-sensory neglect (parietal), and visual field deficits (occipital). Figure 1 represents a common preoperative image of a left frontal convexity meningioma, while Figure 2 demonstrates a similar lesion with hyperostotic bone overlying the tumor. In this case the hyperostotic region contained no tumor, however in some cases there is invasion into the overlying calvarium in which case in situ cranioplasty can be performed [9]. Figure 3 illustrates an occipital convexity meningioma in a patient who presented with headaches and then seizures at which point they elected to undergo surgical resection.

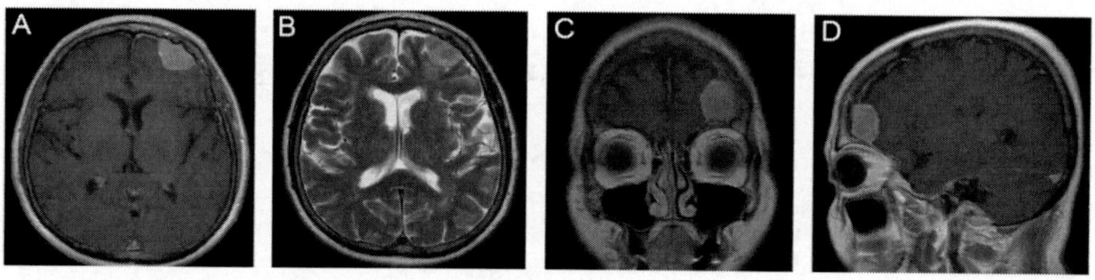


Figure 1. Left frontal convexity meningioma. A. T1-weighted MRI with contrast (A) demonstrates a 2 x 2 x 2 cm left frontal convexity meningioma without associated T2 signal in the adjacent cortex (B) suggesting minimal to no peri-lesional edema. T1-weighted MR with contrast illustrates the lesion in the coronal (C) and sagittal (D) planes. The patient presented with a long history of migraine headaches and was found to have this lesion, which was followed on serial imaging. She developed progressive worsening of her headaches and documented growth of the lesion prompting surgical resection.

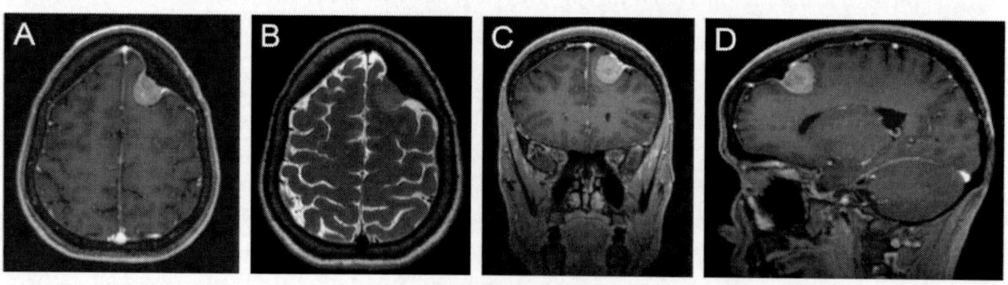


Figure 2. Left frontal convexity meningioma with associated hyperostosis. T1-weighted MRI with contrast in the axial (A) plane demonstrates a 2 x 2 x 2 cm left frontal convexity meningioma with marked hyperostosis of the associated calvarium. T2-weighted MRI (B) shows the lack of peri-lesional edema. T1-weighted MRI with contrast illustrates the lesion in the coronal (C) and sagittal planes (D). The patient presented with dizziness, vertigo, and left earache and was followed by serial imaging until documented growth prompted surgical resection.

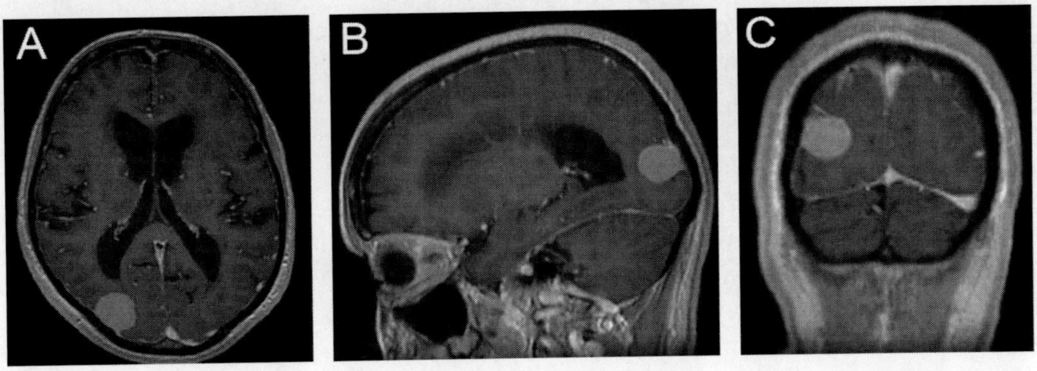


Figure 3. Right occipital convexity meningioma. T1-weighted MRI with contrast demonstrates a 2 x 2 x 2 cm right lateral occipital convexity meningioma in the axial (A), sagittal (B), and coronal (C) planes. The lesion was found during a work-up for chronic headaches and followed with serial imaging until the patient developed seizures and elected to undergo surgical resection of this lesion.

## Initial Management

The appropriate treatment for convexity meningiomas is often complex and must take into account patient age, symptoms, co-morbidities, and tumor anatomy.

Initial strategies may include observation, surgery, radiotherapy/radiosurgery or a combination of these. Despite multiple attempts to describe the natural history of these lesions, predicting the extent and duration of tumor growth is challenging. Two notable preoperative algorithms were developed by Dr. Takeshi Kawase, which is limited to predicting complete resection in skull base meningiomas, and Dr. Joung Lee, whose "CLASS" algorithm predicts the risk of a poor outcome in meningioma patients undergoing surgical treatment [10, 11]. However, the decision to pursue surgery remains complex and cannot be determined by a single algorithm. Among asymptomatic meningiomas, approximately two thirds do not grow and can likely be observed at appropriate intervals. Yano and colleagues found that 63% of asymptomatic meningiomas exhibited no growth and only 6% of all patient went on to develop symptoms over a mean follow-up of nearly 4 years [12]. Additionally, Nakamura reported that 66% of tumors have growth rates less than 1 $cm^3$ per year [13]. Observation is generally acceptable in asymptomatic elderly patients with tumors less than 2.5 cm in diameter and minimal peri-lesional edema.(14) For symptomatic lesions in this age demographic, stereotactic radiosurgery may provide some benefit for tumors less than 2.5 cm in diameter [15].

## Surgical Treatment

### *Preoperative Embolization*

Embolization of feeding arteries has the potential to make surgery safer and easier by reducing intraoperative blood loss and softening tumoral tissue. The optimal timing for surgery after embolization is not completely understood, however one must recognize that occlusion of tumor-feeding arteries only transiently reduces blood flow since collateral flow can develop relatively quickly. Kai and colleagues recommend waiting 7-9 days before proceeding with surgery after embolizing meningiomas that receive more than 50% of their blood supply from the external carotid [16], however there are no randomized studies evaluating this topic and a recent review of literature found that the average time from embolization to craniotomy was less than 2 days, with no significant data to recommend optimal timing between embolization and surgery [17]. Chun et al. found that patients who underwent surgery less than 24 hours after embolization had increased intraoperative blood loss, thus for the largest convexity tumors our practice is to admit patients for embolization followed by surgical resection 72 hours later [18]. Waldron et al. identified an overall angiographic complication rate of 2.5%, however among skull base meningiomas included in the study there were no complications [19].

### *Patient Positioning*

Proper positioning is critical for optimizing exposure and resection of tumor. The patient should be positioned such that the tumor is at the highest point in the surgical field, allowing for the surgeon to operate in a plane parallel to the floor. This promotes visualization of the tumor, allows blood to pool below the resection cavity, and facilitates a comfortable position for the surgeon. In general, patients are placed supine for tumors located anterior to the coronal suture compared to lateral for tumors posterior to the coronal suture or in the occipital convexity. For tumors of the frontal pole, the patient is positioned supine with a bolster under the torso of the opposite side and the head turned so the surgical plane is parallel to the floor. A unilateral or coronal incision is used, depending on how far forward the frontal convexity tumor is, followed by unilateral craniotomy. For meningiomas in the frontotemporal region or lateral sphenoid wing the patient is supine with head turned approximately 60 degrees to the opposite side. A standard pterional incision and two-part pterional craniotomy are used [20]. For posterior temporal or lateral parietal tumors, patients are semi-lateral with a shoulder roll, while occipital tumors are positioned semi- or full-lateral. The problem with aggressive neck rotation or prone positioning is the effect of venous pressures translating to increased venous blood volume and intracranial pressure making the operating environment less than ideal.

### *Surgical Technique*

It is well established that increased extent of resection, defined by the Simpson grade, is associated with increased progression-free and overall survival. Complete resection consists of gross total resection of tumor, dural attachments, and abnormal bone. Therefore, the goal of surgery is to remove both the entire tumor as well as the dural origin with a 1-2 cm margin. The skin incision should be planned to minimize cosmetic deformity and preserve vascular supply to the flap. A two-layer subgaleal dissection is preferred because it allows for harvesting of periosteum, which serves as a valuable dural substitute after resection. The injection of local anesthetic prior to incision improves hemostasis and causes swelling of the underlying tissues, which is particularly helpful in the dissection of subgaleal space. The craniotomy should extend at least a few centimeters beyond the borders of the dural attachment. Intraoperative neuronavigation serves as a valuable adjunct to ensure appropriate and safe margins for the craniotomy. The bone flap should be carefully elevated with minimal manipulation of the meningioma to prevent underlying vessel or cortical injury. In cases where there is a limited or small area of tumor invasion of the inner table, the bone flap may be divided into 2 pieces so that the area of bone involvement can be separated from the tumor under direct visualization. In cases of extensive bony hyperostosis an "in-situ cranioplasty" method may be used [9].

The dural incision should include a 2 cm margin around the tumor to promote complete resection, which Kinjo, Al-Mefty, and Kanaan refer to as a Grade 0 resection [21] Convexity meningiomas often derive their vascular supply from hypertrophied meningeal branches, which must be targeted early to allow for interruption of blood supply and promote clean extra-capsular dissection of the tumor. In extreme examples pre-operative embolization may be employed to reduce blood loss even though meningeal arteries are available with the exposure [18, 19]. Although small lesions can often be removed en-bloc, medium and large tumors generally require internal debulking to facilitate extra-capsular dissection. This can often be performed with an ultrasonic aspirator and proceeds until dissection can proceed in a safe manner with minimal retraction of the underlying brain. Dissection of tumor capsule from underlying pia is done under the operative microscope with care directed towards preserving underlying vascular structures and minimizing manipulation of the underlying brain. Arteries should not be sacrificed unless they are confirmed to feed the tumor. Underlying veins must also be preserved to prevent post-operative venous infarctions. When developing the tumor-arachonid plane, care must be taken to dissect arachnoid from the tumor, not the brain. If there is invasion of tumor into underlying cortex or vascular structures, the decision to pursue further resection will depend on location (eloquence) and tumor grade. In cases of extensive edema on preoperative imaging, the surgeon should expect the lack of an arachnoid plain; in non-eloquent cortex, dissection of the tumor in a sub-pial plain may be well tolerated. Prior to closure, the dura must be inspected to rule out presence of residual tumor. Harvested periosteum can be used to reconstruct the dura, although artificial dural substitutes are also available. If there is minimal invasion of overlying calvarium, the affected area can be drilled away with appropriate margins, however if the invasion is extensive, cranioplasty may be required. A subgaleal drain is left in place to prevent hematoma accumulation.

## Postoperative Management

Patients spend the first post-operative day in the intensive care unit for close neurologic monitoring. Postoperative CT is useful for evaluating an altered patient to rule out hematoma or arterial/venous infarcts. MRI with contrast should be performed within 48 hours to evaluate the extent of resection and can serve as a new baseline. Attention should be paid to areas of restricted diffusion, which may enhance on delayed scans and do not necessarily represent residual or recurrence tumor. Subgaleal drains are continued for 1-2 days until their output tapers to minimize formation of subgaleal hematomas.

### *Seizure Prophylaxis*

The role of antiepileptic agents in patients without prior seizures is unclear and there is an overall paucity of data specific to extra-axial tumors, particularly convexity meningiomas. Sughrue and colleagues reviewed the literature for convexity meningiomas and found no significant difference in post-operative seizure rates in the first month when comparing patients who received 7 days of postoperative antiepileptics compared to those who did not [22]. In a review of supratentorial meningiomas treated over 30 years, Komotar found that perioperative anticonvulstant use was not associated with a difference in early or late postoperative seizures [23]. Unfortunately, there is no level I data to support or reject the use of such therapy and thus, prospective, randomized studies are needed to determine the utility of seizure prophylaxis in the peri- and postoperative period.

### *DVT Prophylaxis*

Meningioma patients carry a high risk of venous thromboembolic events (VTE), with early reports citing an incidence as high as 70% [24]. In recent years, the use of chemoprophylaxis has decreased the incidence VTE among all intracranial meningioma patients to approximately 5%, however the rates for supratentorial and convexity meningiomas are likely even lower [25, 26]. Older age, high BMI, male gender, and non-ambulatory status are known risk factors. Cage and colleagues found that the use of enoxaparin, initiated 24-48 hours post-operatively, was associated with a non-statistically significant decrease in the rate of postoperative DVT/PE without a significant increase in rate of intracranial hemorrhage [27]. Eisenring and colleagues showed that initiation of chemoprophylaxis initiated on the day of surgery combined with intraoperative leg elevation of 10-20° with intermittent pneumatic compression further decreased the risk [28]. Although the timing of initiation remains debatable, all patients should be placed on chemoprophylaxis, preferably low-molecular-weight heparin, until fully ambulatory.

### *Venous Infarcts*

Careful consideration of the venous anatomy both adjacent and within the tumor are critical for safe resection of meningiomas. The exact incidence is not completely understood, however likely varies from 1-7%, with a higher incidence among larger tumors [29]. More superficial locations and tumors close to midline venous sinuses are also more prone to venous infarction due to increased risk of venous injury or sacrifice. The surgical approach is also an important risk factor for venous infarction, with the highest incidence among patients undergoing bifrontal, extended bifrontal, or transpetrosal approaches at 5-6%, while those with convexity approaches are significantly lower at 1-2% [30]. As a precautionary measure, our practice is to keep patients well hydrated in the first 48 hours post-operatively.

### *Surgical Morbidity*

Side effects of surgery depend on patient and tumor factors. While convexity meningiomas are regarded as the most straightforward tumors to remove, care must be taken in each step of the exposure, removal, and closure to ensure a good result. In a report by Sanai et al. of the senior author's experience with convexity meningiomas, the overall complication rate was 10% [7]. Medical complications (deep venous thrombosis and pulmonary embolus) accounted for 4%,while neurosurgical complications (CSF leak, postoperative hematoma, infection) accounted for 6%. The average age in this series was 48 years with an average tumor volume of 146 $cm^3$. Others have reported complication rates of 1.7-4.9% for neurologic deficits and overall complication rate of 9.4-15.3% [8, 31].

### *Residual Disease*

Management of residual disease depends on a variety of factors including patient age, tumor location, and histologic grade. Over 95% of convexity meningiomas undergo gross total resection, which for grade I lesions is considered definitive therapy [8]. Rates of recurrence after gross total resection range from 7-23% at 5 years, 20-39% at 10 years, and 24-60% at 15 years, while recurrence rates with subtotal resection (Simpson grades 4 and 5) range from 37-62% at 5 years, 52-100% at 10 years, and 70% at 15 years [32]. For this small group of subtotally resected grade I tumors, we recommend close imaging follow-up every 6 months for the first two years followed by serial annual scans thereafter. For grade II lesions, most would agree that residual disease requires adjuvant radiation, which can be in the form of stereotactic radiosurgery or fractionated external beam radiotherapy. For grade III tumors all require adjuvant post-operative radiation planned on the post-resection scans. There is also data to suggest that even in cases of gross total resection grade II lesions may warrant adjuvant radiotherapy to improve progression-free survival [33, 34].

## CONCLUSION

Convexity meningiomas represent a subset of lesions with a favorable prognosis and should be treated by surgical resection. Management paradigms are variable, but all decision-making should take into account patient age, symptoms, tumor size and location, radiographic features, and co-morbidities. For asymptomatic or incidentally found lesions in older patients, close observation is likely the best course of action. For young patients with a long life risk exposure, elective early resection may be appropriate. Tumors that enlarge or are symptomatic all warrant intervention. Radiosurgery as a primary treatment is generally reserved for older patients with small tumors who are poor surgical candidates, while young patients with tumors in anatomically favorable locations or large lesions are best served by surgical resection. The goal of surgery is maximal safe resection with minimal to no surgical morbidity. Preservation of underlying neurovascular structures is critical to a safe operation and should include removal of affected dura and bone if possible. Preoperative embolization and intraoperative neuronavigation are useful adjuncts, but are not substitutes for careful examination of the preoperative imaging and meticulous surgical technique.

## REFERENCES

[1] Louis DN, Ohgaki H, Wiestler OD, Cavenee WK, Burger PC, Jouvet A, et al. The 2007 WHO classification of tumours of the central nervous system. *Acta neuropathologica.* 2007;114(2):97-109.

[2] Burger P, Scheithauer B. *Tumors of the Central Nervous System.* Washington, D.C.2007.

[3] S.M. R, Quinones-Hinojosa A, Olivi A. Al-Mefty's Meningiomas. DeMonte F, McDermott MW, Al-Mefty O, editors: *Thieme;* 2011.

[4] F. L, P. B. Principles of Neurological Surgery. Ellenbogen RG, Abdulrauf SI, Sekhar LN, editors: *Elsevier*; 2012.

[5] Sughrue ME, Sanai N, Shangari G, Parsa AT, Berger MS, McDermott MW. Outcome and survival following primary and repeat surgery for World Health Organization Grade III meningiomas. *Journal of neurosurgery.* 2010;113(2):202-9.

[6] Perry A, Dehner LP. Meningeal tumors of childhood and infancy. An update and literature review. *Brain pathology*. 2003;13(3):386-408.

[7] Sanai N, Sughrue ME, Shangari G, Chung K, Berger MS, McDermott MW. Risk profile associated with convexity meningioma resection in the modern neurosurgical era. *Journal of neurosurgery*. 2010;112(5):913-9.

[8] Morokoff AP, Zauberman J, Black PM. Surgery for convexity meningiomas. *Neurosurgery*. 2008;63(3):427-33; discussion 33-4.

[9] Bloch O, McDermott MW. In situ cranioplasty for hyperostosing meningiomas of the cranial vault. *The Canadian journal of neurological sciences Le journal canadien des sciences neurologiques*. 2011;38(1):59-64.

[10] Adachi K, Kawase T, Yoshida K, Yazaki T, Onozuka S. ABC Surgical Risk Scale for skull base meningioma: a new scoring system for predicting the extent of tumor removal and neurological outcome. Clinical article. *Journal of neurosurgery*. 2009;111(5):1053-61.

[11] Lee JH, Sade B. Meningiomas: Diagnosis, Treatment, and Outcome. Lee JH, editor: *Springer*; 2009.

[12] Yano S, Kuratsu J, Kumamoto Brain Tumor Research G. Indications for surgery in patients with asymptomatic meningiomas based on an extensive experience. *Journal of neurosurgery*. 2006;105(4):538-43.

[13] Nakamura M, Roser F, Michel J, Jacobs C, Samii M. The natural history of incidental meningiomas. *Neurosurgery*. 2003;53(1):62-70; discussion -1.

[14] Goutagny S, Bah AB, Henin D, Parfait B, Grayeli AB, Sterkers O, et al. Long-term follow-up of 287 meningiomas in neurofibromatosis type 2 patients: clinical, radiological, and molecular features. *Neuro-oncology*. 2012;14(8):1090-6.

[15] Fokas E, Henzel M, Surber G, Hamm K, Engenhart-Cabillic R. Stereotactic radiotherapy of benign meningioma in the elderly: clinical outcome and toxicity in 121 patients. Radiotherapy and oncology: *Journal of the European Society for Therapeutic Radiology and Oncology*. 2014;111(3):457-62.

[16] Kai Y, Hamada J, Morioka M, Yano S, Todaka T, Ushio Y. Appropriate interval between embolization and surgery in patients with meningioma. *AJNR American journal of neuroradiology*. 2002;23(1):139-42.

[17] Singla A, Deshaies EM, Melnyk V, Toshkezi G, Swarnkar A, Choi H, et al. Controversies in the role of preoperative embolization in meningioma management. *Neurosurgical focus*. 2013;35(6):E17.

[18] Chun JY, McDermott MW, Lamborn KR, Wilson CB, Higashida R, Berger MS. Delayed surgical resection reduces intraoperative blood loss for embolized meningiomas. *Neurosurgery*. 2002;50(6):1231-5; discussion 5-7.

[19] Waldron JS, Sughrue ME, Hetts SW, Wilson SP, Mills SA, McDermott MW, et al. Embolization of skull base meningiomas and feeding vessels arising from the internal carotid circulation. *Neurosurgery*. 2011;68(1):162-9; discussion 9.

[20] Devasagayam S, Benet A, McDermott MW. Two-part pterional craniotomy. *Cureus*. 2012;4(11).

[21] Kinjo T, al-Mefty O, Kanaan I. Grade zero removal of supratentorial convexity meningiomas. *Neurosurgery*. 1993;33(3):394-9; discussion 9.

[22] Sughrue ME, Rutkowski MJ, Chang EF, Shangari G, Kane AJ, McDermott MW, et al. Postoperative seizures following the resection of convexity meningiomas: are

prophylactic anticonvulsants indicated? Clinical article. *Journal of neurosurgery*. 2011;114(3):705-9.

[23] Komotar RJ, Raper DM, Starke RM, Iorgulescu JB, Gutin PH. Prophylactic antiepileptic drug therapy in patients undergoing supratentorial meningioma resection: a systematic analysis of efficacy. *Journal of neurosurgery*. 2011;115(3):483-90.

[24] Sawaya R, Zuccarello M, Elkalliny M, Nishiyama H. Postoperative venous thromboembolism and brain tumors: Part I. Clinical profile. *Journal of neuro-oncology*. 1992;14(2):119-25.

[25] Gerber DE, Segal JB, Salhotra A, Olivi A, Grossman SA, Streiff MB. Venous thromboembolism occurs infrequently in meningioma patients receiving combined modality prophylaxis. *Cancer*. 2007;109(2):300-5.

[26] Hoefnagel D, Kwee LE, van Putten EH, Kros JM, Dirven CM, Dammers R. The incidence of postoperative thromboembolic complications following surgical resection of intracranial meningioma. A retrospective study of a large single center patient cohort. *Clinical neurology and neurosurgery*. 2014;123:150-4.

[27] Cage TA, Lamborn KR, Ware ML, Frankfurt A, Chakalian L, Berger MS, et al. Adjuvant enoxaparin therapy may decrease the incidence of postoperative thrombotic events though does not increase the incidence of postoperative intracranial hemorrhage in patients with meningiomas. *Journal of neuro-oncology*. 2009;93(1):151-6.

[28] Eisenring CV, Neidert MC, Sabanes Bove D, Held L, Sarnthein J, Krayenbuhl N. Reduction of thromboembolic events in meningioma surgery: a cohort study of 724 consecutive patients. *PloS one*. 2013;8(11):e79170.

[29] Jang WY, Jung S, Jung TY, Moon KS, Kim IY. Predictive factors related to symptomatic venous infarction after meningioma surgery. *British journal of neurosurgery*. 2012;26(5):705-9.

[30] Sughrue ME, Rutkowski MJ, Shangari G, Fang S, Parsa AT, Berger MS, et al. Incidence, risk factors, and outcome of venous infarction after meningioma surgery in 705 patients. Journal of clinical neuroscience: *official journal of the Neurosurgical Society of Australasia*. 2011; 18(5):628-32.

[31] Reinert M, Babey M, Curschmann J, Vajtai I, Seiler RW, Mariani L. Morbidity in 201 patients with small sized meningioma treated by microsurgery. *Acta neurochirurgica*. 2006;148(12):1257-65; discussion 66.

[32] Rogers L, Barani I, Chamberlain M, Kaley TJ, McDermott M, Raizer J, et al. Meningiomas: knowledge base, treatment outcomes, and uncertainties. A RANO review. *Journal of neurosurgery*. 2015;122(1):4-23.

[33] Komotar RJ, Iorgulescu JB, Raper DM, Holland EC, Beal K, Bilsky MH, et al. The role of radiotherapy following gross-total resection of atypical meningiomas. *Journal of neurosurgery*. 2012;117(4):679-86.

[34] Park HJ, Kang HC, Kim IH, Park SH, Kim DG, Park CK, et al. The role of adjuvant radiotherapy in atypical meningioma. *Journal of neuro-oncology*. 2013;115(2):241-7.

In: Current Management of Central Nervous System … ISBN: 978-1-63483-856-6
Editors: Steven D. Chang and Anand Veeravagu 

*Chapter 12*

# SURGICAL MANAGEMENT OF SUPRASELLAR MENINGIOMA

***Abdulrazag Ajlan,[1,2,*], MBBS, Allen Ho[1], MD, Sayantan Deb[1], BA and Griffith Harsh[1], MD***

[1]Department of Neurosurgery, Stanford University, Stanford, CA, US
[2]Department of Neurosurgery, King Saud University, Riyadh, KSA

## ABSTRACT

Tuberculum sellae (TS) and Diaphragma sellae (DS) meningiomas account for 5-10% of all intracranial meningiomas. They usually present with slowly progressive symptoms over several months. Many meningiomas have low proliferative rates and are indolent. However, suprasellar tumors have the risk of causing permanent neurological deficits and are thus often treated surgically. The central skull base location of suprasellar meningiomas and their proximity to critical neurovascular structures pose challenges to treatment. Understanding the bony anatomy of the anterior cranial fossa and the sellar region is critical for treating suprasellar meningiomas. In this chapter we will discuss the surgical options, techniques, and indications.

## INTRODUCTION

Intracranial meningiomas represent 36% of all primary brain tumors [32]. Tuberculum sellae (TS) and Diaphragma sellae (DS) meningiomas account for 5-10% of all intracranial meningiomas [3, 7, 20, 40].

In 1938, Cushing used the term suprasellar (SS) meningioma to denote all tumors arising from or around the tuberculum sellae (TS) dura [13] and divided them into four groups depending on their size and symptomatology; this classification did not include the origin of the tumor or its relation to surrounding structures.

* Corresponding author: Abdulrazag M. Ajlan, M.B.B.S. Clinical Instructor, Department of Neurosurgery, Stanford University, California, US. E-mail: a.ajlan@stanford.edu.

This term "suprasellar meningioma" is still in use in the current literature to describe meningiomas arising from the planum sphenoidale (PS), tuberculum sellae (TS), and diaphragma sellae (DS). Olfactory groove meningiomas are not included in this category because of their more anterior location and different clinical presentation [30, 41].

The classification of suprasellar meningiomas according to site of origin into PS, TS, and DS is clinically relevant. Understanding the bony anatomy of the anterior cranial fossa and the sellar region is critical for treating suprasellar meningiomas. The planum sphenoidale is the flat part of the sphenoid bone connecting the two lesser wings of the sphenoid bone. It forms the posterior part of the roof of the sphenoid sinus. The PS is separated anteriorly from the cribriform plate by the sphenoethmoidal suture and posteriorly from the tuberculum sellae by the chiasmatic sulcus (Figure 1). The TS is usually evident as a bony prominence just inferior to the chiasmatic sulcus; it usually corresponds to the tuberculum recess seen from the nasal view [33] (Figure 1 A-B). Although PS meningiomas can be confused with TS and DS meningiomas in clinical evaluation, they can be differentiated radiologically by evaluating the tumor's relationships to surrounding bone and neurovascular structures. The more anterior site of origin of PS tumors leads to posterior and inferior displacement of the optic nerves, optic chiasm, and the anterior cerebral arteries and their communicating artery; in contrast the more posteriorly located TS meningiomas displace the ON, OC, and the ACAs superiorly and posteriorly [2, 20, 31]. These relationships should be evaluated on preoperative imaging.

In a recent radiological evaluation with intraoperative correlation of TS and DS meningiomas, we recognized three distinct subtypes [2]: type A (exclusively tubercular), type B (combined TS-DS meningioma), and type C (exclusively DS) (Figure 1 C-F). In type A tumors, the anterior intercavernous sinus (AIS) was always patent, the DS was not involved by tumor, and the chiasm was posterior or superior-posterior.

In type A meningiomas, the sellar (infra-diaphragmatic) and, more significantly, the suprasellar (supra-diaphragmatic) heights were increased. All type A meningiomas had a clear line of distinction between tumor and pituitary gland on MRI. In type B meningiomas, The AIS was usually occluded, the DS was involved by tumor, the optic chiasm was superior to tumor, the ONs were superior or superior-lateral to tumor, and tumor extension into the canal was seen in 50% of cases.

In type B meningiomas, the increased height was equally divided between sellar and suprasellar components. In our series, only one tumor was a true DS meningioma (type C). True DS meningiomas, arising mainly from the DS are rare. In a series of 67 anterior cranial fossa meningiomas, 25 were classified as TS meningioma and only one as DS meningioma [37]. Al-Mefty et al. classified DS meningiomas into 3 types [21]: type A, originating from the upper leaf of the DS anterior to the pituitary stalk; type B, originating posterior to the pituitary stalk; and type C, originating from the inferior leaf of the DS.

The differentiation between types A and C, both anterior to the stalk, on preoperative imaging can be difficult and among types of large suprasellar meningiomas particularly difficult. The central skull base location of suprasellar meningiomas and their proximity to critical neurovascular structures pose challenges to treatment [7, 18, 29]. Theses tumors can be approached transnasally from "below" or transcranially from "above" [10, 18, 29, 35, 40]. Tumor size, tumor extensions, adjacent neurovascular structures, patients' characteristics and symptomatology, surgical goals, and the surgeon's expertise are important factors in deciding which surgical route to choose. In this chapter we will discuss the surgical options, techniques, and indications.

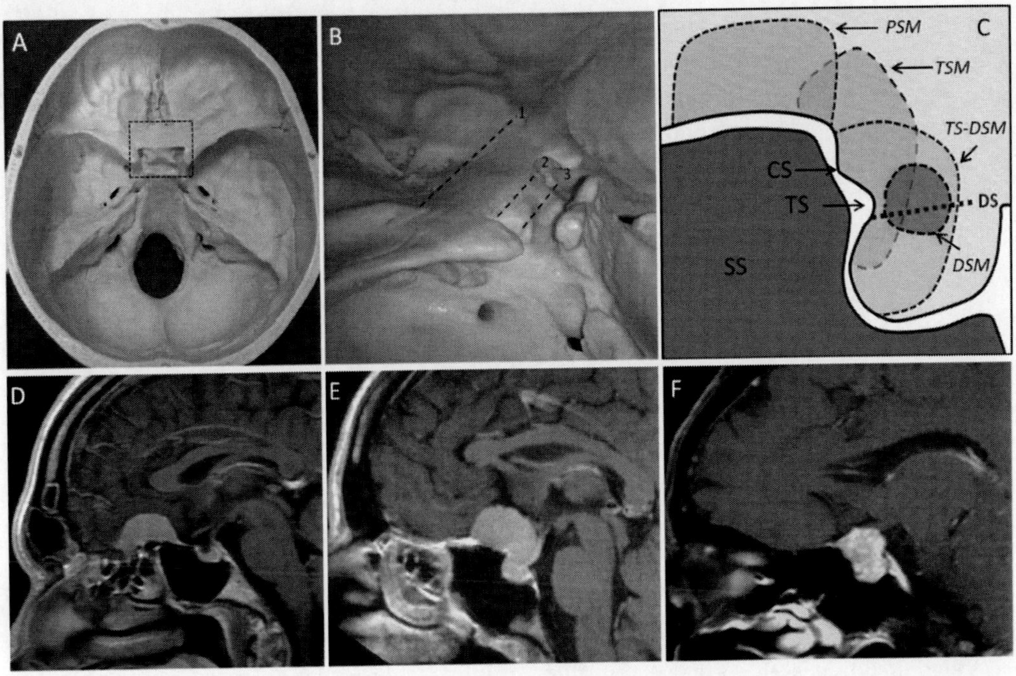


Figure 1. A) Superior view of the skull base; the sellar area is highlighted by a dotted box. B) Lateral view of the sellar demonstrating the sphenoethmoidal suture (line 1) separating the cribriform plate anteriorly from the planum sphenoidale (PS) posteriorly. The chiasmatic sulcus (line 2) separates the PS from the tuberculum sellae (TS). Line 3 represents the highest point of the TS. C) Diagram showing planum sphenoidale meningioma (PSM), tuberculum sellae meningioma (TSM), tuberculum sellae-diaphragma sellae meningioma (TS-DSM), and true diaphragm sellae meningioma (DSM). D) PSM. E) TSM. F) TS-DSM.

## Clinical and Radiological Evaluation

Suprasellar meningiomas usually present with symptoms slowly progressive over months [24, 25]. The most common presenting symptoms are visual disturbance and headache. Ten percent of these lesions are diagnosed incidentally. The visual disturbance is usually asymmetrical and can be unilateral [2, 24, 25]. Ophthalmological consultation and visual field testing should be included in the initial workup for these tumors. The pattern of visual field loss can guide the surgical treatment. Asymmetric field loss usually indicates asymmetrical involvement of the optic canals, which is helpful in determining the surgical goals and optimal surgical approach. Endocrine disturbance, particularly hyperprolactinemia and diabetes insipidus, can occur. Large tumors can present with hypopituitarism [39]; thus global pituitary function should be assessed and deficiencies treated prior to surgical resection. Smell is rarely affected by suprasellar meningiomas, in contrast to olfactory groove meningiomas, but is often threatened by surgical intervention.

Magnetic resonance imaging (MRI) with gadolinium is the gold standard for diagnosing and evaluating SS meningiomas. In most cases, MRI imaging can differentiate between meningiomas and pituitary adenomas, the most common sellar tumors [24]. On a high quality MRI, the optic nerves, optic chiasm, and anterior cerebral arteries can all be identified in relation to tumor.

In thin cut coronal MRIs, the tumor's extension into the optic canals can be recognized. A CT scan is useful for evaluating tumor calcification, which indicates a more solid tumor that might require craniotomy rather than a transnasal approach for resection. CT scans also elucidate the sinonasal anatomy prior to a transnasal approach.

A vascular study such as CTA, MRA or angiogram is indicated in selected cases to rule out uncommon vascular anomalies associated with these lesions [15, 16]. The vascular supply to SS meningiomas originates mainly from the anterior and posterior ethmoidal arteries, both branches of the ophthalmic artery.

The value of preoperative embolization in SS meningiomas is limited because these small branch vessels are technically difficult to occlude [38]. Additionally, the vascular supply can be disconnected before resecting the tumor in both transnasal and transcranial approaches. Thus, endovascular embolizations are rarely performed for SS meningiomas.

## Surgical Considerations

In general, transcranial skull base approaches to SS meningiomas can be challenging. They may require large craniotomies, significant brain retraction, and manipulation of cranial nerves and major vessels. Ventral transnasal midline approaches to these lesions are less invasive, involve less brain manipulation, and diminish the risk of injuring critical neurovascular structures [23].

However, some critics of this approach argue that complete resection of a meningioma, including its dural tall, is less likely to be achieved and cerebrospinal fluid (CSF) leak and infection are more common than with transcranial approaches [6, 14].

A detailed understanding of the anatomic variations among SS meningiomas of differing dural origins is essential to choice of the optimal approach for surgical resection. Most PS meningiomas do not extend below the planum level to involve the diaphragma sellae; they are thus easily exposed by a low subfrontal or pterional craniotomy or an endonasal trans-planum, trans-spheno-ethmoid approach.

In contrast, the more inferior point of origin of TS and DS meningiomas, especially those in which the tuberculum is elongated, require greater inferior dissection below and at an angle perpendicular to the planum sphenoidale. Prior to the use of expanded transphenoidal approaches, tumors inferior to the planum were accessed from above, through craniotomy and opening into the superior-posterior sphenoid sinus [18].

Following the development of advanced neuroimaging, neuronavigation, and neuroendoscopy, as well as improved skull base reconstruction techniques, many surgeons have found this region more accessible using an extended endoscopic transphenoidal approach. Recent reviews comparing transcranial and endoscopic transnasal resection of TS meningiomas failed to show superiority of one approach compared to the other in regard to visual outcomes and found that each approach has its own specific morbidities.

In general, the endoscopic transnasal approach seemed to offer the trade-off of lower complication rates for less complete tumor resection relative to transcranial approaches [3, 9, 11, 19, 22].

## Observation

Many benign meningiomas have low proliferative rates and are indolent. There is little data regarding the natural progression of suprasellar meningiomas as these tumors usually present with a neurological deficit (such as visual impairment) and are therefore treated with surgical resection. However, several studies have shown that left untreated, most such tumors progress slowly but eventually cause permanent neurologic deficits [4]. Many factors are correlated with rate of progression of these meningiomas, including patient age and tumor calcification. Location of the tumor, however, is not a good predictor of progression. Generally, asymptomatic tumors in young patients, symptomatic tumors, and atypical or malignant meningiomas warrant treatment with surgical resection or radiosurgery. Most asymptomatic meningiomas in the elderly have low proliferative potential, and surgical resection, when compared to observation, has not led to significantly better outcomes [4]. However, suprasellar tumors have the risk of causing permanent visual loss and are thus often treated surgically.

## Craniotomy

The multiple transcranial strategies for resecting suprasellar meningiomas vary primarily in the approach to the suprasellar region [28]. Generally, the craniotomy is performed on the side of the eye with the more severe visual loss to minimize the risk of injury to the contralateral optic nerve. The lateral subfrontal approach provides a lateral to medial view of the suprasellar region [26, 28]. The patient is placed in a supine position and the head is rotated to the contralateral side. Placing the head above the heart ensures adequate venous drainage. Finally, to minimize the amount of retraction use during the surgery (and therefore minimize retracted-related injuries), the vertex is tilted down, which allows the frontal lobe to fall away from the frontal base. The approach requires a burr hole at the external orbital angle. This is created using a high-speed drill, in a direction adjusted to prevent opening of the periorbita.

Next, a free bone flap is cut with a craniotome as low as possible frontally along the supraorbital rim while avoiding the lateral border of the frontal air sinus and as anteriorly as possible across the medial sphenoid wing. Some may prefer to include the superior-lateral orbital rim. If the air sinus is opened, it should be exenterated of mucosa, filled with fat or temporalis muscle, and covered with a pericranial flap to prevent CSF rhinorrhea.

Next, the dura is opened in a curvilinear fashion and reflected anteriorly, over the supraorbital rim. The Sylvian fissure and related arachnoid cisterns are opened to drain CSF and separate frontal and temporal lobes.

The pterional/frontotemporal approach uses a patient position similar to that of the frontolateral approach [28] with the exception that the head is usually rotated 30-40 degrees versus 10-20 degrees. The burr hole is placed in a similar location.

However, the craniotomy exposes more of the anterior-superior temporal lobe, removes more of the sphenoid wing, and opens more of the Sylvian fissure. Depending on the size of the tumor, the lesser wing of the sphenoid can be resected to the superior orbital fissure; this provides greater visibility with less brain retraction.

For the bifrontal approach, the patient is placed supine, and a bicoronal skin incision extends from one preauricular region to the other, passing posterior to the frontal hair line. Next, the scalp flap, including pericranium, is reflected anteriorly, and a bur hole is placed in each external orbital angle. The craniotomy is carried along the superior rim. Its posterior border is placed above the forehead for favorable cosmesis.

The basal cut likely opens the frontal air sinus; it is exenterated of mucosa and then filled with temporalis muscle and covered by pedicled pericranium. The dura is incised low, parallel to the base; the proximal superior sagittal sinus is coagulated, sutured and cut, and the falx is transected.

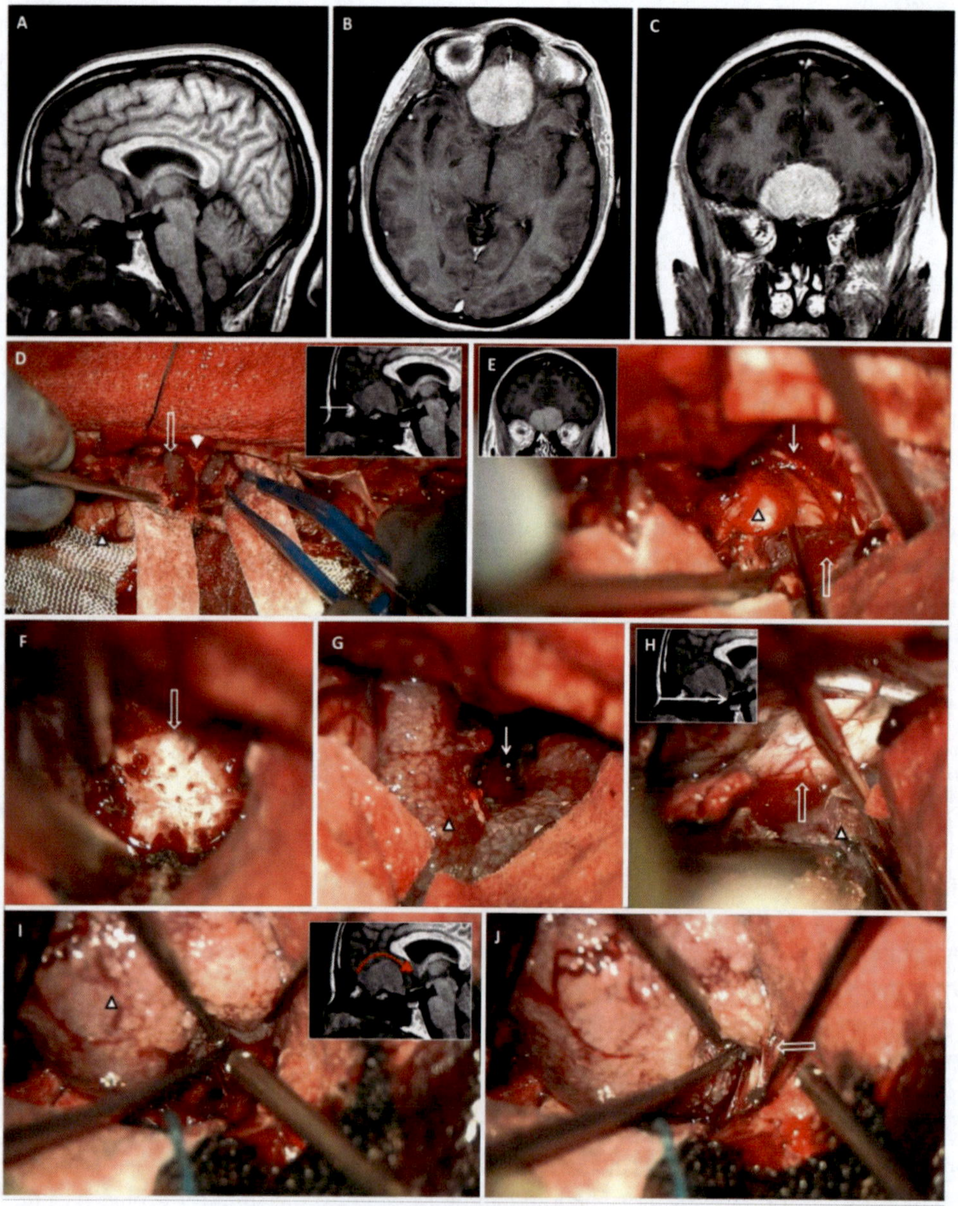


Figure 2. (Continued)

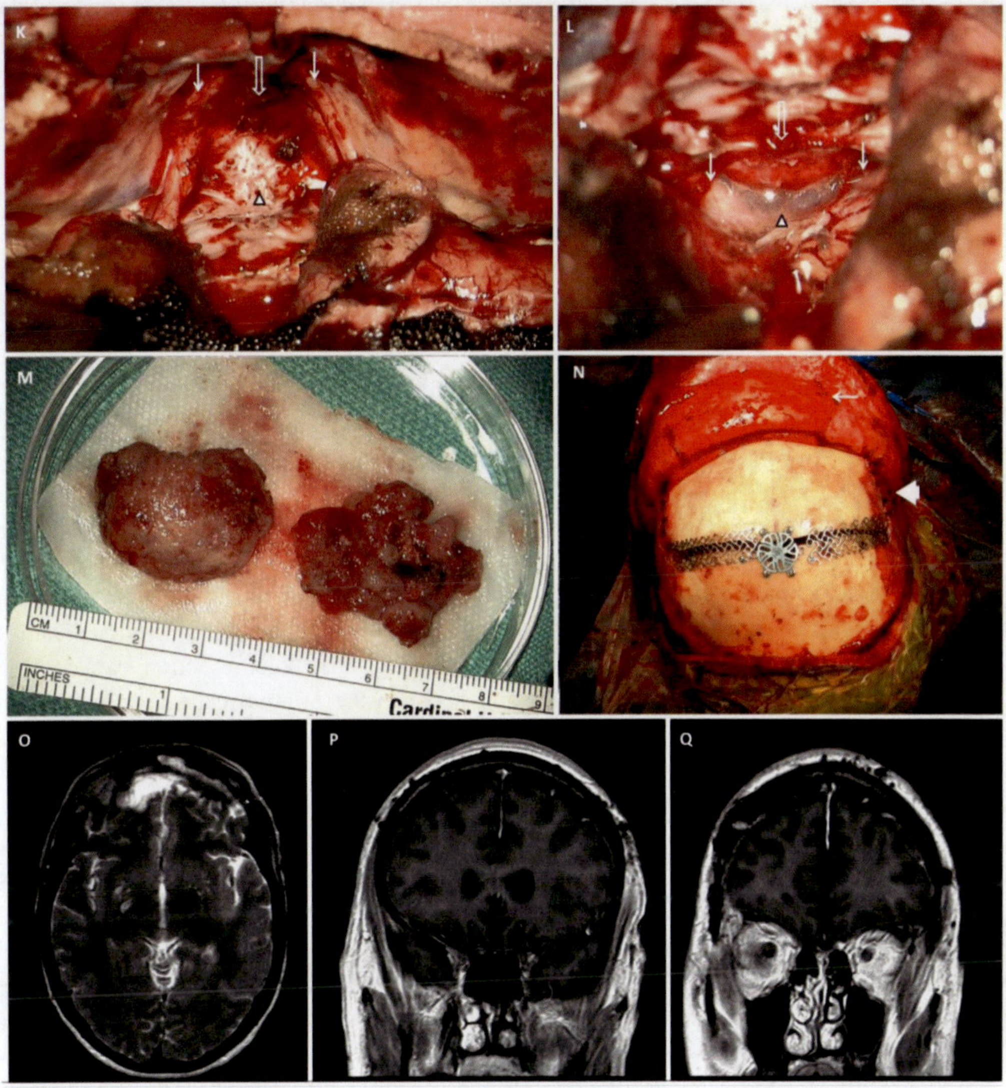


Figure 2. 48-year-old woman who presented with anosmia (A-C). Her MRI showed dural based anterior extra-axial enhancing lesion consistent with an olfactory groove (OG) meningioma. The tumor was resected electively via a bifrontal craniotomy utilizing a subfrontal approach. The skin incision was made behind the hairline. Sharp dissection was used to separate the skin flap from the temporal fascia which was left intact. The *periosteum* was elevated and left attached to the scalp flap. To preserve the frontal branch of the facial nerve bilaterally, subfascial dissection and release of the anterior-superior attachment of the temporalis muscle exposed the most anterior portion of the sphenofrontal suture where two anterior bur holes were placed. The Craniotomy extended 5 cm above the glabella from the frontal floor. The dura was opened on both sides of the superior sagittal sinus and the sinus was ligated proximally (D). The falx was coagulated using bipolar cautery at its most inferior attachment to the crista galli (arrow). The tumor was detached from the dura to interrupt its blood supply (open arrow). Minimal retraction was applied to the frontal lobes (triangle) (E). The tumor (open arrow) was separated from its dural attachment (triangle) and the right olfactory nerve (ON) was identified and preserved (arrow) (F). The tumor's attachment to the frontal bone was exposed after separating the tumor from the dural attachment and resecting the dura. Bone wax was used to control bone bleeding and to prevent postoperative cerebrospinal fluid (CSF) leak (G). At this point, the tumor was relatively avascular; central debulking (arrow) facilitated later extracapsular dissection (H). The tumor (triangle)

was completely separated from the dura back to its most posterior dural attachment. Dura covering the planum sphenoidale more posteriorly was then visible (open arrow) (I, J). Dissection separating tumor (triangle) from frontal lobe was achieved utilizing the arachnoid plane (open arrow) (K). At this stage, the tumor and its dural attached were completely resected. The tumor attachment site (triangle), crista galli (open arrow), bilateral ONs (arrow were then visible (L). Enlarged view of the field demonstrating the PS (open arrow), bilateral optic nerves (arrows), suprachiasmatic cistern (triangle) (M). The resected tumor (N). The temporalis fascia was sutured (arrow head) bilaterally, the frontal sinus was cranialized and packed with a small periostial vascularized flap (arrow) which was dissected at the end of the case just before closure to prevent flap dehydration (O-Q). Postoperative MRI demonstrated complete tumor resection and minimal frontal lobe change. The patient recovered well from the surgery with no new postoperative deficits or CSF leak. The sense of smell was stable at base line compared to preoperative evaluation.

After gaining access to the surgical field using any of the approaches described above, the tumor is resected microsurgically [26, 28]. First, its dural base is exposed and its feeding arteries are coagulated. The ipsilateral optic nerve is exposed. The capsule is separated from the medial aspect of the nerve.

Next, the tumor is debulked in order to decompress the optic nerve. Resection is continued till the optic chiasm and the contralateral optic nerve are visible. Care must be taken to preserve vascular supply to the optic nerve and the chiasm during the dissection. The basal dura is resected and tumor resection continues posteriorly until the pituitary stalk is visible and can be safely preserved. For larger meningiomas, the resection can continue around the posterior communicating artery, and between the internal carotid artery and the occulomotor nerve. Hyperostotic bone is removed with a high speed drill.

To minimize recurrence, ideally all tumor and dura of origin should be removed and adjacent dura coagulated.

The majority of published reports utilizing a craniotomy to resect suprasellar meningiomas report high rates of gross total resection; this is not always achieved with endoscopic approaches [23]. The most common complications of craniotomy are anosmia (13.8%), CSF leak (4.3%), and hemorrhage (5.8%). Reviews have also shown a 2% perioperative mortality rate. The froto-lateral and the pterional approaches have lower operative morbidity and mortality and better visual improvement than the bifrontal approach. Craniotomies have rates of postoperative complications similar to those which follow endoscopic surgical approaches. Most craniotomies result in visual improvement or stability (58.7% and 27.1% respectively). However, 14.2% are followed by deterioration of visual function. This is not significantly different from the visual outcomes achieved by the endoscopic transnasal approach. The open craniotomy approach has also been reported to have a 6% tumor recurrence rate [23].

# Surgical Approaches

## Transnasal

The advantages and risks of an endoscopic transnasal approach to surgical removal of a suprasellar meningioma differ from those of transcranial approaches. Many argue that the endoscopic approach is safer because it allows devascularisation of the basal tumor's origin prior to tumour resection [11].

Importantly, the endoscopic route avoids brain retraction and approaches the optic nerves only after much if the tumor has been removed. Furthermore, the arachnoid plane between the tumor and the vascular supply to the optic apparatus is protective. The major limitation of this approach is tumor size, since larger tumors are more difficult to access in their entirety through this approach.

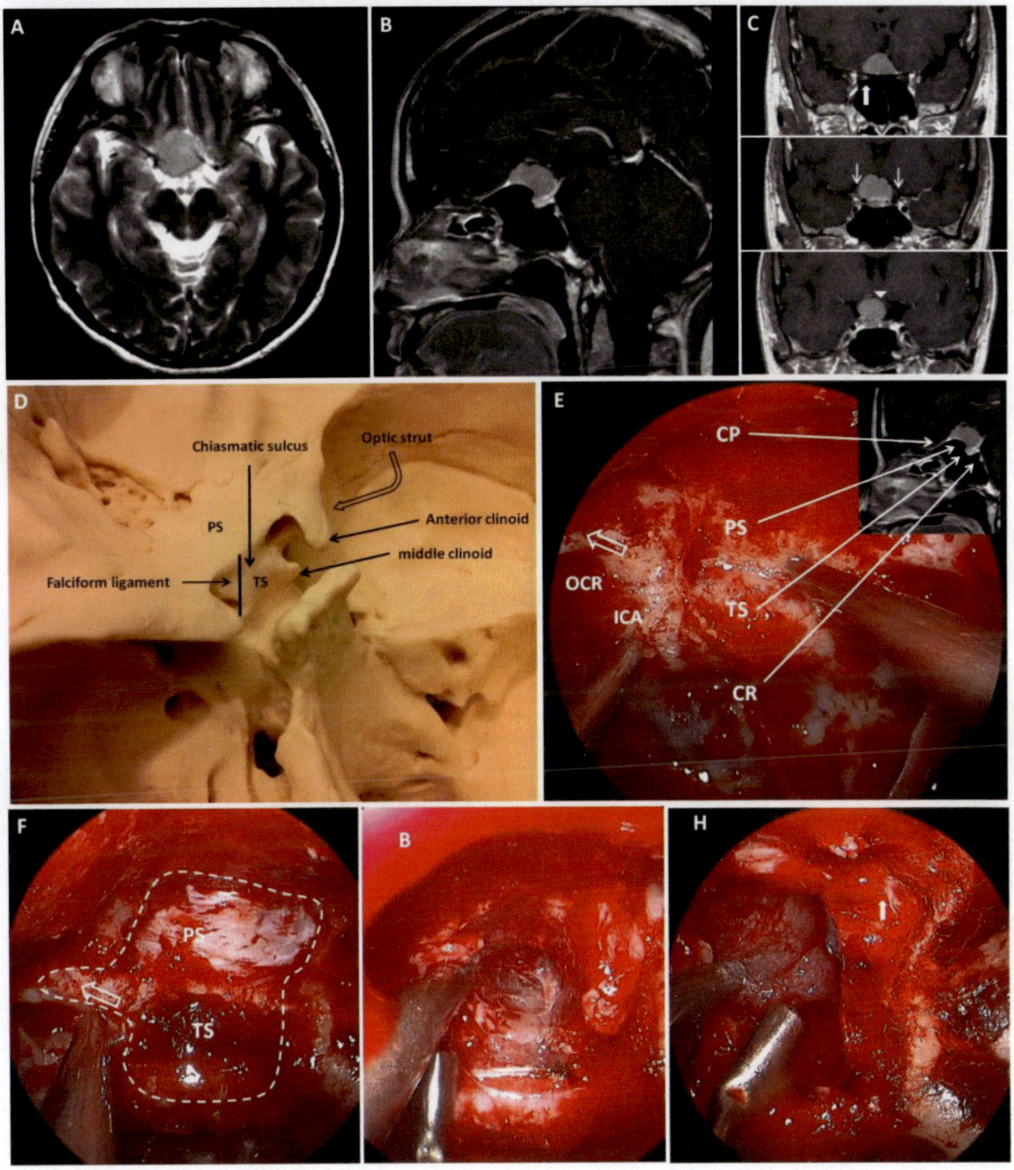


Figure 3. (Continued)

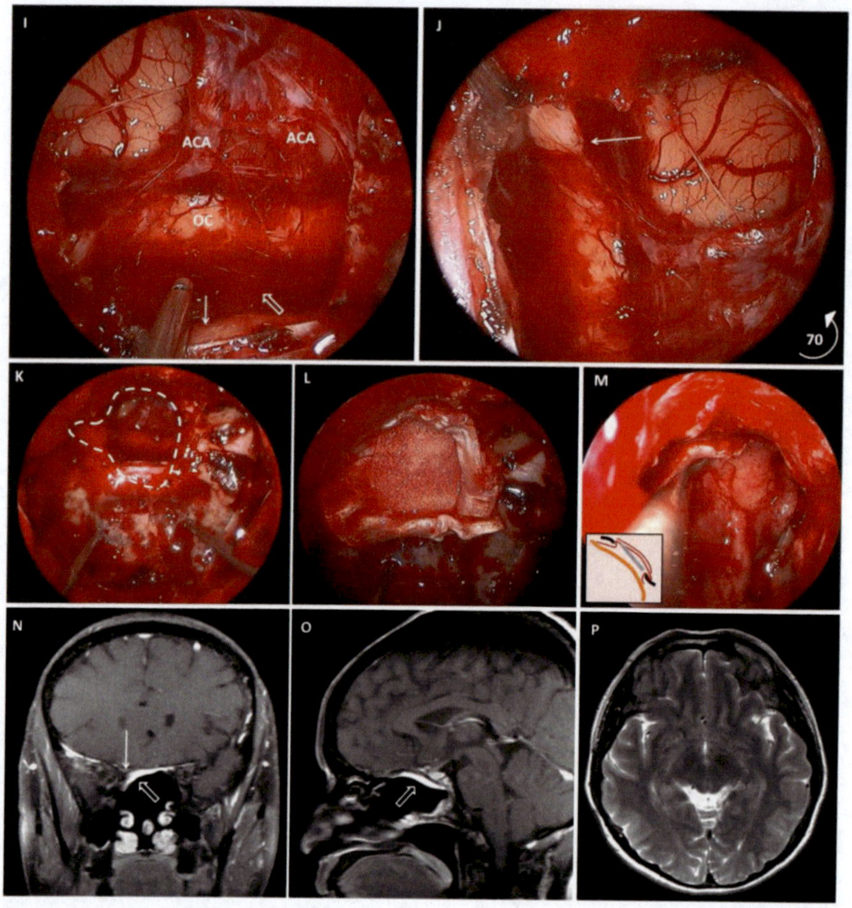


Figure 3. 53-year-old female who presented with right eye visual impairment (A). T2-weighted MRI and (B) T-1 weighted gadolinium enhanced MRI demonstrate a suprasellar lesion consistent with Tuberculum Sellae (TS) meningioma (C). The optic nerves (ON) are displaced laterally (arrow), the optic chiasm (OC) displaced posteriorly (triangle), and the tumor extends to the right optic canal (D). Superolateral view of the sellar and parasellar bone. The chiasmatic sulcus (CS) separates the planum sphenoidale (PS) from the tuberculum sellae (TS). The falciform ligament is the dura stretching from the PS to the tip of the anterior clinoid forming the most proximal part of the optic canal roof. We elected to proceed with an endoscopic transnasal resection of her tumor (E). Intraoperative endonasal view revealing the cribriform plate, PS, TS, and the clival recess (CR). The right optico-carotid recess (OCR) between the cavernous internal carotid artery (ICA) and the bony prominence representing the optic canal (arrow). The PS, TS, and superior sellar bone is removed exposing dura. The arrow designates the optic canal dura after removing the bone (G). The dura is coagulated and opened above the anterior intercavernous sinus (AIS), the diaphragma sellae is kept intact (DS). Central debulking at this point facilitates extracapsular dissection (H). Extracapsular dissection utilizing the arachnoid plane (I). Most of the tumor has been removed at this point. The anterior cerebral arteries are shown. We can see the pituitary stalk (open arrow) and the preserved DS (arrow) (J). A 45° endoscope is used to visualize the tumor in the OC, and the remaining tumor is detached from the ON using sharp dissection (arrow) (K). The dural defect after the tumor resection (L, M). The sellar floor reconstruction using two layers of fasica lata (red) and gasket-seal technique using synthetic bone substitute Medpor (Stryker, Hamilton, OH) (L), and the nasoseptal flap (orange) (M). Perioperative lumbar drainage diverted CSF for 2 days after surgery (N-P). Postoperative MRI showing complete resection of tumor with no tumor in the optic canal (arrow). The nasoseptal flap is enhancing (open arrow). No evidence of brain injury is seen. Postoperatively, the patient's vision improved but did not completely. No CSF leak was observed in the follow-up period.

The surgery begins with the patient under general anesthesia and the placement of a lumbar CSF drain [10, 34]. After decongestion of the nasal mucosa, the middle and superior turbinates are resected or retracted to visualize the sphenoid ostia. Next, the nasal septum is fractured and displaced from the rostrum of the sphenoid, and the posterior 1 cm of the nasal septum is resected. This allows for more access to the region of interest through both nostrils, and provides a bilateral panoramic view of the sphenoid sinus rostrum and ostia. Next the mucosa of the sphenoid sinus and the intersinus sphenoid septa are removed, which brings the posterior wall of the sphenoid sinus into view. The posterior ethmoid sinuses are also removed, thus giving access to the tuberculum sellae, the planum sphenoidale, the sellar floor, and the optic protuberances.

To gain access to the meningioma, the tuberculum sellae, the planum sphenoidale, the upper third of the sellar face, and the medial portions of the optic protuberances are removed. The meningioma is identified, and the base is coagulated. Next, the dura is opened above and below the intercavernous sinus, which is cauterized and transected, exposing the basal tumor. Internal decompression of the tumor is carried out, avoiding the optic nerve and carotid arteries laterally, which are protected by an arachnoid layer separating the tumor and these structures. Once the decompression is complete, the tumor can be progressively mobilized and resected. Vascular attachments, usually branches of the superior hypophyseal arteries and the anterior cerebral and anterior communicating arteries are dissected off the tumor capsule under direct vision as the decompressed capsule is turned medially and inferiorly. The arachnoidal plane is preserved in dissecting the tumor from the optic nerve, optic chiasm and pituitary stalk. Next the surgical field is visualized with an angled lens endoscope to confirm complete resection of the tumor. Specifically, any dura that might seem thickened by tumor involvement should be removed if possible. Furthermore, the optic canal must be opened and any tumor of its anterior-inferior dura resected. Tumor extending supero-laterally and posterior to the optic nerves in their canals may be inaccessible. Larger tumors, particularly those extending in these directions, may warrant craniotomy or a combined approach. In closing, the resected dura is replaced with an inlay graft of fascia lata or dural substitute and a vascularized mucosal flap is mobilized and rotated to cover the bone defect to minimize the risk of CSF leak and meningitis. Posterior nasal septal flaps are used most frequently, though middle and inferior turbinate pedicled flaps, palatal flaps and temporoparietal fascia flaps can also be used.

Compared to transcranial approaches, the endoscopic endonasal approach has a lower, though not statistically significant, rate of gross total resection [23]. The endoscopic approach has a higher rate of subtotal or partial resections. The endoscopic approach has a complication rate of about 21%, which is not significantly different from transcranial approaches. The most common complication of the endoscopic approach is CSF leak (21.3%), which is significantly higher with this approach than with transcranial approaches. Other complications include anosmia (5.3%, a rate similar to that of transcranial approaches).

Perioperative mortality rate has been reported to be 3%. 69.1% of patients undergoing tumor removal through the endoscopic approach experienced improvement of vision, 18.2% had visual stability and 12.7% suffered visual deterioration. These visual outcomes were similar to m those seen after transcranial surgery [23].

Overall, for small tumors, the endoscopic approach has the potential of achieve high rates of gross total resection and visual improvement or stability, similar to those following craniotomy [14]. Historically, a high incidence of CSF leak and meningitis has been a major deterrent to use of this technique, but use of vascularized mucosal flaps has reduced this problem significantly. Craniotomy is still preferred for tumors that envelop the optic nerves or chiasm or the supraclinoid internal carotid arties or their branches.

## Mini Burr Hole Surgery

Although the endonasal transphenoid approach to resecting suprasellar tumors allows minimal retraction of the brain and avoids manipulation of important optic and vascular structures, it is limited in its scope, especially for tumors that extend laterally beyond the supraclinoid carotid arteries and the optic nerves. The mini-bur hole eyebrow approach, or the supraorbital minicraniotomy, allows access to more of the parasellar area with minimal brain retraction [42]. However, there is less maneuverability because the small bone and skin openings.

The patient is positioned supine with the head rotated 10-30 degrees towards the contralateral side [27, 36, 42]. The head is extended such that the frontal lobe falls away from the floor of the anterior fossa, obviating the need for retraction. The ipsilateral eye is taped or sutured shut to protect the cornea. Then the incision is marked. The position of the incision is critical to preserve the supraorbital nerve and avoiding entering the frontal sinus and. To this end, the supraorbital notch is palpated to identify the medial border of the incision. The incision extends inferiorly and laterally to the end of the eyebrow. The incision is carried through the skin superficial to the supraorbital nerve. It can be extended up to 1 cm beyond the eyebrow.

Next, the skin flap is retracted superiorly with fishhooks, preserving the pericranium. The pericranium is then incised along the superior border of the skin flap, in a U-shape. The pericranial flap extends laterally to the superior temporal line and into the fascia. The flap is reflected over the orbital rim, and a portion of the temporalis fascia along with muscle is dissected at the superior temporal line to expose the keyhole where a burr hole is made. Next, a standard craniotomy in the shape of a half-moon is made, with the inferior border flush with the orbital roof. The flap is usually 2-2.5 cm wide and 1.5-2 cm high. Bony protuberances on the floor of the opening are also drilled away to create a clear trajectory to the parasellar areas.

The dura is opened to create a C-shaped flap with the base extending to the orbital rim, over which it is reflected [27, 36, 42]. Care must be taken to keep the dura under tension and moist throughout the surgery to minimize shrinkage and ensure a watertight closure. Incisions are made in the arachnoid layer at the dural opening to allow for CSF egress.

Under the microscope, the olfactory tract can be visualized though this opening and followed back to the carotid cistern and the optic nerve. The next incisions are made in the arachnoid layer at the opticocarotid and optico-occulomotor cisterns to allow for CSF drainage. This critical step allows sufficient brain relaxation to open surgical corridors and allow access to the parasellar areas, while avoiding retraction of the frontal lobe. Following brain relaxation, there should be a clear path to the suprasellar areas, and the tumor is then removed using standard microdissection techniques.

First, the dura around the tumor at the tuberculum sellae or the planum sphenoidale is coagulated to interrupt the blood supply, devascularizing the meningioma [27]. Smaller tumors (<2 cm in diameter) can usually be removed in their entirety while preserve critical structures such as the optic chiasm and nerve. Medium-sized tumors (2-4 cm diameter) can often encapsulate or involve these critical structures, so the tumor must be partially internally debulked before proceeding with the dissection around arteries and nerves. For tumors greater than 4 cm in diameter, the initial internal debulking is performed to make space to reach the dura in the surrounding areas for further coagulation and devascularization of the meningioma. Micro Doppler is often used to locate critical vasculature of the area (ACA, MCA, ICA, and their branches, etc.) during tumor resection. Larger craniotomies should be used for larger and more calcified tumors to permit exposure and safer manipulation of critical structures. After tumor removal has been completed, the dura is closed in watertight fashion and stitched to the inferior edge of the craniotomy [27, 36, 42]. A collagen sponge that extends beyond the boundary of the bone flap can be placed on top of the dura. The bone flap is then replaced and fixed with titanium plates. The temporalis fascia and muscles are then replaced and the pericranium and galea are closed. Any frontal sinus opening can be repaired with collagen sponge and bone flap if the opening is small or with abdominal fat supported by collagen and then bone or pericranial flap if the defect is large. The skin is closed in a cosmetically aesthetic fashion.

Common complications of this approach include forehead numbness from supraorbital nerve injury and frontalis weakness due to stretching or injury of the frontalis branch of the facial nerve [27, 36, 42]. These are usually transient. Lasting paresis has been reported in 5.5% of patients [42]. CSF rhinorrhea can occur if the frontal sinus is breached during the surgery and inadequately repaired. Ineffective dural closure can also lead to pseudomeningocele formation. While both the endonasal and supraorbital approaches provide minimally invasive access for meningioma removal, the supraorbital approach is preferred for larger tumors and those with considerable lateral extension [17].

## RADIOSURGERY

Radiosurgery has emerged as a primary treatment option for certain kinds of meningiomas depending on the size and location of the tumor, as well as adjuvant therapy following partial meningioma resection [8, 12]. Radiosurgery involves radiation delivered in a focused beam to an intracranial target [5]. MRI or CT is used to identify the location of the tumor in treatment planning. A computer program aids in designing the dose and fractionation scheme. This considers tumor volume, past history of radiation, visual deterioration, nearby critical structures, and other factors. Patients are usually followed for nine or more months after the procedure to document tumor regression.

Suprasellar meningiomas are unique in their location close to the optic apparatus. Historically, radiosurgery has been contraindicated in perioptic meningiomas because the visual apparatus is sensitive to radiation; for radiation doses greater that 10-12 Gy, the procedure carries significant risk of visual impairment [1, 12, 36].

However, lower doses of radiotherapy have been historically inefficient in treating the tumor. Stereotactic radiosurgery, however, has made it possible to deliver smaller doses of radiation to a specific target, over multiple sessions, thus rendering the technique more effective than traditional methods of radiation treatment, while sparing critical visual structures exposure to large doses [8, 12].

Although few studies specifically analyze the effect of stereotactic radiosurgery on suprasellar meningiomas, there have been multiple studies of radiosurgery of perioptic meningiomas. These studies have limited sample sizes but have reported promising results. A 2015 study of 64 cases of perioptic meningiomas treated with stereotactic radiosurgery combining retrospective and prospective data reported no visual deterioration and impressive progression-free survival. In the retrospective group (25 cases), the study reported that 20% of patients had improved visual acuity after surgery, but 8% of the patients suffered from trigeminal neuralgia lasting 6 to 12 months. The retrospective group followed patients up to 3 years after radiosurgery. In the prospective group (39 cases), no patient reported visual deterioration and 18% had visual improvement.

No tumor progression was reported in this group with up to 4 year follow-up, and 28% of the patients had shrinkage of tumor. 7.7% of the patients did report trigeminal neuralgia that lasted 6 to 12 months [12].

## Conclusion

Surgical treatment of suprasellar meningiomas is often essential for preservation of critical neurologic function including vision. Surgical resection can be challenging, and the optimal approach to these lesions is highly dependent on their dural site of origin and relationships with the bony and neurovascular anatomy of the anterior cranial fossa. Recent develops in minimally invasive mini-burrhole and endoscopic transphenoidal and extended endonasal approaches, along with advances in anterior skull base reconstruction techniques have expanded their indications for treatment of suprasellar meningiomas and aided in achieving decreased morbidity, with comparable degrees of resection, and acceptably low levels of CSF leak. The addition of fractionated, multi-session radiosurgery to the neurosurgeon's armamentarium has demonstrated promising tumor control results without significant damage to the optic apparatus. Thus, as a result of continued advancements in neurosurgical techniques, surgical intervention continues to be the mainstay of treatment for suprasellar meningiomas to limit progression and preserve vision and other essential neurologic function.

## References

[1] Adler, J. R., Jr., Gibbs, I. C., Puataweepong, P., Chang, S. D. Visual field preservation after multisession cyberknife radiosurgery for perioptic lesions. *Neurosurgery* 62 Suppl. 2:733-743, 2008.

[2] Ajlan, A. M., Choudhri, O., Hwang, P., Harsh, G. Meningiomas of the tuberculum and diaphragma sellae. *J. Neurol. Surg. B Skull Base* 76:74-79, 2015.

[3] Al-Mefty, O., Holoubi, A., Rifai, A., Fox, J. L. Microsurgical removal of suprasellar meningiomas. *Neurosurgery* 16:364-372, 1985.

[4] Bindal, R., Goodman, J. M., Kawasaki, A., Purvin, V., Kuzma, B. The natural history of untreated skull base meningiomas. *Surgical Neurology* 59:87-92, 2003.

[5] Buatti, J. M., Friedman, W. A., Meeks, S. L., Bova, F. J. The radiobiology of radiosurgery and stereotactic radiotherapy. *Medical Dosimetry* 23:201-207, 1998.

[6] Cappabianca, P., Kelly, D. F., Laws, E. R., Jr. Endoscopic transnasal versus open transcranial cranial base surgery: the need for a serene assessment. *Neurosurgery* 63: 240-241; discussion 241-243, 2008.

[7] Chan, R. C., Thompson, G. B. Morbidity, mortality, and quality of life following surgery for intracranial meningiomas. A retrospective study in 257 cases. *J. Neurosurg.* 60:52-60, 1984.

[8] Choi, C. Y., Soltys, S. G., Gibbs, I. C., Harsh, G. R., Jackson, P. S., Lieberson, R. E. et al. Cyberknife stereotactic radiosurgery for treatment of atypical (WHO grade II) cranial meningiomas. *Neurosurgery* 67:1180-1188, 2010.

[9] Chokyu, I., Goto, T., Ishibashi, K., Nagata, T., Ohata, K. Bilateral subfrontal approach for tuberculum sellae meningiomas in long-term postoperative visual outcome. *J. Neurosurg.* 115:802-810, 2011.

[10] Chowdhury, F. H., Haque, M. R., Goel, A. H., Kawsar, K. A. Endoscopic endonasal extended transsphenoidal removal of tuberculum sellae meningioma (TSM): an experience of six cases. *Br. J. Neurosurg.* 26:692-699, 2012.

[11] Clark, A. J., Jahangiri, A., Garcia, R. M., George, J. R., Sughrue, M. E., McDermott, M. W. et al. Endoscopic surgery for tuberculum sellae meningiomas: a systematic review and meta-analysis. *Neurosurg. Rev.* 36:349-359, 2013.

[12] Conti, A., Pontoriero, A., Midili, F., Iatì, G., Siragusa, C., Tomasello, C., et al. CyberKnife multisession stereotactic radiosurgery and hypofractionated stereotactic radiotherapy for perioptic meningiomas: intermediate-term results and radiobiological considerations. *SpringerPlus* 4:37, 2015.

[13] Cushing, H. Meningioms. *Their classification, regional behavior, life history, and surgical end results*. Springfield, Illinois: C.C. Thomas, 1938.

[14] de Divitiis, E., Esposito, F., Cappabianca, P., Cavallo, L. M., de Divitiis, O. Tuberculum sellae meningiomas: high route or low route? A series of 51 consecutive cases. *Neurosurgery* 62:556-563; discussion 556-563, 2008.

[15] Dolenc, V. V., Pregelj, R., Slokan, S., Skrbec, M. Anterior communicating artery aneurysm associated with tuberculum sellae meningioma-case report. *Neurol. Med. Chir.* (Tokyo) 38:485-488, 1998.

[16] Dumitrescu, B. G. M. Giant tuberculum sellae meningioma with unruptured anterior communicating artery aneurysm encased. *Romanian Neurosurgery* 18:533-540, 2011.

[17] Fatemi, N., Dusick, J. R., de Paiva Neto, M. A., Malkasian, D., Kelly, D. F. endonasal versus supraorbital keyhole removal of craniopharyngiomas and tuberculum sellae meningiomas. *Neurosurgery* 64:ons269-ons287, 2009.

[18] Fernandez-Miranda, J. C., Pinheiro-Nieto, C., Gardner, P. A., Snyderman, C. H. Endoscopic endonasal approach for a tuberculum sellae meningioma. *J. Neurosurg.* 32 Suppl. E8, 2012.

[19] Hayhurst, C., Teo, C. Tuberculum sella meningioma. *Otolaryngol. Clin. North Am.* 44: 953-963, viii-ix, 2011.

[20] Jallo, G. I., Benjamin, V. Tuberculum sellae meningiomas: microsurgical anatomy and surgical technique. *Neurosurgery* 51:1432-1439; discussion 1439-1440, 2002.

[21] Kinjo, T., al-Mefty, O., Ciric, I. Diaphragma sellae meningiomas. *Neurosurgery* 36: 1082-1092, 1995.

[22] Komotar, R. J., Starke, R. M., Raper, D. M., Anand, V. K., Schwartz, T. H. Endoscopic endonasal versus open transcranial resection of anterior midline skull base meningiomas. *World Neurosurg*. 77:713-724, 2012.

[23] Komotar, R. J., Starke, R. M., Raper, D. M. S., Anand, V. K., Schwartz, T. H. Endoscopic Endonasal versus Open Transcranial Resection of Anterior Midline Skull Base Meningiomas. *World Neurosurgery* 77:713-724, 2012.

[24] Kwancharoen, R., Blitz, A. M., Tavares, F., Caturegli, P., Gallia, G. L., Salvatori, R. Clinical features of sellar and suprasellar meningiomas. *Pituitary* 17:342-348, 2014.

[25] Leu, C. H., Hu, T. L., Shen, C. C., Wang, Y. C. Tuberculum sellae meningiomas: clinical manifestation, radiologic diagnosis, surgery and visual outcome. *Zhonghua Yi Xue Za Zhi* (Taipei) 61:1-7, 1998.

[26] Li-Hua, C., Ling, C., Li-Xu, L. Microsurgical management of tuberculum sellae meningiomas by the frontolateral approach: Surgical technique and visual outcome. *Clinical Neurology and Neurosurgery* 113:39-47, 2011.

[27] McLaughlin, N., Ditzel Filho, L. F., Shahlaie, K., Solari, D., Kassam, A., Kelly, D. The Supraorbital Approach for Recurrent or Residual Suprasellar Tumors. *Minim. Invasive Neurosurg*. 54:155-161, 2011.

[28] Nakamura, M., Roser, F., Struck, M., Vorkapic, P., Samii, M. tuberculum sellae meningiomas. *Neurosurgery*:1019???1029, 2006.

[29] Nakamura, M., Roser, F., Struck, M., Vorkapic, P., Samii, M. Tuberculum sellae meningiomas: clinical outcome considering different surgical approaches. *Neurosurgery* 59:1019-1028; discussion 1028-1019, 2006.

[30] Nakamura, M., Struck, M., Roser, F., Vorkapic, P., Samii, M. Olfactory groove meningiomas: clinical outcome and recurrence rates after tumor removal through the frontolateral and bifrontal approach. *Neurosurgery* 60:844-852; discussion 844-852, 2007.

[31] Nanda, A., Ambekar, S., Javalkar, V., Sharma, M. Technical nuances in the management of tuberculum sellae and diaphragma sellae meningiomas. *Neurosurg. Focus* 35:E7, 2013.

[32] Ostrom, Q. T., Gittleman, H., Farah, P., Ondracek, A., Chen, Y., Wolinsky, Y. et al. CBTRUS statistical report: Primary brain and central nervous system tumors diagnosed in the United States in 2006-2010. *Neuro Oncol*. 15 Suppl. 2:ii1-56, 2013.

[33] Peris-Celda, M., Kucukyuruk, B., Monroy-Sosa, A., Funaki, T., Valentine, R., Rhoton, A. L. Jr. The recesses of the sellar wall of the sphenoid sinus and their intracranial relationships. *Neurosurgery* 73:ons117-131; discussion ons131, 2013.

[34] Prosser, J., Vender, J., Alleyne, C., Solares, C. Expanded Endoscopic Endonasal Approaches to Skull Base Meningiomas. *Journal of Neurological Surgery Part B: Skull Base* 73:147-156, 2012.

[35] Prosser, J. D., Vender, J. R., Alleyne, C. H., Solares, C. A. Expanded endoscopic endonasal approaches to skull base meningiomas. *J. Neurol. Surg. B Skull Base* 73:147-156, 2012.

[36] Romani, R., Laakso, A., Kangasniemi, M., Niemelä, M., Hernesniemi, J. Lateral Supraorbital Approach Applied to Tuberculum Sellae Meningiomas. *Neurosurgery* 70:1504-1519, 2012.

[37] Rubin, G., Ben David, U., Gornish, M., Rappaport, Z. H. Meningiomas of the anterior cranial fossa floor. Review of 67 cases. *Acta Neurochir*. (Wien) 129:26-30, 1994.

[38] Sartor, K. A., K. G.; Atzor, R. *Diagnostic and Interventional Neuroradiology*. New York, NY: Thieme New York, 2002.

[39] Sathananthan, M., Sathananthan, A., Scheithauer, B. W., Giannini, C., Meyer, F. B., Atkinson, J. L. et al. Sellar meningiomas: an endocrinologic perspective. *Pituitary* 16: 182-188, 2013.

[40] Soni, R. S., Patel, S. K., Husain, Q., Dahodwala, M. Q., Eloy, J. A., Liu, J. K. From above or below: the controversy and historical evolution of tuberculum sellae meningioma resection from open to endoscopic skull base approaches. *J. Clin. Neurosci*. 21:559-568, 2014.

[41] Spektor, S., Valarezo, J., Fliss, D. M., Gil, Z., Cohen, J., Goldman, J. et al. Olfactory groove meningiomas from neurosurgical and ear, nose, and throat perspectives: approaches, techniques, and outcomes. *Neurosurgery* 57:268-280; discussion 268-280, 2005.

[42] Wilson, D. A., Duong, H., Teo, C., Kelly, D. F. The Supraorbital Endoscopic Approach for Tumors. *World Neurosurgery* 82:S72-S80, 2014.

In: Current Management of Central Nervous System … ISBN: 978-1-63483-856-6
Editors: Steven D. Chang and Anand Veeravagu 

*Chapter 13*

# RADIATION THERAPY AND STEREOTACTIC RADIOSURGERY FOR INTRACRANIAL MENINGIOMAS

***Ching-Jen Chen, MD, I. Jonathan Pomeraniec, BSc, Dale Ding, MD and Jason Sheehan, MD PhD***
Department of Neurological Surgery,
University of Virginia Health System, Charlottesville, Virginia, US

## ABSTRACT

Meningiomas are common intracranial tumors in the adult population. The management of intracranial meningiomas depends on specific patient factors and tumor characteristics. When treatment is deemed necessary, surgical resection remains the primary intervention, with gross total resection (GTR) representing the gold standard. When GTR cannot be safely achieved without a significant risk of neurological compromise, residual tumor can be treated with fractionated radiation therapy or stereotactic radiosurgery (SRS) depending on the location and volume of residual disease. The contemporary therapeutic landscape has paved way for SRS as an integral therapeutic modality for patients with meningioma.

SRS was initially confined to the setting of recurrent or residual skull base meningiomas. With broadened experience and progressively successful outcomes for these types of meningiomas, the indications for SRS have gradually expanded to include parasagittal, parafalcine, and convexity meningiomas. SRS can also serve as an upfront treatment for patients presenting with clinical and radiographic features consistent with a benign (WHO grade I) meningioma. SRS has enjoyed particular efficacy as a primary or adjunctive treatment for grade I meningiomas, primarily those tumors located at the skull base, where the operative morbidity is particularly high with aggressive resection [1-3].

The majority of contemporary SRS series of patients with WHO grade I meningiomas report tumor control rates in excess of 85%. The role of SRS for WHO grade II and III meningiomas remains less established, with relatively sparse literature describing radiosurgical outcomes for these uncommon, aggressive tumors [4, 5]. Nevertheless, nascent reports suggest that SRS may play an important role in the management of residual or recurrent grade II and III meningiomas [6]. Futures studies will hopefully further delineate this role.

As with any modern surgical technique, potential benefits are not devoid of complications. While complications can occur, neurological function is generally preserved. Longitudinal follow-up including neurologic and radiologic assessment is required for an effective radiosurgical therapeutic regimen. Single and multisession stereotactic radiosurgery will likely play an expanding role in the treatment of patients with meningiomas going forward.

## INTRODUCTION

Meningiomas are one of the most common intracranial tumors in adults [7]. The majority are benign (WHO grade I) tumors [7-9]. In concordance with the prevailing pathological framework, up to 35% of all intracranial meningiomas can be classified as either atypical (WHO grade II) or malignant (WHO grade III) [10]. WHO grade I meningiomas are frequently discussed in literature due to their relatively high incidence and long-term survival afforded by contemporary management protocols. In contrast, atypical and malignant meningiomas tend to follow significantly poorer natural histories exhibited by recurrence, invasion and even distant metastasis [11, 12].

Surgical resection has traditionally been the treatment of choice for meningiomas and continues to play a significant role in the modern management of these patients. The benefits of resection include histological confirmation, relief of mass effect on adjacent neurovascular structures and, in instances of gross total resection (GTR), an opportunity for cure. Tumor control rates vary depending upon the extent of resection. Following GTR – excision of tumor with any attendant dural attachment and/or abnormal bone – tumor recurrences at 5, 10, and 15 years are 5, 10, and 30%, respectively [13].

However, advantages of resection must still be weighed against the risk, morbidity and feasibility of surgery. For example, tumors involving major venous structures, such as the superior sagittal sinus, or cranial nerves may render safe GTR unachievable. In cases not conducive to GTR, a subtotal resection (STR) may be performed to relieve mass effect and decrease tumor volume in anticipation of subsequent observation or radiotherapy. Recent work by Sughrue et al. challenges the long-term utility of achieving Simpson grade I or II resection for patients with WHO grade I meningiomas; the 5-year progression-free survival rates for all patients who underwent Simpson grades I, II, III, and IV resections were 95, 85, 88, and 81%, respectively, without any significant difference between Simpson grades [14]. Stereotactic radiosurgery and fractionated radiation therapy are effective adjuvant treatments for residual or recurrent WHO grade I meningiomas in a modern era where GTR may not be as essential to long-term survival as during Simpson's time.

The application of radiation oncology, including conventional fractionated external beam radiotherapy (EBRT), intensity modulated radiotherapy (IMRT), and fractionated stereotactic radiotherapy (FSRT) are prominent in the management of meningiomas. Using doses of 50 to 55 Gray (Gy) in 1.8 to 3 Gy per fractions, EBRT has achieved local tumor control rates of 70 to 95% at 10 years [15, 16].

Improved precision in radiation delivery can be obtained via IMRT and FSRT, thereby limiting radiation exposure to normal brain structures. IMRT serves as a three-dimensional conformal treatment approach and the intensities of radiation can be modulated across target volumes near important structures using subfields created by a multi-leaf collimator. While the rates of tumor control and radiation-induced adverse effects are generally acceptable with IMRT and FSRT, these approaches are typically reserved for patients with larger tumor volume or diffuse meningiomas that are not amenable to radiosurgical targeting.

Over the past two decades, SRS has become an increasingly integral part of the treatment regimen for meningioma patients. SRS should be considered for meningiomas abutting critical neurovascular structures and for residual disease following STR. Radiosurgical management may also be offered to patients with significant medical comorbidities precluding them from surgical intervention as well as to those who refuse surgery. Meningiomas often demonstrate uniform enhancement on contrasted imaging and are thus well-defined on neuroimaging. With increasingly precise and accurate diagnostic technologies, meningiomas are typically detected at a small to moderate volume (<10 cc). Benign meningiomas tend to displace rather than invade normal brain structures. The combination of these attributes renders meningiomas appealing targets for SRS.

## History of Radiosurgery

Stereotactic radiosurgery, both in concept and design, was initially envisaged by Lars Leksell in his quest to obliterate intracranial targets through an intact skull. Leksell witnessed firsthand successes and failures of open neurosurgical techniques as a pupil of Olivecrona and consequently found purpose in trying to dampen the operative morbidity and mortality which accompanied such procedures. His conceptualization of the stereotactic method – introduced in the laboratory by Clarke and Horsley [17] and applied in the clinical setting by Spiegel and associates [18] – spawned a practical foundation for a minimally invasive neurosurgical approach. In his autobiography, Brain Fragments, Leksell penned: "I have in my hand a new type of brain surgery, an operative system, a more sophisticated and less risky surgical procedure based on progressively improving imaging of the brain and on mechanical accuracy and modern physics, a necessary addition to classical bloody surgery" [19]. Leksell ultimately promoted a stereotactic system of his own for open interventions and adapted a center of arc device in the creation of the Gamma Knife.

Since its inception by Leksell, SRS has since expanded in both breadth and depth. As a minimally invasive approach, SRS has transcended beyond the original operating framework of the Leksell model U Gamma Knife and can now be delivered with an increasing scope of devices (e.g., Gamma Knife Perfexion, Novalis, Cyberknife, Tomotherapy, and Trilogy). As of December 2013, Gamma Knife SRS had been used to treat 112,703 patients with meningiomas worldwide [Leksell Gamma Knife Society, Cumulative Indications 1991-2013; http://www.elekta.com/healthcare_international_treatment_statistics.php]. Many additional patients have been treated with LINAC-based SRS devices.

Furthermore, radiosurgical management as a clinical discipline has blossomed into an inherently interprofessional pursuit that encourages intimate collaboration between specially trained neurological surgeons, radiation oncologists and medical physicists.

# DETAILED ACCOUNT OF RADIOSURGICAL MANAGEMENT

## The Radiobiology of Radiosurgery

SRS employs a mixture of stereotaxis, image guidance and ionizing beams from multiple vantage points to deliver a high dose of radiation to a single target. The purpose and effect of this combination is to inactivate cells contained within the target volume while simultaneously minimizing radiation to surrounding tissue. The mathematical analog of SRS would be the step function (i.e., a piecewise constant function), although SRS merely approaches such a theoretical absolute.

Since the biological construct of SRS is not entirely understood, the classic 4 R's of radiation therapy (repair, reassortment, repopulation, and reoxygenation) probably reside with much less gravity. In fact, the linear quadratic formula of radiation oncology, predicated on a single radiation track to induce double-stranded DNA breaks, fails to predict SRS outcomes [20]. The cellular responses differ markedly with radiation doses in excess of 5Gy compared to lower doses [21]. SRS does share similarities to fractionated EBRT, though, including of the deployment of the same single- and double-stranded DNA breaks. The radiobiological effectiveness of SRS may also be fashioned by vascular changes within the targeted volume [21]. In Gamma Knife radiosurgery, dose heterogeneity from "hot spots" has also been posited to confer radiobiological advantages over EBRT for the treatment of small to moderately sized tumors [22].

Meningiomas, classically considered late responding tissue, can be exploited in radiosurgery by a higher biologically equivalent dose (BED) delivered to these tumors than what might be afforded by conventional EBRT. Provided a steep enough dose fall-off to surrounding structures, the higher BED should translate to a greater rate of local tumor control while still affording a low rate of complications.

## Radiosensitivity of Cranial Nerves

Meningiomas frequently reside adjacent to cranial nerves, particularly when localized to the skull base. Radiation injury to cranial nerves likely results from small vessel and protective Schwann cell damage. Radiation tolerance of a cranial nerve is likely dependent upon the dose per volume delivered and the neurological condition of the nerve prior to SRS. In particular, cranial nerves with dysfunction at the time of SRS are generally regarded less tolerant of radiation than their counterparts without dysfunction. Interestingly, there also appear to exist a differential tolerance of various cranial nerves: sensory nerves (optic and acoustic cranial nerves) have the lowest tolerance to radiation while the facial nerves and other lower cranial nerves exhibit relatively higher radiation tolerance. This phenomenon may in fact be explained by virtue of both optic and acoustic nerves comprising central nervous system fiber tracts that carry more complex data. Moreover, clinical experience dictates that these cranial nerves do not possess much potential for recovery from any form of injury such as mechanical from surgery, compressive from a tumor or ionizing from radiation.

The radiosensitivities of cranial nerves often limit the dose of radiation that can safely be delivered to tumors in close proximity. Although the precise dose tolerance of cranial nerves remains undetermined, the anterior visual pathways seem to be able to tolerate a single dose of radiation in the range of 8 to 12 Gy [23-25]. Hence the distance between nerve and tumor in the case of parasellar and tuberculum meningiomas must be carefully assessed. The risk of visual dysfunction is associated with the volume of the optic apparatus receiving radiation dose [26-29]. A distance of 5 mm between meningioma and optic apparatus (i.e., optic nerves and chiasm) can achieve an optimal dose fall-off, but a distance of 1-2 mm may still be tolerable due to shielding capabilities of modern radiosurgical devices and multisession approaches.

Experiences outlining tolerance to radiation of cranial nerves are more readily available for the trigeminal and facial nerves. In an institutional series of 151 patients who underwent SRS for trigeminal neuralgia, 12 patients (8%) developed new-onset facial numbness following treatment [30]. The risk factors associated with facial and trigeminal nerve dysfunction appears to be associated with the length of nerve irradiated in contrast to the volume of tumor or maximal dose, as observed by Norén et al. in a cohort of patients with vestibular schwannomas treated using SRS doses between 12 and 20 Gy [31].

Moving along the spectrum of sensitivity to radiation, cranial nerves contained within the cavernous sinus appear to be more radioresistant though their maximal radiation tolerance remains unclear. In the brainstem, radiation tolerance likely varies between 12 to 15 Gy or higher when that radiation is delivered to a small volume. Thus, brainstem doses do not typically pose major obstacles in the blueprint planning of radiosurgical treatment of petroclival, foramen magnum, or cerebellopontine angle meningiomas.

SRS is becoming more widely accepted as a treatment option for benign, deep-seated intracranial lesions. Patients with parasellar and sellar tumors have been treated with doses between 20-30 Gy delivered to parasellar cranial nerves with only rare complications. Tishler et al. noted that SRS appeared to be relatively safe in treating lesions within or near the cavernous sinus for 29 patients after LINAC SRS and 33 patients after Gamma Knife SRS (GK): 12 new neuropathies were observed from 3-41 months that were related to the nerves in the parasellar region, but the development of these complications did not show a clear relationship to the maximum dose in the range of 10-40 Gy. Doses up to 40 Gy have been shown to be relatively safe for nerves in the parasellar region [32].

## Stereotactic Radiosurgery Approach

SRS, by nature, contains many intricate components that are perhaps optimally synthesized and operated by a specialized, multidisciplinary team using specifically tailored and rigorously tested devices capable of sub-millimeter accuracy and precision. The actual technique varies with stereotactic device but this does not preclude a shared set of fundamental steps for all such procedures. First and foremost, a careful and comprehensive assessment of the patient, including a detailed neurological and radiological assessment, should be performed and reviewed. Depending on the location of the tumor, neuro-ophthalmologic, endocrine and/or otolaryngologic assessments may also be warranted. If a patient underwent prior microsurgery, the appropriate operative and histopathological reports should be scrutinized and fat suppression imaging protocols may be necessary.

Once a radiosurgical regimen has been deemed an appropriate treatment modality by both patient and physician, appropriate stereotactic image datasets should be acquired. This image acquisition is typically performed with some degree of target immobilization through rigid frame fixation or aquaplast mask. The tumor, along with any surrounding structures at risk, can be contoured in order to render and balance an ideal dose to the tumor margin (typically 12 to 16 Gy for grade I meningiomas) with a safe dose to eloquent brain structures.

The Models U, B, C, 4C, or Perfexion Gamma Knife units are commonly employed depending on the available technology at particular treatment centers. The radiosurgery procedure begins with the application of the Leksell Model G stereotactic frame (Elekta AB, Stockholm, Sweden) after applying a local anesthetic supplemented by any additional sedation as appropriate. Following frame placement, high-resolution stereotactic MRI with gadolinium contrast is performed. In cases in which MRI is not feasible or when MRI distortion raises concerns, stereotactic contrasted CT can be performed instead. Dose planning is subsequently performed by a team of neurosurgeons, radiation oncologists and medical physicists. LINAC-based systems may use frame or mask immobilization coupled with on-board imaging (e.g., CT or X-ray). Dose selection is based on an empirical algorithm that considers tumor volume, proximity to critical structures such as the cranial nerves and brainstem, preexisting neurological deficits and history of previous treatment with fractionated EBRT. Radiosurgical treatment parameters (e.g., margin dose, treatment isodose) are thus individualized for each patient. The radiosurgical treatment should be delivered with utmost precision and accuracy and any additional precautionary measures, such as perioperative corticosteroids, should remain at the discretion of specific treatment centers and matched to individual patient characteristics.

Clinical and imaging evaluations are typically performed during regular follow-up in the outpatient setting with a generally recommended schedule of MRIs at 6 month intervals for the first 2 years after radiosurgery. In patients demonstrating no evidence of tumor growth and/or new neurological findings, follow-up intervals can be lengthened. Neuroimaging can thereafter be performed at annual intervals until year five, and then on a biannual basis in perpetuity. Clinical follow-up should parallel radiologic examinations.

## Radiosurgical Complications

As mentioned earlier, radiosurgery is not immune to risk or complication. The radiosurgical procedure itself does not appear to be associated with any particular immediate or upfront risks. Patients sometimes experience nausea and/or headaches during or following frame-based procedures, though infections of pin sites and perioperative seizures are extremely rare complications. Patients who develop seizures usually have supratentorial tumors and a history of epilepsy and so patients with pre-existing seizures should be maintained within normal therapeutic ranges of antiepileptic medications both pre- and post-operatively. For those with new-onset seizures following meningioma SRS, follow-up neuroimaging yields clinically significant information and enables one to exclude peri-tumoral edema, intra-tumoral hemorrhage, venous infarction, tumor growth and/or necrosis.

Overall, complications associated with meningioma SRS have been reported in 3 to 40% of cases, depending upon the series reviewed. The majority of reported complications are around8% with approximately 5% being permanent and 3% being transient. Complications include neurological deficits associated with adverse post-radiosurgical changes observed on follow-up neuroimaging (e.g., edema, necrosis, etc.) and partial or complete cranial nerve dysfunction, most commonly seen in patients with parasellar or other skull base meningiomas. Kondziolka et al. reported a 9% complication rate in 972 patients, with 6.3% morbidity including visual decline, CN VI neuropathy, and trigeminal neuropathy for those with parasellar meningiomas [33]. The optic apparatus appears to be able to tolerate radiation dose of 8 to 12 Gy to a 1% volume. A distance of 2 to 3 mm between the tumor and the adjacent optic apparatus is usually required for the delivery of a tumor margin dose of 15Gy using modern radiosurgical techniques while limiting the radiation dose to the optic apparatus to less than 12Gy.

Radiation induced changes in the surrounding brain parenchyma following meningioma treatment are well described. The most commonly observed post-radiosurgical change is peri-tumoral edema, which was observed in 24.7% of meningioma patients in a series reported by Cai et al. [34]. Post-treatment peri-tumoral edema may be asymptomatic or manifest with neurological sequelae. T2-weighted and post-contrast changes on MRI can be reversible and are often associated with edema and increased permeability of the blood brain barrier. These radiologic changes can typically be adequately managed with a short course of steroids. For those with steroid-refractory or worsening edema, surgical resection of the lesion is frequently warranted. Risk factors for edema following radiosurgery include age greater than 60 years, peri-tumoral edema prior to radiosurgery, no previous surgical resection, larger treatment volume (e.g., >10 cc), tumor location in the anterior cranial fossa and higher margin dose (e.g., >15 Gy) [35].

In contrast to the aforementioned reversible changes, irreversible changes elucidated on MRI are often associated with necrosis. T1 and T2 changes on MRI may provide a simple means of differentiation between tumor growth and adverse radiation effects. Lesions poorly defined on T2-weighted sequences compared to the contrast-enhancing margin on T1 (i.e., T1/T2 mismatch) were found to correlate with adverse radiation effects [36]. PET, perfusion and SPECT imaging can be utilized to discern tumor progression from radiation induced necrosis [37]. Unfortunately, despite advances in resolution and analytics, neuroimaging results do not always yield clear or definitive diagnoses. Therefore, surgical biopsy and/or resection may be required to distinguish between tumor growth and radiation necrosis. As a brief aside, bevacizumab (Avastin) has been used to manage some patients with persistent peri-tumoral edema or necrosis following radiation therapy for whom resection does not appear a viable option [38, 39].

## Radiosurgery-Induced Neoplasia

Cahan et al. [40] defined the criteria for a radiation induced tumor as follows: 1) the tumor must occur in the radiation field; 2) it cannot be present prior to irradiation; 3) the primary tumor must differ histologically from the induced tumor; and 4) there should be no genetic predisposition for occurrence of a secondary malignancy or tumor progression. Based on the literature, the incidence of radiosurgery-induced neoplasia ranges between 0 and 3 per 200,000 patients [41]. In 2007, Rowe et al. cross-referenced the results of patients treated with SRS in Sheffield against England's national mortality and cancer databases [42]. Among a cohort of 4,896 patients in this study with more than 30,000 patient-years of data, only two patients were identified to have new malignant brain tumors. The investigators concluded that the risk of SRS-induced malignancy did not appear to rise above the natural incidence of cancer in the general population. Although the risk of SRS-induced tumor seems quite low, the risk is not negligible and must be taken into consideration when treating patients with benign tumors such as WHO grade I meningiomas who have a long life expectancy. In general, the risks of open surgery or conservative management of patients with meningiomas outweigh the small risk of SRS-induced neoplasia.

# DISCUSSION

## Radiosurgical Outcomes for Skull Base Meningiomas

SRS has become more widespread as a therapeutic modality offered at meningioma treatment centers (Figure 1). SRS has most commonly been utilized in the setting of skull base meningiomas, which tend to neighbor or envelope neurovascular structures and extend beyond one cranial fossa. Given the difficulty requisite with achieving complete resection, many of these tumors represent ideal targets for radiosurgery. More recently, SRS has become a primary treatment option for small- to medium-sized skull base meningiomas (less than 3 cm in diameter).

With adoption of SRS for skull base meningiomas, larger case series have documented excellent actuarial tumor control rates. In a large GK series of 972 patients with mostly skull base meningiomas treated using a median dose of 13Gy, the 5-, 10-, and 15-year tumor control rates were 93%, 87%, and 87%, respectively [33]. In an earlier report from the same group on patients with cavernous sinus meningiomas, the 5-and 10-year tumor control rates were both 93%. Of 159 cavernous sinus meningiomas treated with SRS, 3% markedly decreased in size, 60% remained stable and 6% increased in size [43]. Another large series of 200 patients with skull base meningiomas reported even higher control rates of 98.5 and 97% at 5 and 10 years following SRS, respectively [44]. Other studies of LINAC-based or GK have reported comparable tumor control rates for grade I meningiomas.

In contemporary practice, presumptive diagnoses of skull base meningiomas can be rendered based on radiographic characteristics even without definitive histologic confirmation. In a group of meningiomas primarily diagnosed by imaging which were treated with SRS, Spiegelmann et al. demonstrated a 98% tumor control rate at mean 67 months [45]. In another series of similarly diagnosed tumors, SRS for 219 skull base meningiomas resulted in tumor control rate of 93.2% at 5 years [46]. At the University of Virginia, 206 patients with skull base meningiomas treated with GK (142 with residual or recurrent meningiomas after prior resection and 64 with SRS as the primary treatment) exhibited an overall tumor control rate of 89% at follow-up spanning up to 6 years [2].

Cyberknife SRS (CK) utilizes a modified LINAC positioned on a robotic arm, which can be moved to different nodes that deliver beams of radiation. In a series of 199 predominately skull base meningiomas, 93.5% of patients exhibited local tumor control at 5 years following CK [47]. CK has also been utilized in the treatment of peri-optic meningiomas by the Stanford group [48]. In their experience, visual function appeared to be preserved in the vast majority of patients undergoing multisession CK. Other technologies such as Novalis TX or GK Extend have been used to deliver multi-session SRS to peri-optic meningiomas with reasonable safety [49].

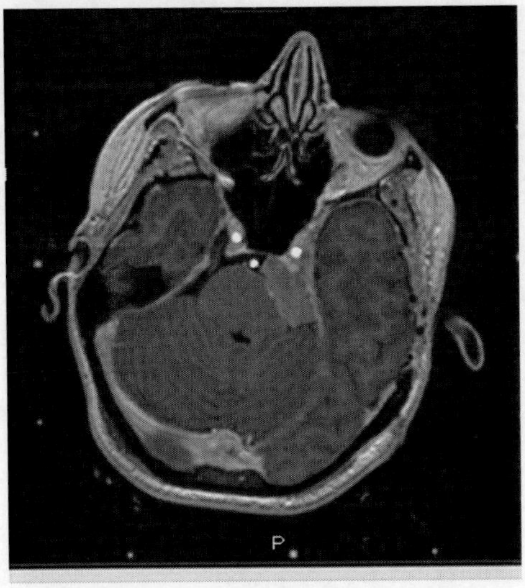


Figure 1. Pre-operative MRI; axial view.

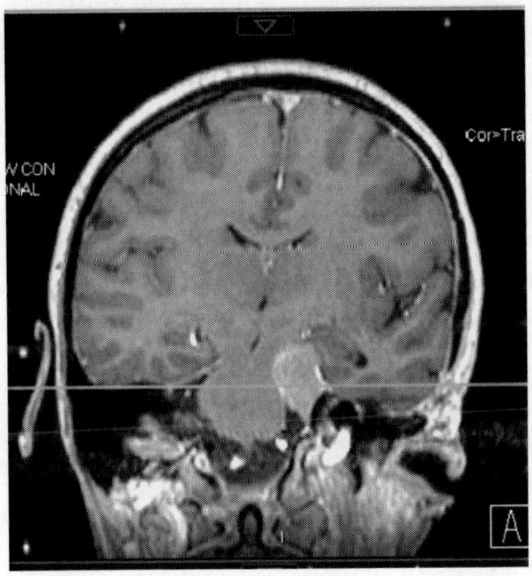


Figure 2. Pre-operative MRI; coronal view Patient was treated with single session SRS with a tumor margin dose of 15 Gy. Follow up coronal MRI (Figure 3) at four years following SRS demonstrate a marked regression of the tumor. The patient's trigeminal nerve dysfunction began to improve approximately six months after SRS.

SRS has also been frequently adopted to treat meningiomas of the posterior fossa and foramen magnum. Despite innate risks of irradiating near the brainstem, tumor control rates for posterior fossa and foramen magnum meningiomas are nevertheless high with acceptably low complication rates. A multicenter study of 254 patients with a benign petroclival meningioma and mean follow up of 71 months showed that tumor volumes increased in 9% of tumors, remained stable in 52% and decreased in 39%. At last clinical-follow up, 93.6% of patients demonstrated no change or improvement in their neurological condition and 6.4% of patients experienced progression of symptoms [50]. Another multicenter cohort study of 177 patients with benign cerebellopontine angle (CPA) meningiomas with mean clinical follow-up of 46 months showed actuarial rates of progression-free survival of 93% and 77% at 5 and 10 years, respectively (median tumor volume and prescription dose were 3.6 cc and 13 Gy, respectively) [51]. Nicolato et al. reported radiosurgical treatment of 62 meningiomas located in the posterior fossa [52]. On neuroimaging evaluation over a follow-up of 6 to 64.3 months (median 28.7 months), the meningioma either disappeared or reduced in size in 34 of 62 (55%), remained stable in 25 of 62 (40%), and progressed in 3 of 62 (5%) of cases. Two patients died from tumor progression and 6.5% of patients experienced transient complications due to post-radiosurgical edema.

A review of 222 patients with a meningioma in the posterior fossa treated with GK at the University of Virginia analyzed long-term outcomes over a mean follow-up for six years with median tumor volume of 6.8 cc and marginal dose of 12 Gy (range 10-15) [53]. Among five patients with foramen magnum meningiomas, 80% of patients achieved tumor control during follow-ups ranging from 4 to 13 years.

The fifth patient achieved stabilization following initial progression and subsequent treatment with repeat radiosurgery. Despite the inherent risks, no radiation-induced adverse effects to the brainstem or spinal cord were observed in these patients.

Time and institutional experience have aided in the refinement of effective radiosurgical margin doses, which have actually reduced to more appropriately balance tumor control rates and adverse effects. The reduction in margin dose to 12Gy appears to achieve that delicate balance. In a series of 97 patients with meningiomas of mean tumor volume 15.9 cc, a mean dose of 12Gydelivered to tumor margins yielded a 2-year progression free survival of 100%, and only three patients suffered from adverse radiation effects [54]. However, with margin doses below 12 Gy, long-term tumor control appears less durable [2].

In the recent literature, reports of skull base tumor reduction following radiosurgery vary from 16% to 69%, a fairly wide variation likely attributable to different study populations, treatment parameters and follow-up lengths. In reality, most meningiomas and other benign tumors will either increase or decrease in size over the course of adequate follow-up. There is utility in distinguishing benefits attributable to SRS (i.e., growth cessation) from that of tumors that simply do not grow as manifestations of their underlying natural histories, like many meningiomas. Tumor stability may result from SRS or could in fact represent limited period of follow-up. The result from tumor reduction or stability in size maybe improvement in neurological functioning [2].

Other factors such as age, tumor location, gender and baseline neurological status have not been consistently reported to affect radiologic control. In contrast, tumor volume and margin dose (12 Gy or higher) have been identified as factors that directly correlate to long-term tumor control. DiBiaise et al. demonstrated 5-year local tumor control of 92% in meningiomas less than 10 cc compared to 68% in those larger than 10 cc [55]. Another team led by Kondziolka reported diminished local tumor control with larger tumor volume [33].

## Radiosurgical Outcomes for Convexity Meningiomas

Convexity meningiomas have traditionally been managed by microsurgical resection, which allows for curative opportunity by extirpating the tumor and any involved dura. With the ongoing success of SRS for skull base meningiomas, SRS has been recently applied to convexity meningiomas in selected cases. Contemporary series of convexity meningiomas have reported tumor control rates comparable to those observed in skull base series (i.e., >85% tumor control rate).

The SRS-induced risks for convexity and skull base meningiomas are different and more frequently involve post-treatment cerebral edema [48, 52, 54, 55]. In a series of 125 patients with convexity meningiomas treated at the University of Pittsburgh, tumors treated with upfront SRS achieved a tumor control rate of 92% and those with prior resection had a tumor control rate of 97%. Overall morbidity was observed in9.6% of cases with 5% developing edema or adverse radiation effects [56]. This morbidity rate associated with radiosurgical treatment of convexity meningiomas is comparable to the 10% complication rate in a recent microsurgical series of convexity meningioma patients [57]. Girvigian et al. reported a lower rate of complications for convexity and parasagittal meningiomas treated with smaller target volumes and margin doses less than 14 Gy [58].

With respect to meningiomas involving the superior sagittal sinus, Pamir et al. reported a series of 43 patients with median follow-up of 46 months and treated with a margin dose of 15 Gy. Tumor size decreased in 51% of cases, remained stable in 37% and increased in 12%. For patients with larger tumors, these colleagues advocated resection without violation of the sinus and major cortical draining veins followed by SRS for residual or recurrent tumor [59]. In 2005, Kim et al. reported a series of 23 patients with 26 superficially located meningiomas over a mean follow-up of 32 months. The investigators observed that 25 of 26 tumors (96%) exhibited tumor control following GK and reported a complication rate of 43% with worsening edema as the most common complication (all of these patients experienced relief with perioperative steroids).

The group did note that those patients with symptomatic signal intensity changes on post-radiosurgical MRI were more likely to exhibit tumor shrinkage at latest follow-up [60]. Given this reasonable balance between tumor control and complications following SRS, this approach continues to gain favor as a reasonable alternative to resection in the treatment of convexity meningiomas.

Parasagittal and parafalcine (PSPF) meningiomas represent the second most common location for intracranial meningiomas. These tumors can involve the superior sagittal sinus or deep draining veins and thus prevent safe operative resection. Radiosurgery can offer a minimally invasive treatment modality for these types of meningiomas with good tumor control rates and low complication rates compared to most surgical series. A recent institutional review identified 65 patients with 90 WHO Grade I parasagittal (59%) and parafalcine (41%) meningiomas with median initial tumor volume of 3.7 $cm^3$ and median prescription dose of 15 Gy [1].

Over a follow-up period of 56.6 months, actuarial tumor control rates were 85% and 70% at three and five years, respectively. Parasagittal location, young age, and no prior resection were found to be independent predictors of tumor progression-free survival.

## Radiation-Induced Meningiomas

EBRT and SRS can both induce formation of meningiomas after a latency period of approximately 30 years [61-63]. The incidence of radiation-induced meningiomas appears to be higher with EBRT than SRS, although differences in follow-up duration may bias the comparison. These meningiomas may demonstrate a different underlying genetic composition and have actually been shown to under-express NF2 [64]. Radiosurgery has been shown to be highly effective for the treatment of some radiation induced meningiomas [65, 66].

## Radiosurgical Outcomes for WHO Grade II and III Meningiomas

A recent literature review of approximately 600 Grade II and III meningiomas treated with SRS showed a wide variation in outcomes [6]. The progression-free survival (PFS) rates at 5 years were 25%–83% for Grade II tumors (median 59%) and 0%–72% for Grade III tumors (median 13%). The median SRS-related complication rate was 8% (range 0%–62%). Despite significant statistical limitations due to small patient and tumor numbers, a myriad of factors influenced PFS, disease-specific survival or overall survival including patient age, tumor volume, WHO grade, mitotic index, radiosurgical margin and maximum dose, conformality index, timing of treatment, prior EBRT, and number of tumor recurrences prior to treatment [67-72].

SRS for Grade II and III meningiomas and any reliable measure of efficacy remains relatively elusive secondary to variations in patient populations, tumor characteristics and outcome measures. Investigators of some series have combined Grade I tumors with Grade II and III tumors without reporting outcomes differentiated by grade [4, 73-75]. Others did not report whether patients received prior EBRT, which has been previously shown to predict poorer radiosurgical tumor control [5]. Comparisons across different meningioma SRS series has been further complicated by the change in WHO diagnostic criteria for Grade II meningiomas in 2007, which drastically increased the proportion of meningiomas diagnosed as atypical [8, 10, 76]. Therefore, the Grade II meningiomas defined by previous WHO criteria may represent lesions histologically and biologically disparate from those defined by the revised criteria.

Many high grade meningioma patients present for SRS after failed EBRT (median 39%). In these cases, tumors may have acquired resistance to radiation-based therapies or may represent inherently more aggressive lesions. In addition, patients with a history of EBRT often require lower SRS doses which, when coupled with an unknown optimal timing of postoperative radiation, can potentially muddle optimal care delivery.

Despite the multitude of uncertainties that plague a robust understanding of radiosurgical outcomes for patients with Grade II and III meningiomas, current literature suggests that SRS provides some degree of tumor control for the majority of patients. For this very reason, prolonged efforts in basic science, translational and clinical research, as well as prospective clinical trials outlining the risk-benefit profile of conservative management, EBRT and radiosurgery in the setting of residual and recurrent disease, are warranted to improve outcomes for this subset of aggressive tumors [77]. However, due to the relatively low prevalence of Grade II and III meningiomas compared to their Grade I counterparts, prospective trials will be unlikely to accrue statistically powerful populations of patients. Thus, multicenter registries may be the best available tool for accruing evidence for SRS outcomes for non-benign meningiomas.

Radio-sensitizing agents may potentiate lower margin doses of EBRT or SRS, thereby more effectively sparing normal brain tissue and minimizing radiation-induced adverse effects. Improved understanding of the molecular biology of meningiomas and promoters of tumor progression may develop avenues for the discovery and implementation of targeted agents or immunotherapies [78].

While there are currently no chemotherapeutic regimens that effectively treat meningiomas, agents such as bevacizumab are being evaluated for the treatment of Grade II and III meningiomas [79, 80]. Finally, hypo-fractionated SRS delivery systems, such as the CK or GK Extend (Elekta AB) may expand the versatility of SRS and ultimately result in better outcomes for patients harboring Grade II and III meningiomas [81].

## FUTURE DIRECTIONS

SRS has emerged as an effective primary or adjuvant treatment for meningiomas. Despite a steep radiation dose gradient inherent to the radiosurgical platform, eloquent structures within 2-5mm of the traditional single-session high-dose radiation target are at risk. Recent studies have suggested that hypo-fractionation via multi-session SRS may help overcome some of the limitations of single-session SRS [48, 82, 83].

Preliminary data culled from patient reviews demonstrate promising results with reasonable tumor control and complication rates. Multisession SRS may lead to more routine treatment of lesions in close proximity to radiosensitive and/or eloquent structures, large lesions, and lesions that may require staged treatments [49].

Because of the increase in radiation dose to normal brain that is associated with larger tumor volumes, the general guidelines for single-session SRS are lesions smaller than 3cm in diameter [41, 84]. However, multi-session SRS may be able to overcome the obstacle of tissue toxicity via some degree of fractionation [83].

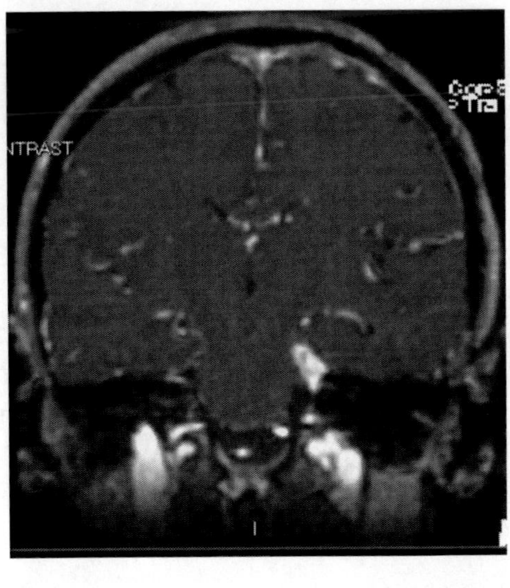


Figure 3. Follow up MRI; coronal view.

## CONCLUSION

SRS occupies an important role in the management of intracranial meningiomas and affords a high and durable rate of tumor control. SRS can be used as an upfront treatment for some meningiomas or reserved for those with recurrent or residual lesions following previous surgical resection. Complications resulting from SRS tend to be uncommon, but they are typically manageable and temporary. For many patients with meningiomas, the risk to benefit profile of SRS is favorable in comparison to the alternatives of microsurgical resection or tumor progression.

The management of atypical and malignant meningiomas includes initial resection with or without adjuvant radiation therapy in the form of EBRT or SRS, depending on the preferences and experience of the treating physician and institution. While WHO Grade I meningiomas may be successfully managed by GTR alone, Grade II and III meningiomas are significantly more difficult to control without adjuvant radiation therapy. Despite multimodality management, including resection, EBRT, and SRS, the long-term survival for patients harboring these lesions (particularly Grade III) remains relatively poor. Furthermore, the combined neurological morbidity from multiple treatment regimens accumulates over time. SRS appears to enhance tumor control and overall survival in this patient population, but its specific role in the management of Grade II and III meningiomas is not well-defined. Additional studies are required to bolster our understanding of SRS and improve our decisions regarding safety, efficacy and optimal timing in relation to surgical resection and EBRT.

### Case Study

The patient presented with a progressive left petroclival meningioma. Figures 1 and 2 (below) demonstrate the T1 post contrast axial and coronal views, respectively. He had trigeminal nerve pain and numbness.

## REFERENCES

[1] Ding D, Xu Z, McNeill IT, Yen CP, Sheehan JP. Radiosurgery for parasagittal and parafalcine meningiomas. *Journal of neurosurgery,* 2013;119 (4):871-7.

[2] Sheehan JP, Williams BJ, Yen CP. Stereotactic radiosurgery for WHO grade I meningiomas. *Journal of neuro-oncology,* 2010;99(3):407-16.

[3] Starke RM, Williams BJ, Hiles C, Nguyen JH, Elsharkawy MY, Sheehan JP. Gamma knife surgery for skull base meningiomas. *Journal of neurosurgery,* 2012;116(3):588-97.

[4] Hakim R, Alexander E, 3rd, Loeffler JS, Shrieve DC, Wen P, Fallon MP, et al. Results of linear accelerator-based radiosurgery for intracranial meningiomas. *Neurosurgery,* 1998;42(3):446-53; discussion 53-4.

[5] Pollock BE, Stafford SL, Link MJ, Garces YI, Foote RL. Stereotactic radiosurgery of World Health Organization grade II and III intracranial meningiomas: treatment results on the basis of a 22-year experience. *Cancer,* 2012;118(4):1048-54.

[6] Ding D, Starke RM, Hantzmon J, Yen CP, Williams BJ, Sheehan JP. The role of radiosurgery in the management of WHO Grade II and III intracranial meningiomas. *Neurosurgical focus,* 2013;35(6):E16.

[7] Deltour I, Johansen C, Auvinen A, Feychting M, Klaeboe L, Schuz J. Time trends in brain tumor incidence rates in Denmark, Finland, Norway, and Sweden, 1974-2003. *Journal of the National Cancer Institute,* 2009;101(24):1721-4.

[8] Louis DN, Ohgaki H, Wiestler OD, Cavenee WK, Burger PC, Jouvet A, et al. The 2007 WHO classification of tumours of the central nervous system. *Acta neuropathologica,* 2007;114(2):97-109.

[9] Kleihues P, Louis DN, Scheithauer BW, Rorke LB, Reifenberger G, Burger PC, et al. The WHO classification of tumors of the nervous system. *Journal of neuropathology and experimental neurology,* 2002;61 (3):215-25; discussion 26-9.

[10] Pearson BE, Markert JM, Fisher WS, Guthrie BL, Fiveash JB, Palmer CA, et al. Hitting a moving target: evolution of a treatment paradigm for atypical meningiomas amid changing diagnostic criteria. *Neurosurgical focus,* 2008;24(5):E3.

[11] Durand A, Labrousse F, Jouvet A, Bauchet L, Kalamarides M, Menei P, et al. WHO grade II and III meningiomas: a study of prognostic factors. *Journal of neuro-oncology,* 2009;95(3):367-75.

[12] Rosenberg LA, Prayson RA, Lee J, Reddy C, Chao ST, Barnett GH, et al. Long-term experience with World Health Organization grade III (malignant) meningiomas at a single institution. International journal of radiation oncology, biology, *physics,* 2009;74(2):427-32.

[13] Simpson D. The recurrence of intracranial meningiomas after surgical treatment. *Journal of neurology, neurosurgery, and psychiatry,* 1957;20 (1):22-39.

[14] Sughrue ME, Kane AJ, Shangari G, Rutkowski MJ, McDermott MW, Berger MS, et al. The relevance of Simpson Grade I and II resection in modern neurosurgical treatment of World Health Organization Grade I meningiomas. *J Neurosurg.,*

[15] Minniti G, Amichetti M, Enrici RM. Radiotherapy and radiosurgery for benign skull base meningiomas. *Radiation oncology,* 2009;4:42.

[16] Elia AE, Shih HA, Loeffler JS. Stereotactic radiation treatment for benign meningiomas. *Neurosurgical focus,* 2007;23(4):E5.

[17] Clarke RH, V. One method of investigating the deep ganglia and tracts of the central nervous system (cerebellum). Br Med J. 1906;2:1799-800.

[18] Spiegel E, Wycis, H., Marks, M., Lee, A. Stereotaxic apparatus for op¬erations on the human brain. *Science,* 1947;106:349-50.

[19] Leksell L. Brain fragments in radiosurgery. In: Steiner L, editor. Radiosurgery: Baseline and Trends. New York: Raven Press; 1992. p. 623-92.

[20] Kirkpatrick JP, Meyer JJ, Marks LB. The linear-quadratic model is inappropriate to model high dose per fraction effects in radiosurgery. *Seminars in radiation oncology,* 2008;18(4):240-3.

[21] Garcia-Barros M, Paris F, Cordon-Cardo C, Lyden D, Rafii S, Haimovitz-Friedman A, et al. Tumor response to radiotherapy regulated by endothelial cell apoptosis. *Science,* 2003;300(5622):1155-9.

[22] Ma L, Larson D, Petti P, Chuang C, Verhey L. Boosting central target dose by optimizing embedded dose hot spots for gamma knife radiosurgery. *Stereotactic and functional neurosurgery,* 2007;85(6):259-63.

[23] Jagannathan J, Sheehan JP, Pouratian N, Laws ER, Steiner L, Vance ML. Gamma Knife surgery for Cushing's disease. *Journal of neurosurgery,* 2007;106(6):980-7.

[24] Leber KA, Bergloff J, Langmann G, Mokry M, Schrottner O, Pendl G. Radiation sensitivity of visual and oculomotor pathways. *Stereotactic and functional neurosurgery,* 1995;64 Suppl 1:233-8.

[25] Leber KA, Bergloff J, Pendl G. Dose-response tolerance of the visual pathways and cranial nerves of the cavernous sinus to stereotactic radiosurgery. *Journal of neurosurgery,* 1998;88(1):43-50.

[26] Chen JC, Giannotta SL, Yu C, Petrovich Z, Levy ML, Apuzzo ML. Radiosurgical management of benign cavernous sinus tumors: dose profiles and acute complications. *Neurosurgery,* 2001;48(5):1022-30; discussion 30-2.

[27] Lim YL, Leem W, Kim TS, Rhee BA, Kim GK. Four years' experiences in the treatment of pituitary adenomas with gamma knife radiosurgery. *Stereotactic and functional neurosurgery,* 1998;70 Suppl 1:95-109.

[28] Sheehan JM, Vance ML, Sheehan JP, Ellegala DB, Laws ER, Jr. Radiosurgery for Cushing's disease after failed transsphenoidal surgery. *Journal of neurosurgery,* 2000;93(5):738-42.

[29] Witt TC, Kondziolka D, Flickinger JC, Lunsford LD. Gamma Knife Radiosurgery for Pituitary Tumors. In: Lunsford LD, Kondziolka D, Flickinger J, editors. Gamma Knife Brain Surgery Progress in Neurological Surgery. 14. Basel: Karger; 1998. p. 114-27.

[30] Sheehan J, Pan HC, Stroila M, Steiner L. Gamma knife surgery for trigeminal neuralgia: outcomes and prognostic factors. *Journal of neurosurgery,* 2005;102(3):434-41.

[31] Noren G, Greitz D, Hirsch A, Lax I. Gamma knife surgery in acoustic tumours. *Acta neurochirurgica Supplementum,* 1993;58:104-7.

[32] Tishler RB, Loeffler JS, Lunsford LD, Duma C, Alexander E, 3rd, Kooy HM, et al. Tolerance of cranial nerves of the cavernous sinus to radiosurgery. *International journal of radiation oncology, biology, physics,* 1993;27(2):215-21.

[33] Kondziolka D, Mathieu D, Lunsford LD, Martin JJ, Madhok R, Niranjan A, et al. Radiosurgery as definitive management of intracranial meningiomas. *Neurosurgery,* 2008;62(1):53-8; discussion 8-60.

[34] Cai R, Barnett GH, Novak E, Chao ST, Suh JH. Principal risk of peritumoral edema after stereotactic radiosurgery for intracranial meningioma is tumor-brain contact interface area. *Neurosurgery,* 66(3): 513-22.

[35] Kollova A, Liscak R, Novotny J, Jr., Vladyka V, Simonova G, Janouskova L. Gamma Knife surgery for benign meningioma. *Journal of neurosurgery,* 2007;107(2):325-36.

[36] Kano H, Kondziolka D, Lobato-Polo J, Zorro O, Flickinger JC, Lunsford LD. T1/T2 matching to differentiate tumor growth from radiation effects after stereotactic radiosurgery. *Neurosurgery,* 66(3):486-91; discussion 91-2.

[37] Jain R, Narang J, Sundgren PM, Hearshen D, Saksena S, Rock JP, et al. Treatment induced necrosis versus recurrent/progressing brain tumor: going beyond the boundaries of conventional morphologic imaging. *J. Neurooncol.,*

[38] Liu AK, Macy ME, Foreman NK. Bevacizumab as therapy for radiation necrosis in four children with pontine gliomas. International journal of radiation oncology, *biology, physics,* 2009;75(4):1148-54.

[39] Levin VA, Bidaut L, Hou P, Kumar AJ, Wefel JS, Bekele BN, et al. Randomized Double-Blind Placebo-Controlled Trial of Bevacizumab Therapy for Radiation Necrosis of the Central Nervous System. *Int. J. Radiat. Oncol. Biol. Phys.,*

[40] Cahan WG, Woodard HQ, Higinbotham NL, Stewart FW, Coley BL. Sarcoma arising in irradiated bone: report of eleven cases. 1948. *Cancer,* 1998;82(1):8-34.

[41] Ganz JC. Gamma knife radiosurgery and its possible relationship to malignancy: a review. *Journal of neurosurgery,* 2002;97(5 Suppl):644-52.

[42] Rowe J, Grainger A, Walton L, Silcocks P, Radatz M, Kemeny A. Risk of malignancy after gamma knife stereotactic radiosurgery. *Neurosurgery,* 2007;60(1):60-5; discussion 5-6.

[43] Lee JY, Niranjan A, McInerney J, Kondziolka D, Flickinger JC, Lunsford LD. Stereotactic radiosurgery providing long-term tumor control of cavernous sinus meningiomas. *Journal of neurosurgery,* 2002;97(1):65-72.

[44] Kreil W, Luggin J, Fuchs I, Weigl V, Eustacchio S, Papaefthymiou G. Long term experience of gamma knife radiosurgery for benign skull base meningiomas. *J. Neurol. Neurosurg. Psychiatry,* 2005;76(10):1425-30.

[45] Spiegelmann R, Cohen ZR, Nissim O, Alezra D, Pfeffer R. Cavernous sinus meningiomas: a large LINAC radiosurgery series. *J. Neurooncol.,* 98(2):195-202.

[46] Flickinger JC, Kondziolka D, Maitz AH, Lunsford LD. Gamma knife radiosurgery of imaging-diagnosed intracranial meningioma. International journal of radiation oncology, biology, *physics.,* 2003;56 (3):801-6.

[47] Colombo F, Casentini L, Cavedon C, Scalchi P, Cora S, Francescon P. Cyberknife radiosurgery for benign meningiomas: short-term results in 199 patients. *Neurosurgery,* 2009;64(2 Suppl):A7-13.

[48] Adler JR, Jr., Gibbs IC, Puataweepong P, Chang SD. Visual field preservation after multisession cyberknife radiosurgery for perioptic lesions. *Neurosurgery,* 2006;59(2):244-54; discussion -54.

[49] Nguyen JH, Chen CJ, Lee CC, Yen CP, Xu Z, Schlesinger D, et al. Multisession gamma knife radiosurgery: a preliminary experience with a noninvasive, relocatable frame. *World neurosurgery,* 2014;82(6):1256-63.

[50] Starke R, Kano H, Ding D, Nakaji P, Barnett GH, Mathieu D, et al. Stereotactic radiosurgery of petroclival meningiomas: a multicenter study. *Journal of neuro-oncology,* 2014;119(1):169-76.

[51] Ding D, Starke RM, Kano H, Nakaji P, Barnett GH, Mathieu D, et al. Gamma knife radiosurgery for cerebellopontine angle meningiomas: a multicenter study. *Neurosurgery,* 2014;75(4):398-408; quiz

[52] Nicolato A, Foroni R, Pellegrino M, Ferraresi P, Alessandrini F, Gerosa M, et al. Gamma knife radiosurgery in meningiomas of the posterior fossa. Experience with 62 treated lesions. Minimally invasive neurosurgery : MIN. 2001;44(4):211-7.

[53] Starke RM, Nguyen JH, Reames DL, Rainey J, Sheehan JP. Gamma knife radiosurgery of meningiomas involving the foramen magnum. *Journal of craniovertebral junction & spine,* 2010;1(1):23-8.

[54] Ganz JC, Reda WA, Abdelkarim K. Gamma Knife surgery of large meningiomas: early response to treatment. *Acta neurochirurgica,* 2009; 151(1):1-8.

[55] DiBiase SJ, Kwok Y, Yovino S, Arena C, Naqvi S, Temple R, et al. Factors predicting local tumor control after gamma knife stereotactic radiosurgery for benign intracranial meningiomas. *International journal of radiation oncology, biology, physics,* 2004;60(5):1515-9.

[56] Kondziolka D, Madhok R, Lunsford LD, Mathieu D, Martin JJ, Niranjan A, et al. Stereotactic radiosurgery for convexity meningiomas. *J. Neurosurg.,* 2009;111(3):458-63.

[57] Sanai N, Sughrue ME, Shangari G, Chung K, Berger MS, McDermott MW. Risk profile associated with convexity meningioma resection in the modern neurosurgical era. *J. Neurosurg.,* 112(5):913-9.

[58] Girvigian MR, Chen JC, Rahimian J, Miller MJ, Tome M. Comparison of early complications for patients with convexity and parasagittal meningiomas treated with either stereotactic radiosurgery or fractionated stereotactic radiotherapy. *Neurosurgery,* 2008;62(5 Suppl):A19-27; discussion A-8.

[59] Pamir MN, Peker S, Kilic T, Sengoz M. Efficacy of gamma-knife surgery for treating meningiomas that involve the superior sagittal sinus. *Zentralblatt fur Neurochirurgie,* 2007;68(2):73-8.

[60] Kim DG, Kim Ch H, Chung HT, Paek SH, Jeong SS, Han DH, et al. Gamma knife surgery of superficially located meningioma. *Journal of neurosurgery,* 2005;102 Suppl:255-8.

[61] Umansky F, Shoshan Y, Rosenthal G, Fraifeld S, Spektor S. Radiation-induced meningioma. *Neurosurgical focus,* 2008;24(5):E7.

[62] Sheehan J, Yen CP, Steiner L. Gamma knife surgery-induced meningioma. Report of two cases and review of the literature. *Journal of neurosurgery,* 2006;105(2):325-9.

[63] Pettorini BL, Park YS, Caldarelli M, Massimi L, Tamburrini G, Di Rocco C. Radiation-induced brain tumours after central nervous system irradiation in childhood: a review. Child's nervous system : ChNS : *official journal of the International Society for Pediatric Neurosurgery,* 2008;24 (7):793-805.

[64] Lillehei KO, Donson AM, Kleinschmidt-DeMasters BK. Radiation-induced meningiomas: clinical, cytogenetic, and microarray features. *Acta neuropathologica,* 2008;116(3):289-301.

[65] Kondziolka D, Kano H, Kanaan H, Madhok R, Mathieu D, Flickinger JC, et al. Stereotactic radiosurgery for radiation-induced meningiomas. *Neurosurgery,* 2009;64(3):463-9; discussion 9-70.

[66] Jensen AW, Brown PD, Pollock BE, Stafford SL, Link MJ, Garces YI, et al. Gamma knife radiosurgery of radiation-induced intracranial tumors: local control, outcomes, and complications. *International journal of radiation oncology, biology, physics.,* 2005;62(1):32-7.

[67] Attia A, Chan MD, Mott RT, Russell GB, Seif D, Daniel Bourland J, et al. Patterns of failure after treatment of atypical meningioma with gamma knife radiosurgery. *Journal of neuro-oncology,* 2012;108(1): 179-85.

[68] Choi CY, Soltys SG, Gibbs IC, Harsh GR, Jackson PS, Lieberson RE, et al. Cyberknife stereotactic radiosurgery for treatment of atypical (WHO grade II) cranial meningiomas. *Neurosurgery,* 2010;67(5):1180-8.

[69] Harris AE, Lee JY, Omalu B, Flickinger JC, Kondziolka D, Lunsford LD. The effect of radiosurgery during management of aggressive meningiomas. *Surgical neurology,* 2003;60(4):298-305; discussion

[70] Kano H, Takahashi JA, Katsuki T, Araki N, Oya N, Hiraoka M, et al. Stereotactic radiosurgery for atypical and anaplastic meningiomas. *Journal of neuro-oncology,* 2007;84(1):41-7.

[71] Kim JW, Kim DG, Paek SH, Chung HT, Myung JK, Park SH, et al. Radiosurgery for atypical and anaplastic meningiomas: histopathological predictors of local tumor control. *Stereotactic and functional neurosurgery,* 2012;90(5):316-24.

[72] Ojemann SG, Sneed PK, Larson DA, Gutin PH, Berger MS, Verhey L, et al. Radiosurgery for malignant meningioma: results in 22 patients. *Journal of neurosurgery,* 2000;93 Suppl 3:62-7.

[73] Kondziolka D, Lunsford LD, Flickinger JC. The application of stereotactic radiosurgery to disorders of the brain. *Neurosurgery,* 2008;62 Suppl 2:707-19; discussion 19-20.

[74] Mattozo CA, De Salles AA, Klement IA, Gorgulho A, McArthur D, Ford JM, et al. Stereotactic radiation treatment for recurrent nonbenign meningiomas. *Journal of neurosurgery,* 2007;106(5):846-54.

[75] Stafford SL, Pollock BE, Foote RL, Link MJ, Gorman DA, Schomberg PJ, et al. Meningioma radiosurgery: tumor control, outcomes, and complications among 190 consecutive patients. *Neurosurgery,* 2001;49 (5):1029-37; discussion 37-8.

[76] Rogers L, Gilbert M, Vogelbaum MA. Intracranial meningiomas of atypical (WHO grade II) histology. *Journal of neuro-oncology,* 2010;99 (3):393-405.

[77] Vogelbaum MA, Leland Rogers C, Linskey MA, Mehta MP. Opportunities for clinical research in meningioma. *Journal of neuro-oncology,* 2010;99(3):417-22.

[78] Choy W, Kim W, Nagasawa D, Stramotas S, Yew A, Gopen Q, et al. The molecular genetics and tumor pathogenesis of meningiomas and the future directions of meningioma treatments. *Neurosurgical focus,* 2011;30 (5):E6.

[79] Chamberlain MC, Tsao-Wei DD, Groshen S. Temozolomide for treatment-resistant recurrent meningioma. *Neurology,* 2004;62(7):1210-2.

[80] Gupta V, Su YS, Samuelson CG, Liebes LF, Chamberlain MC, Hofman FM, et al. Irinotecan: a potential new chemotherapeutic agent for atypical or malignant meningiomas. *Journal of neurosurgery,* 2007;106 (3):455-62.

[81] Schlesinger D, Xu Z, Taylor F, Yen CP, Sheehan J. Interfraction and intrafraction performance of the Gamma Knife Extend system for patient positioning and immobilization. *Journal of neurosurgery,* 2012;117 Suppl: 217-24.

[82] Kim JW, Im YS, Nam DH, Park K, Kim JH, Lee JI. Preliminary report of multisession gamma knife radiosurgery for benign perioptic lesions: visual outcome in 22 patients. *Journal of Korean Neurosurgical Society,* 2008;44(2):67-71.

[83] Tuniz F, Soltys SG, Choi CY, Chang SD, Gibbs IC, Fischbein NJ, et al. Multisession cyberknife stereotactic radiosurgery of large, benign cranial base tumors: preliminary study. *Neurosurgery,* 2009;65(5):898-907; discussion

[84] Ganz JC. Role of radiosurgery in the management of intracranial malignancies. *Acta neurochirurgica Supplement,* 2013;116:61-2.

In: Current Management of Central Nervous System …
Editors: Steven D. Chang and Anand Veeravagu
ISBN: 978-1-63483-856-6


*Chapter 14*

# MENINGIOMAS: ENDOVASCULAR EMBOLIZATION, APPLICATIONS AND LIMITATIONS

***Michael Galgano MD, David J. Padalino MD, Hoon Choi MD MS and Lawrence S. Chin MD***
Department of Neurosurgery, SUNY Upstate Medical University, US

## ABSTRACT

Meningiomas are often highly vascularized benign tumors that harbor a dural based arterial blood supply. Such vascular characteristics in addition to the pathoanatomical growth of meningiomas have shaped the evolution of various endovascular approaches to meningioma treatment. Skull base locations and involvement of the dural venous sinus, particularly, can present significant surgical challenges. The purpose of this chapter is to review endovascular treatment options, with a particular focus on preoperative embolization, when used as an adjunct to surgical resection in the treatment of meningiomas.

## INTRODUCTION

The use of endovascular intervention in neurological surgery has in many ways improved the safety and clinical outcome of difficult to treat vascular pathology. Neurosurgical oncology has increasingly crossed paths with the endovascular field over the last few decades. Surgical resections of tumors laden with high vascularity prompted neurosurgeons to find effective ways of reducing operative blood loss. Similar to tumors such as hemangioblastomas and renal cell carcinoma, meningiomas often have a rich vascular supply that is specific to their location within the central nervous system. At times, this complicates their resection, with large operative blood loss. Pre-operative embolization of meningiomas was first described by Manelfe in France during the 1970's. It has since become commonly utilized, but not without controversy. In this chapter, we focus on endovascular applications and the supporting evidence available for these techniques. The utilization of endovascular technique as an adjunct to the treatment of meningiomas will be discussed, with an emphasis on pre-surgical embolization.

## Vascular Anatomy

Dural arteries course along the outer covering of the brain. These vessels often provide major contributions to the arterial vascular supply of meningiomas. Specific branches of the external carotid artery (ECA), such as the middle meningeal artery (MMA), ascending pharyngeal artery, accessory meningeal artery, and occipital transmastoid perforating branches, are often implicated as the common primary feeding arteries for meningiomas. Depending on the location, other vessels such as the tentorial and inferolateral trunk branches of the internal carotid artery (ICA) and the posterior meningeal branch of the vertebral artery may be involved. Meningiomas may also develop a dual, or secondary supply, often from smaller pial vessels that normally supply the brain parenchyma. Diagnostic cerebral angiography is utilized if pre-operative embolization is being considered. This allows the surgeon to understand the arterial supply to the meningioma, while also providing information regarding the patency of dural sinuses, should they also be involved by the tumor [1].

Various branches of the ECA typically serve as the primary blood supply for tumors of the anterior fossa, while tumors of the posterior fossa are often supplied by branches of the vertebral artery, such as the posterior tentorial artery branch. Tumors of the middle fossa are most frequently supplied by ECA branches but can also derive their arterial supply from posterior circulation artery branches. Meningiomas located at the convexity of the calvarium most often receive their primary blood supply from the MMA and are easily devascularized by ligating the MMA, as well as other superficial dural arteries that may supply the tumor, during the dural resection portion of the operation.

Therefore, pre-operative embolization of these tumors is rarely needed, unless the major blood supply to the tumor arises from deeper pial branches. This is because they are not encountered superficially upon exposure of the tumor, but rather are encountered only after the tumor has been debulked or resected. Additionally, these arteries can lead to significant blood loss during the tumor resection. A major caveat to endovascular embolization is that tumor vessels capable of being embolized tend to have relatively few feeding pedicles and the diameter of the vessel must be large enough to accommodate the microcatheter that will be used for the embolization.

When the wall of a dural sinus is involved with the meningioma, one needs to determine if sacrifice of the sinus is an appropriate surgical option. In cases such as tumor involvement of the anterior third of the superior sagittal sinus, or involvement of an already hypoplastic transverse sinus, the decision is relatively easy as these locations are generally able to be sacrificed to allow for complete resection of the tumor tissue. However, when the tumor involves the posterior portion of the superior sagittal sinus to the torcula, or compromises a dominant transverse/sigmoid sinus or internal jugular vein at the bulb, then sacrifice of these venous conduits may not be feasible. Sacrificing may lead to issues with venous outflow obstruction, including venous strokes. It is often safer to intentionally leave some tumor behind in these situations and treat these regions with radiation therapy, such as Gamma Knife stereotactic radiosurgery.

## Applications of Endovascular Embolization

Not all meningiomas can be embolized nor should they be embolized pre-operatively. The rationale behind pre-surgical meningioma embolization is multifactorial. Diminishing intra-operative blood loss during resection is beneficial for both thc patient and surgeon. After embolization, the possibility of reduced surgical blood loss can subsequently result in reduced need for blood transfusions during or shortly after surgical resection of the tumor. This becomes most important when operating on individuals experiencing forms of chronic vascular compromise. Patients with coronary artery disease or severe carotid artery stenosis are more likely to be at increased risk of vascular events taking place when the hemoglobin level drops below a critical threshold. It is important to optimize the hemoglobin and hematocrit levels in these patients to maximize the oxygen delivery to areas already affected by some degree of baseline chronic ischemia. A study by Zhang and Jin showed that pre-operative embolization of meningiomas allowed for significantly reduced intra-operative blood loss and thus diminished need for blood transfusions [2]. Less bleeding also results in improved visualization of the operative field for and may aid in improved tumor resection.

Numerous agents have been utilized for pre-surgical meningioma embolization. Liquid embolic agents include fibrin glue, NBCA (*N*-butyl cyanoacrylate), and Onyx (ethylene vinyl alcohol copolymer dissolved in dimethyl sulfoxide) (Covidien/eV3, Irvine, CA). Particulate embolizing agents include both small and large polyvinyl alcohol (PVA) particles and microspheres as well as cellulose beads [3]. Absorbable gelatin sponge has also been successfully used in particular cases [4].

Studies have been reported over the last four decades using various embolic agents, but without a clear consensus on the most efficacious benefit-complication profile. Embolization with PVA particles continues to be the most commonly used [5].

According to certain studies, smaller-sized PVA particles (45-150 μm) tend to be more effective in pre-operative meningioma devascularization as opposed to larger-sized particles (150-250 μm). The reason for this appears to be that distal penetration of smaller particles into the tumor-feeding capillaries can result in relatively improved devascularization of tumor tissue. This is compared with the more proximal vessel embolization using larger particles or platinum coils or liquid embolic agents delivered at the arterial pedicle alone [3, 6]. Success has been seen with pre-operative embolization with Onyx for tumors of the brain and spine, including meningiomas, and particularly when use of the liquid embolic agent results in robust distal vessel penetration within the tumor tissue [7]. Liquid embolic agents often have the benefit of superior distal penetration. Despite the success seen with Onyx, some authors report that it may increase the risk of cranial nerve palsies and is therefore not widely used for pre-operative meningioma embolization procedures [8].

Reflux of injected embolic material into unintended vessels may result in cerebral ischemic events. This includes the possibility of stroke if the embolic material enters the intracranial circulation to normal brain parenchyma. Such events may be prevented in part through balloon-assisted embolization whereby a balloon is inflated proximal to the catheter tip to prevent the reflux of embolic material into a normal intracranial artery. When using a liquid embolic agent, balloon-assisted embolization proximal to the feeding arterial pedicle may improve penetration into smaller distal vessels as it allows for greater anterograde delivery of the agent [9].

Pre-surgical meningioma embolization is almost always performed with the intent of a post-embolization surgical resection. However, there have been instances of meningioma embolization as a stand-alone procedure without subsequent tumor resection [10, 11]. This may be utilized in situations where the patient is a poor operative candidate and surgical intervention would be contraindicated.

The patient would need to be closely followed with frequent imaging to ensure that the tumor is not progressing [12]. Additionally, the risks of post-embolization tumor necrosis and subsequent increases in edema are significant in tumor embolization alone.

This tends to be seen more in larger tumors and is a major reason why embolization alone without subsequent surgical resection is not commonly performed.

## HISTOPATHOLOGY OF EMBOLIZED MENINGIOMAS

Embolized meningiomas display various features when examined histopathologically. They reveal the presence of emboli and thrombi within the tumor and dural vasculature. Tumor cells display changes consistent with ischemia and infarction.

There is often an associated inflammatory response to the tumor necrosis that results in significantly increased peri-tumor edema. The necrosis observed is typically diffuse or nodular, and the cells that survive form isolated clusters [13]. Histological grading of embolized meningiomas may pose significant problems for the pathologist. Higher grade tumors generally have a tendency to display areas of necrosis. This can be confusing to the physician making the histological diagnosis, as embolized meningiomas display features similar to necrosis due to the embolization procedure and not necessarily due to the underlying tumor grade. Differentiating an embolized low grade meningioma from a higher grade tumor can be quite challenging in this situation. To avoid overgrading the meningioma, it is suggested to look for abrupt and well demarcated borders of necrosis since this indicates the likelihood of pre-surgical embolization [14].

## OTHER ENDOVASCULAR APPLICATIONS

The less utilized endovascular applications for the management of meningiomas include venous stenting and angioplasty. Some meningiomas present themselves in technically challenging areas for resection, such as the jugular bulb. Zilani and colleagues have described deploying a balloon-expandable renovascular stent in the jugular bulb for a petrous meningioma, which causes significant venous outflow obstruction with associated symptoms [15]. Parasagittal meningiomas can also present a significant challenge, especially when they involve the posterior two-thirds of the superior sagittal sinus. Ganesan et al. reported on a successful case of superior sagittal sinus stenting in a patient with a presentation of benign intracranial hypertension and a parasagittal meningioma [16]. Chivoret et al. reported on a similar case [17].

Some locations of meningiomas and their intimate involvement of vital vasculature make a complete resection unobtainable. In a case such as a medial sphenoid wing meningioma with cavernous carotid vessel wall invasion, total resection is not safe. As a result of the vessel wall invasion, symptomatic carotid stenosis may ensue. Heye and colleagues reported on a case regarding successful endovascular intra-arterial stent placement when the tumor burden resulted in significant encasement and vessel wall invasion of the cavernous carotid artery, and in turn, severe symptomatic stenosis [18]. Other reports of vessel re-expansion after meningioma have related severe symptomatic stenosis through pre-operative angioplasty [19]. A gross total tumor resection at the expense of one of the carotid arteries would potentially leave the patient with considerable and unacceptable deficits, specifically if the patient does not tolerate a carotid artery balloon test occlusion study [18, 20, 21].

Carotid artery balloon test occlusion studies can be performed to determine if it is reasonable to consider carotid artery sacrifice as a part of the tumor resection plan if the tumor encases this artery and would otherwise be unresectable. The stent procedures noted above would be considered for patients who do not tolerate the balloon test occlusion. The placement of a stent often requires dual anti-platelet agent therapy for the first few months, at minimum, to prevent in-stent thrombosis. Thus, this strategy would not typically be used in a patient who requires surgical resection immediately after stent placement.

The carotid artery balloon test occlusion is described using a variety of protocols. The protocol most used by this author and colleagues includes inducing hypotension to 20% below baseline systolic or mean blood pressure while performing serial neurological exams as the balloon is inflated and causes occlusion of the particular cervical ICA that is being tested over 10-20 minutes.

The technical details of the balloon test occlusion procedure are beyond the scope of this chapter.

## EMBOLIZATION AND SPINAL MENINGIOMAS

Although cranial meningiomas are more frequently encountered than their spinal counterparts, spinal meningiomas can pose significant surgical challenges given their intimate proximity to the spinal cord and potential for a shared blood supply. Low thoracic meningiomas can be especially challenging, given their close proximity to the artery of Adamkiewicz. Spinal angiography should be considered prior to surgical intervention in the case of lower thoracic meningiomas [22]. Both the lumbar and sacral spinal cord derive their blood supply primarily from the artery of Adamkiewicz. This is the largest known anterior segmental medullary artery. The artery of Adamkiewicz is most commonly located between T8 and L3, and at T9 or T10 in about 50% of cases and 75% of the time, it originates from the left side [23]. The unintentional interruption of this artery during lower thoracic meningioma resection has the potential to cause ischemia to the ventral commissura, the sympathetic centers of the intermediolateral region, and the ventral horn of the spinal cord.

Clinically, this can manifest as pain and temperature sensory loss, incontinence of bowel and bladder functions, and distal paraplegia. Pre-surgical spinal angiography affords the surgeon topographical knowledge of the artery of Adamkiewicz. Pre-surgical awareness of this artery's location may alter the surgical approach, either by attempting a resection from the contralateral side, or employing another selective surgical technique [24]. Pre-surgical angiography can also be used for embolization of spinal meningiomas. Some spinal meningiomas can be hypervascular, at times revealing signs of blood products on imaging. Resection of such hypervascular tumors can complicate the surgery secondary to field obliteration and the need for blood transfusions [25].

## LIMITATIONS OF ENDOVASCULAR EMBOLIZATION

Although pre-operative meningioma embolization can have significant benefits, it does not come without potential complications and limitations. Some authors have cited complication rates as high as 21%. This represents a time when techniques were not as refined as they are today, however [26]. Newer data have revealed overall complication rates on the lower end at 6% [27, 28]. Hemorrhage, stroke, tumor edema, and cranial nerve palsies are feared complications that can be encountered post-procedure [29–31]. They can be disastrous for the patient, and often will require urgent surgical decompression in the cases of significant intratumoral hemorrhage and edema. Although two separate studies demonstrated essentially no incidence of post-embolization hemorrhage [32, 33], it has been reported in the literature [34–36], albeit rather infrequently. It is easy to classify these hemorrhages as interventional "complications", but there may be merit to attributing an intrinsic risk factor to tumor-related characteristics. It has been postulated that some of the vessels proximal to the site of embolization are quite fragile. This essentially makes them more prone to rupture from episodes of higher blood pressure, such as during endovascular vessel occlusion [34–36]. Risk factors associated with post-embolization hemorrhage include large meningiomas (6-8 cm) that have either a cystic or necrotic component [29, 34, 35]. Radiographic evidence of any of these features should alert the interventionalist prior to embolization. Although cranial neuropathies caused by occlusion of the nerve's vasa nervorum are not necessarily as life-threatening as hemorrhage and edema, there is a significant associated morbidity depending on which cranial nerve is affected [3, 37].

As mentioned earlier, smaller embolization particles are typically able to achieve better distal penetration into the tumor. However, they have been the subject of criticism secondary to their higher risk of complications such as post-embolization hemorrhage and cranial neuropathies. Another potential complication of this procedure is an iatrogenic carotid-cavernous fistula, by perforation with the guidewire [38]. Anomolous intracranial and extracranial anastomoses are known to exist in some individuals. Embolization of a MMA feeder that has an ophthalmic artery anastomosis may be one of the etiological risk factors for post-procedure blindness through retinal emboli [39]. Ischemia of the temporalis muscles may be another complication related to an unintended vessel being embolized, resulting in lockjaw [40]. Scalp necrosis has been reported to result from meningioma embolization. This can cause a significant cosmetic defect, with subsequent poor wound healing, and the eventual necessity of plastic surgical intervention [41–44]. Although exceedingly rare, *Clostridium perfringens* has been reported in the literature as a complication of pre-surgical meningioma embolization. This bacterium has the potential to invade the tumor itself, causing intratumoral gas and associated surrounding edema. This will eventually lead to a rapid clinical decline of the patient's neurological status [45]. Inherent risks do exist related to tumor location, vascular supply and anastomoses, embolic agent of choice, and experience of the interventionalist. It is difficult to classify individual risks to patients given the variability of the multiple confounding factors found in each isolated case [8].

## Technical and Clinical Pearls

Proper technique with care taken at every step of the embolization procedure may aid in the prevention of complications. The speed and force with which the interventionalist performs the injection of either the particulate matter or liquid embolic material may play a role in causing or preventing reflux, stroke and/or hemorrhage. If a meningioma is fed by the ophthalmic artery, slow injection to avoid reflux into the central retinal artery is warranted [46]. Low pressure delivery of embolic particles can also aid in the avoidance of intratumoral hemorrhage [34]. As discussed earlier, improper manipulation of the guidewire can cause an arterial wall puncture with subsequent formation of an arteriovenous fistula. The MMA has a sharp bend, and it is suggested to avoid introducing the microcatheter beyond this area to prevent a vessel wall violation [47]. When manipulating around the ophthalmic artery, and when concern about retinal artery embolization exists, provocation tests with lidocaine or sodium amytal prior to embolization may hold merit. They can help identify arterial feeder branches that have branches or small collateral anastomoses to normal intracranial arteries that supply the functional tissue of the brain or eye. This pre-embolization testing technique can offer the interventionalist the opportunity to avoid embolization of arterial feeders, which show clinical deficit symptoms upon testing [30, 48].

Tumor edema is a potential consequence of embolization. Some authors have suggested the use of steroids prior to embolization to help minimize this effect [6]. The timing of surgery after an embolization has always been debatable [49]. It has been observed histopathologically that embolized meningiomas exhibit necrosis, apoptosis and cell cycle arrest [50]. Although apoptosis occurs only until six days after embolization, arrest of meningioma growth may be longer [51]. In vivo proton spectroscopy may be used to detect tumor necrosis and help determine the optimal post-embolization day for surgical resection [52]. Some authors have suggested waiting at least one week after embolization for surgical resection. This has proven in some studies to significantly reduce transfused blood volume during surgery. A shorter time interval from embolization to surgery has been linked to a longer surgery and more transfusions. As mentioned earlier, histologic interpretation and the determination of grade should be done with extreme caution in embolized meningiomas. The embolization may cause tumor cells to appear rhabdoid cell-like, papillary cell-like, or clear cell-like [53, 54]. This can be falsely interpreted as a higher grade meningioma, causing unnecessary adjuvant therapy for the patient. Chun et al. have published a retrospective case series of 50 patients who had meningioma tumor resection after pre-operative embolization (28 operations within 24 hours after embolization and 22 operations > 24 hours after embolization, ranging from 2-7 days, mean 2.5 days) and they showed a statistically significant reduction in blood loss in the delayed surgery group. 29% of the early surgery group had blood loss of > 1000 mL, while 100% of patients in the delayed surgery group had blood loss of < 700 mL [55]. Cessation of adequate blood flow to the meningioma is the rationale behind embolization, but it must be remembered that complication avoidance rather than devascularization of the tumor should be the primary goal of the interventionalist [56].

## Clinical Outcomes

Evidence for preoperative embolization of meningiomas exists largely in the form of case reports and retrospective studies. Major studies are summarized in Table 1. The study sample size ranges from 18 to 199, with eight studies having more than 100 patients. The mean age of patients studied is in the mid-50's, reflective of the patient population who commonly presents with meningioma. The rate of neurologic complications from embolization appears to have decreased over time. Earlier studies in the 1980's and 1990's reported neurologic complication rates ranging from 10% to 44.1% [6, 31, 57], whereas a 2014 clinical study reports a 2.3% rate of neurologic complication.(58) Minor complications are rare, with the most common being scalp necrosis [57–59]. Death was rarely reported [27, 28, 32]. The most popular embolization agents are 1) PVA particles, 50-500 μm (Boston Scientific, MA; Cook Medical, IN), used alone or in conjunction with coils and/or Gelfoam, and 2) Embosphere/EmboGold Microspheres 40-300 μm (Merit Medical Systems, Inc, UT). Liquid embolic agents, such as NBCA and Onyx (Covidien/eV3), have been used as adjuncts to the particle embolic agents.

In the current literature, there are no standardized indications or protocols for endovascular embolization of meningiomas, with the interventionalist's own preferences and experiences dictating most management decisions. However, the authors generally agree on the following as relative indications: large tumor size (generally exceeding 3-4 cm in largest dimension), high tumor vascularity, intraoperatively inaccessible or difficult to access arterial feeders, challenging skull base tumor locations, and significant ECA feeders easily accessible by endovascular means. Conditions that result in higher risk of complications with endovascular embolization have less of a consensus, but can include significant comorbid medical risk factors for and pertinent medical history of stroke and peripheral vascular disease, significant tumor-associated edema (that can worsen after embolization and lead to herniation syndromes, especially when combined with large tumor size), involvement of venous sinuses, and risk of scalp necrosis.

Many studies concluded that pre-operative endovascular arterial feeder tumor vessel embolization resulted in decreased operative blood loss and consequently led to a reduced need for blood transfusion, greater extent of resection, shortened surgical time, and reduced surgical complications [32, 57, 60–62]. However, in the absence of a large prospective randomized controlled trial, it is difficult to definitively and consistently show the benefits of embolization with statistical significance. Dean and colleagues [61] published a case-control study in which the results in patients with meningioma resection surgery along with pre-operative endovascular embolization were compared with 18 matched control patients who had similar kinds of meningiomas resected without the pre-operative embolization. This review showed that embolization decreased blood loss, the need for transfusion, and surgical complications. Bendszus and colleagues [60] reported on a small prospective study with 30 patients, showing a reduction in operative blood loss only with complete tumor devascularization by embolization. One of the more long-term studies related to pre-surgical embolization of meningiomas was undertaken by Gruber and colleagues over a 17-year period from 1982-1998. 60.3% of their patients experienced total or subtotal devascularization of the tumor. The remaining 39.7% had partial tumor devascularization for various reasons [32]. Borg and colleagues reviewed 117 consecutive patients with pre-operative meningioma embolization (with the use of glue and particles) with a low complication rate. There was not a statistically significant difference in the degree of tumor devascularization between the types of embolic agent used [59].

Because of a relatively low incidence of large meningiomas suitable for embolization, operator variability in experience and preference and different institutional protocols for embolization have made it difficult to design and perform a randomized controlled trial. Although a number of studies suggest a number of benefits of embolization, the literature mainly consists of retrospective studies, representing level 3 evidence.

## Discussion

The use of endovascular pre-surgical embolization of highly vascularized tumors, such as large skull base meningiomas, has advanced dramatically and has become more widely accepted since the technique was initially proposed in the 1970's. However, there remains significant controversy regarding the specific indications for this intervention. Complication rates have diminished over the years.

This is likely due to the greater experience in embolization of these tumors and technological advancements in endovascular equipment. Microcatheters have become more flexible and trackable into smaller vessels with greater tortuosity. This allows for better distal penetration of embolic materials being delivered while minimizing the potential for embolic material inadvertently entering a collateral anastomosis, or reflux of the embolic material into a parent vessel, thus leading to a stroke. Although the use of PVA particles remains the standard embolic material of choice, the introduction and refinement of liquid embolic agents has provided a significant advancement to allow for safer embolization of smaller target vessels.

Other techniques, which are not as well described, include venous stenting for those cases that have a significant venous outflow obstruction as a result of tumor invasion or obstruction by mass effect of a large dural sinus. In the properly selected patient, this can be a useful treatment strategy, but it is very difficult to develop large studies on the very small patient population who would qualify for treatment with this technique. There is simply not much in the literature beyond occasional case reports and small case series of these patients.

Varying complication rates could be reflective of the level of expertise and prior training of the interventionalist as we learn more about treating these kinds of patients with the available technology. Additionally, as technological advancements are being made with the endovascular equipment and embolic agents available, complications from these interventions seem to become lower. Future prospective studies are needed.

# ILLUSTRATIVE CASES

## Case 1

A 57-year-old male was found by his wife bleeding at the mouth from a bite injury to the tongue and with urinary incontinence, with reports of "personality changes" in the months leading up to this new onset seizure event. A CT scan of the head was performed at a local hospital and showed a hyperdense extra-axial mass at the midline anterior fossa skull base with surrounding vasogenic edema of the bilateral frontal lobes and mass effect on the bilateral frontal lobes (Figure 1).

The patient was transferred to the University Hospital for a higher level of care. An MRI of the brain with and without gadolinium contrast was performed and confirmed this large extra-axial anterior fossa mass with a homogeneous enhancement pattern, which is consistent with an olfactory groove meningioma (Figure 2).

This patient is known to have uncontrolled type 2 diabetes mellitus and he does not take his prescribed medications. His physical exam revealed a temperature of 37.9 degrees Celsius, blood pressure of 164/82, heart rate of 108, respiratory rate of 32, oxygen saturation on non-rebreather mask of 97%. His general appearance indicated respiratory distress and oral obstruction from a swollen tongue secondary to the bite injury. The pertinent neurologic exam findings included general lethargy and were consistent with a post-ictal state, with a GCS of 13 because he did not follow commands at the time of the initial evaluation. However, no focal motor or sensory deficit was seen.

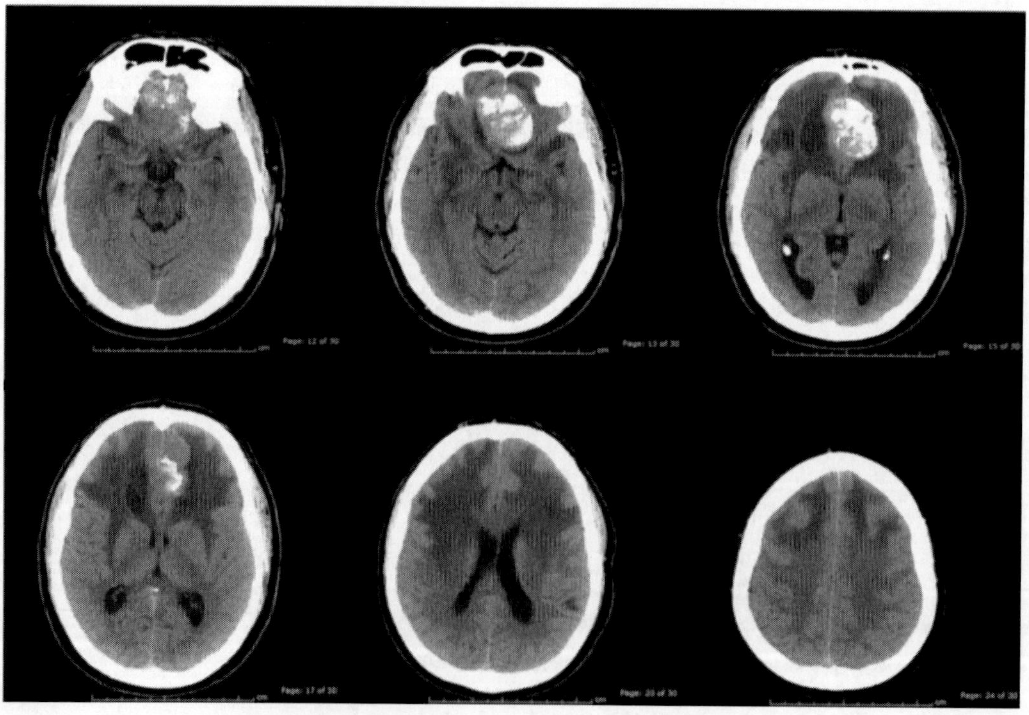

Figure 1. Pre-operative CT scan of the head without contrast showing a large olfactory groove meningioma with bifrontal peritumoral edema.

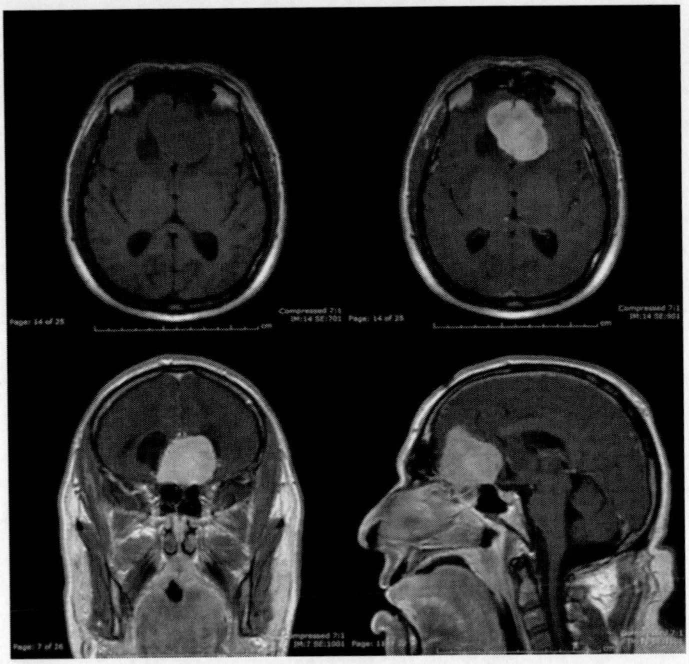

Figure 2. Pre-operative T1-weighted MRI of the brain with and without contrast showing a large olfactory groove meningioma with bifrontal peritumoral edema.

The patient was started on dexamethasone 6 mg IV q6h and 3% NaCl for hyperosmolar therapy to treat the vasogenic edema and levetiracetam for seizures. After a discussion with the patient's family about the treatment options, it was decided that the treatment of choice would be a surgical excision of the tumor with pre-operative endovascular embolization of the blood supply to the tumor.

*Description of the procedure:* The patient was properly identified and placed in the supine position. The right groin site was prepped and draped in usual sterile fashion.

The right femoral arteriotomy was performed using the standard modified Seldinger technique, and a 6 French right femoral sheath was placed without difficulty. A 6 French MPC Envoy (Cordis, Miami, FL) guide catheter was inserted over a glidewire and a complete cerebral angiogram was performed to identify all visible feeding arteries that were large enough for microcatheter access and embolization. The right ECA was selectively catheterized and cerebral angiography revealed that the right MMA provided a relatively large contribution to the tumor blood supply. This vessel was accessed by superselective microcatheter placement using an Echelon-10 microcatheter (Covidien/eV3) and 0.014" Synchro 2 soft microwire (Stryker, Kalamazoo, MI). Microcatheter cerebral angiography confirmed that the right MMA was large enough for catheterization and embolization (Figure 3A and 3B). PVA particle embolization of the tumor through the right MMA was performed using 100-300 μm embospheres (Merit Medical, South Jordan, UT) mixed in a 50:50 ratio with Omnipaque-300 (iohexol) (GE Healthcare, Waukesha, WI) contrast material to visualize the injection of the PVA particles through the microcatheter to the main supplying arterial pedicle feeding branch to the tumor from this vessel (Figure 3C and 3D). Using road-mapping techniques to watch for reflux of the embolic material, the PVA particles were slowly injected until anterograde flow of contrast was significantly slowed. A post-embolization angiogram revealed significantly reduced blood flow to the tumor from the embolized feeding pedicle (Figure 3E and 3F). The left ICA angiogram showed left anterior cerebral artery (ACA) vessels supplying the tumor. An attempt was made to catheterize these vessels for embolization. They were too small to catheterize with the Echelon-10 microcatheter over a Synchro 2 soft microwire and further embolization attempts were abandoned because it was determined that attempted embolization would not provide a significant enough benefit for the operation over the potential risk of this procedure. After the embolization procedure, the patient was taken to the operating room for a craniotomy for tumor resection. The patient was intubated, intravenous lines, arterial line and Foley catheter were placed. The patient was put in the lateral position for placement of the lumbar drain, which was placed at approximately the L4-5 level, by the iliac crest and bony landmarks. Then the patient was positioned supine on the operating room table with the head stabilized in a Mayfield head clamp and slightly flexed forward. The patient was given pre-operative antibiotics per routine surgical protocol. The patient was also given dexamethasone and mannitol during the operation. A standard bicoronal incision was made for exposure, and burr holes were placed for the craniotomy flap.

The dura was very adherent to the bone and this was separated using a #3 Penfield. The durotomy was performed to expose the bilateral frontal lobes, and the anterior portion of the superior sagittal sinus involved with the tumor was ligated and cut. Microdissection of the tumor from the brain was performed in standard fashion under the operating microscope. All the feeding vessels into the tumor were gradually coagulated using the bipolar and cut with microscissors.

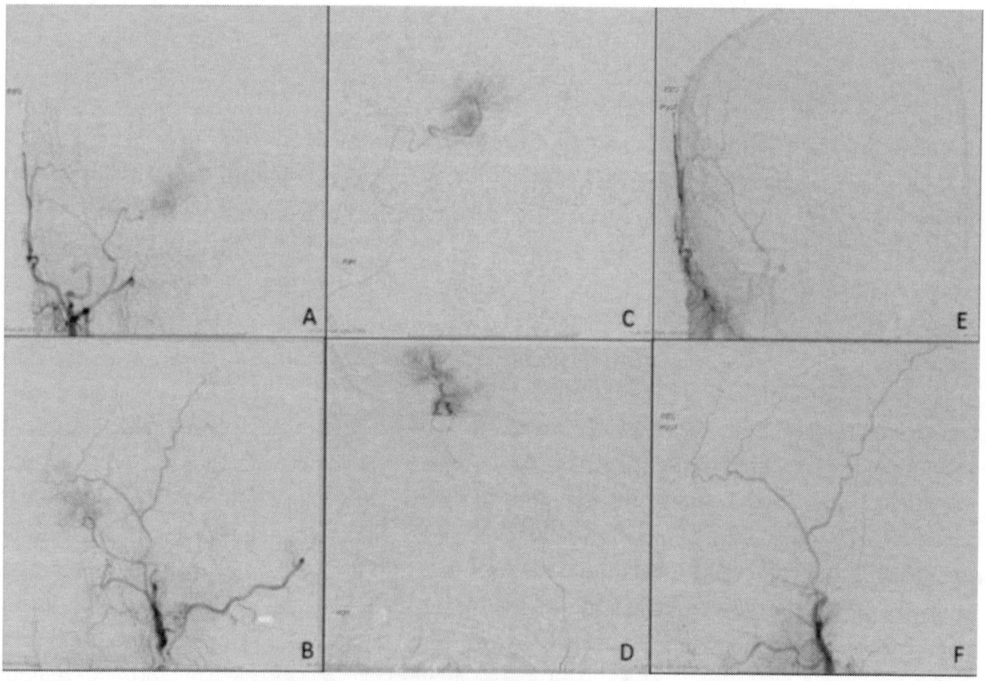


Figure 3. (A,B) Pre-embolization right ECA cerebral angiogram (A, anterior-posterior (AP); B, lateral). (C,D) Microcatheter cerebral angiogram of feeding pedicle to the tumor from the right MMA branch (C, AP; D, lateral). (E, F) Post-embolization right ECA cerebral angiogram (E, AP; F, lateral) showing complete embolization of the right MMA branch arterial supply to the tumor.

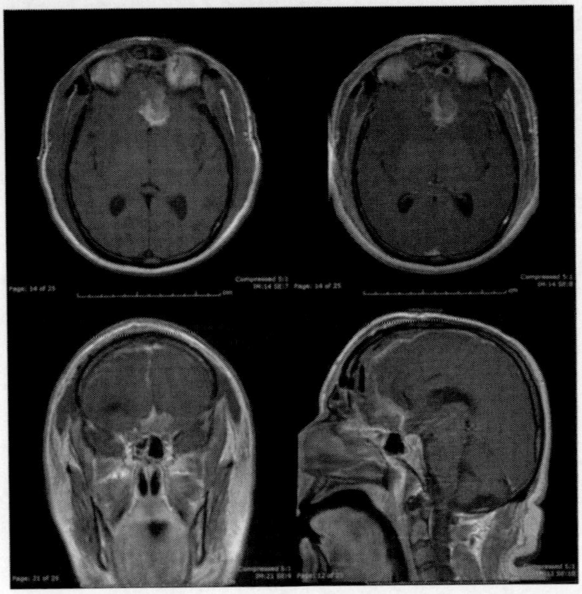

Figure 4. Post-operative T1-weighted MRI of the brain with and without contrast showing only small residual tumor at the anterior fossa floor.

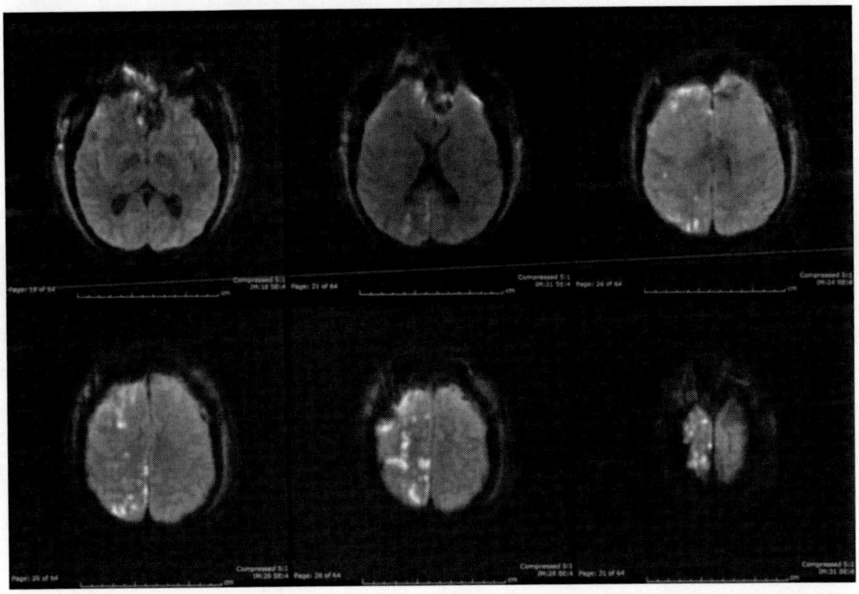

Figure 5. Post-operative DWI sequence MRI of the brain showing right ACA territory scattered infarcts.

The entire tumor was initially debulked using the ultrasonic tissue dessicator within the tumor capsule and then the capsule and portions of the tumor adherent to the skull base were resected. The craniotomy was closed in standard fashion after hemostasis was obtained. Blood loss was noted to be approximately 1,000 mL.

Post-operatively, the patient had difficulty with arousal and difficulty moving the left leg. Post-operative MRI brain study showed resection of the majority of the tumor, with only a small residual at the anterior fossa floor on T1-weighted sequences with and without contrast (Figure 4).

On DWI sequences, right ACA territory strokes were seen (Figure 5). The embolization catheter had never accessed the right ICA territory and the embolization was limited to the right MMA. It is unclear these sequelae were due to PVA particles traveling through collateral vessels to the ICA territory.

## Case 2

Case 2 was a 53-year-old female with a medical history significant for hypertension and hyperlipidemia, who had a history of several months of dull, throbbing and often intense headaches in the left occipital region without significant relief upon taking over the counter headache medications. She had occasional blurry vision, but was asymptomatic for nausea or emesis. An MRI of the brain with and without gadolinium contrast was obtained and showed a large 8 cm × 6 cm homogeneously enhancing parasagittal tumor consistent with a meningioma (Figure 6).

Her physical exam revealed a temperature of 36.1 degrees Celsius, blood pressure of 143/69, pulse of 69, respirations of 18 and oxygen saturation of 100% on room air. Her general appearance was calm, comfortable and in no apparent distress. The neurologic exam was normal without motor, sensory, coordination, or visual deficits.

The patient was started on dexamethasone for peritumoral edema and levetiracetam for seizure prophylaxis. After a discussion with the patient's family about the treatment options, it was decided that the treatment of choice would be a surgical excision of the tumor with pre-operative endovascular embolization of the blood supply to the tumor.

*Description of the procedure:* The patient was properly identified and placed in the supine position and the right groin site was prepped and draped in usual sterile fashion. A right femoral arteriotomy was performed using the standard modified Seldinger technique, and a 6 French right femoral sheath was placed without difficulty. A 4 French angled glide catheter (Terumo, Somerset, NJ) was used to perform a complete diagnostic cerebral angiogram, which showed bilateral MMA supply to the tumor (Figure 7A-D), and no blood supply to the tumor from the posterior circulation.

The catheter was then exchanged for a 6 French MPC Envoy (Cordis) guide catheter over a glidewire to access the left ECA. An attempt was then made to navigate an Echelon-10 microcatheter and Synchro 2 soft microwire into the distal left MMA, but it was not able to pass beyond the proximal portion of this vessel due to the arterial tortuosity. A smaller diameter Marathon microcatheter and Mirage microwire (both from Covidien/eV3) were then used in an attempt to navigate more distally. Because of the vessel tortuosity and hairpin loops, it was not possible to navigate the catheter any further distally than in the attempt with the initial microcatheter. Due to the potential risk of extracranial-intracranial collateral circulation with the ophthalmic artery and skull base branches, the use of PVA particles in this vessel was felt to be unsafe.

This microcatheter was then pre-flushed with dimethyl sulfoxide (DMSO), and then Onyx 18 (Covidien/eV3) liquid agent was injected to embolize this left MMA branch. The post-embolization angiogram confirmed that this vessel was completely embolized (Figure 7H and 7I).

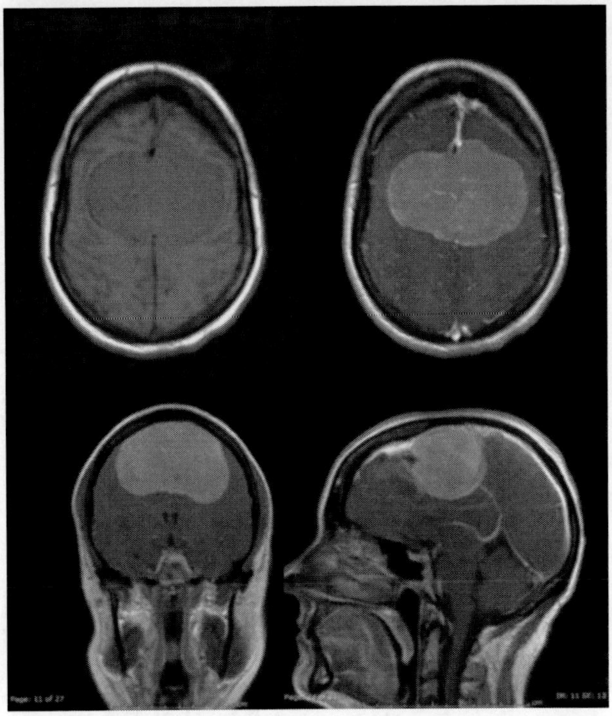

Figure 6. Pre-operative T1-weighted MRI of the brain with and without contrast showing a large parasagittal meningioma with encasement of the superior sagittal sinus.

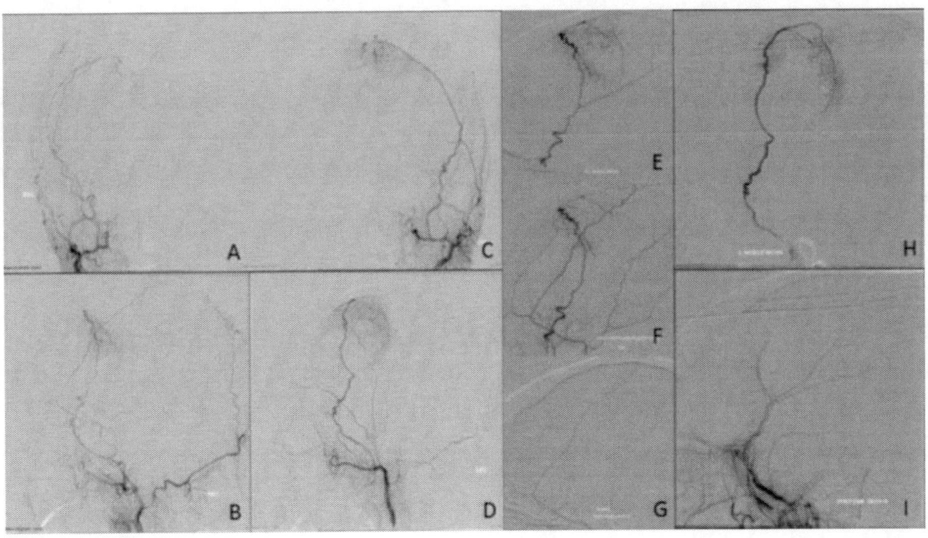


Figure 7. (A, B) Pre-embolization right ECA cerebral angiogram showing a right MMA branch supplying the tumor (A, AP; B, lateral). (C, D) Pre-embolization left ECA cerebral angiogram showing a left MMA branch supplying the tumor (C, AP; D, lateral). (E) Microcatheter cerebral angiogram of right MMA feeding pedicle (lateral). (F) Right ECA lateral cerebral angiogram post-microsphere embolization showing reduced tumor blush. (G) Right ECA lateral cerebral angiogram post-Onyx 18 embolization showing complete occlusion of the right MMA feeding pedicle to the tumor. (H) Pre-embolization lateral microcatheter cerebral angiogram of the left MMA feeding pedicle to the tumor. (I) Post-embolization left ECA cerebral angiogram after Onyx 18 embolization of the left MMA.

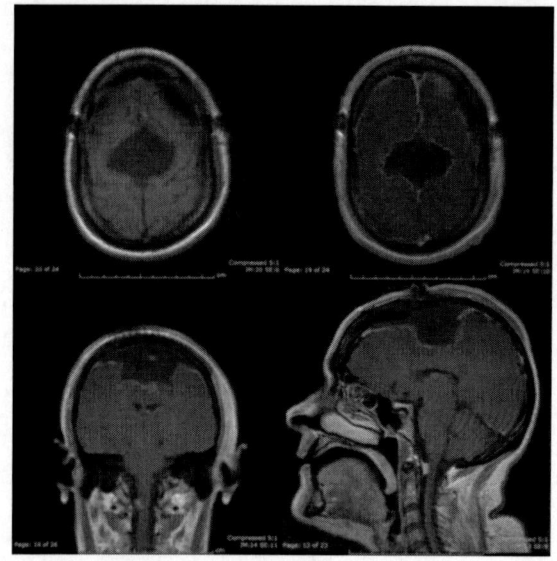

Figure 8. Post-operative T1-weighted MRI of the brain with and without contrast showing gross total resection of the tumor.

The right ECA was then selectively catheterized. Using the Echelon-10 microcatheter and Synchro 2 soft microwire, this right MMA was catheterized distally enough for injection of 700-900 μm diameter embosphere PVA particles mixed 50:50 with iohexol contrast, using road mapping techniques, until the contrast did not flow as rapidly in an anterograde manner. Cerebral angiography revealed that the right MMA supply to the tumor was significantly diminished after PVA particle injection.

The Onyx 18 liquid embolic agent was injected after the microcatheter was pre-flushed with DMSO and the follow-up post-embolization cerebral angiogram showed complete occlusion of the right MMA (Figure 7E-G). The patient was also given 10 mg of dexamethasone IV at the end of the embolization procedure in anticipation of possible increased edema associated with the embolization.

The next day the patient was taken to the operating room for a craniotomy for tumor resection. The patient was intubated, intravenous lines, arterial line and Foley catheter were placed, and the patient was then positioned supine on the operating room table with the head stabilized in a Mayfield head clamp and slightly flexed forward. The patient was given pre-operative antibiotics per routine surgical protocol. The patient was also given dexamethasone and mannitol during the operation. A standard bicoronal incision was made for exposure, and burr holes were placed for the craniotomy flap. Microdissection of the tumor from the brain was performed in standard fashion under the operating microscope. All the feeding vessels into the tumor were gradually coagulated using the bipolar and cut with microscissors. The entire tumor was initially debulked within the tumor capsule using the ultrasonic tissue dessicator, and then the tumor capsule was resected. The craniotomy was closed in standard fashion after hemostasis was obtained. Blood loss was noted to be approximately 1,000 mL.

Post-operatively the patient had an MRI of the brain with and without contrast study (Figure 8) showing gross total resection of the tumor and no radiographic complications. The patient did develop a *Staphylococcus epidermidis* wound infection and required removal and subsequent replacement of the cranial flap at future operations. The tumor has not recurred on follow-up MRI brain studies.

## CASE DISCUSSION

The use of pre-operative endovascular embolization of meningiomas remains controversial, although studies have shown that the potential for blood loss is reduced with this procedure [57, 60, 61]. Chun et al. [55] examined the timing of surgical tumor resection after endovascular embolization within the same day or delayed by at least 24 hours (mean 2.5 days, range 2-7 days), and there was a correlation between delaying surgical resection and significantly reducing blood loss during surgery. Other described techniques include open surgical ligation of the ethmoidal artery pre-operatively since this is a commonly involved feeding artery to anterior fossa skull base meningiomas [63]. However, this open surgical approach would not allow for ligation of other arteries supplying the tumor. If the ligation is performed 24 hours before the tumor resection, this would mean that the patient would undergo two separate general anesthesia procedures within 1-2 days. Endovascular embolization can be performed with PVA microspheres, detachable platinum coils, or liquid embolic agents, such as Onyx, with desired results. However, the potential for inadvertent embolization with these materials through naturally occurring extracranial-intracranial anastomoses is a distinct potential complication of these interventions.

The patient in Case 1 developed right-sided ACA territory strokes that appeared to be multiembolic, and could have occurred as a result of embolization with PVA microspheres through collateral anastomoses from the right MMA branch. It is impossible to tell how this occurred, but this case emphasizes the point that stroke is a potential complication of embolization and surgical resection of these kinds of tumors.

The patient in Case 2 had a successful pre-operative embolization as well as surgical resection of the tumor, and eventually developed a *Staphylococcus epidermidis* wound infection. It was noted by Yen et al. that post-operative *Clostridium perfringens* infection is possible when performing pre-operative embolization, although rare [45]. This case appears to be most consistent with a common skin flora related- infection source.

In both of these cases, arterial feeding branches were identified and could be catheterized and embolized. However, there were also smaller vessels that supplied the tumors that we were unable to catheterize and safely embolize. The blood loss of these two isolated cases was near 1000 mL, which seems to be consistent with literature-reported blood loss for resection of these skull base meningiomas, even with pre-operative embolization [57, 60, 61]. Both of these operations were performed the day after the endovascular embolization, although the operations were performed very close to 24 hours post-embolization. Both patients received pre-operative dexamethasone and levetiracetam for vasogenic edema and seizure control, respectively.

PVA microspheres were the embolic material of choice in both of these cases, however, the patient in Case 2 did not have as significant a reduction in tumor blush with the microsphere injection alone. This was then followed with Onyx liquid embolization of the feeding pedicle, which completely occluded this vessel. The use of Onyx liquid embolic agent alone is an option, but is reserved by the authors for cases when it has been determined that PVA particles cannot be safely used.

## Conclusion

Many of the advancements in treating large and highly vascularized tumors, such as large skull base meningiomas, over the past three decades has revolved around pre-operatively reducing blood flow to the tumor with arterial embolization. There are also case reports of improving drainage of compromised dural venous sinuses by means of stent and angioplasty techniques. Further advancements in endovascular technology may help to provide safer and more effective adjuncts to surgical resection of large, complex and highly vascular meningiomas. However, surgical resection remains the only effective potential cure. Perhaps endovascular chemotherapy or other treatments delivered by endovascular means, including newer nanotechnology that has shown some promise in other areas of oncology research, can be useful. Further understanding of meningioma pathology is needed to develop more effective treatment strategies. Additionally, current tumor embolization techniques appear to be safe, reducing potential blood loss and need for blood product transfusion, however, they still remain controversial since patient outcomes and length of hospital stay have not been affected by pre-operative embolization. Larger prospective clinical trials are needed to determine statistical significance of these factors.

## References

[1] Dowd CF, Halbach VV, Higashida RT. Meningiomas: the role of preoperative angiography and embolization. Neurosurg Focus. 2003 Jul 15;15(1):E10.

[2] Zhang X, Jin Z. [Clinical application of presurgical embolization of meningiomas]. Zhongguo Yi Xue Ke Xue Yuan Xue Bao. 2003 Apr;25(2):168–71.

[3] Singla A, Deshaies EM, Melnyk V, Toshkezi G, Swarnkar A, Choi H, et al. Controversies in the role of preoperative embolization in meningioma management. Neurosurg Focus. 2013 Dec;35(6):E17.

[4] Alberione F, Iturrieta P, Schulz J, Masenga G, del Giudice G, Ripoli M, et al. [Preoperative embolisation with absorbable gelatine sponge in intracranial meningiomas]. Rev Neurol. 2009 Jul 1;49(1):13–7.

[5] Kominami S, Watanabe A, Suzuki M, Mizunari T, Kobayashi S, Teramoto A. Preoperative embolization of meningiomas with N-butyl cyanoacrylate. Interv Neuroradiol J Peritherapeutic Neuroradiol Surg Proced Relat Neurosci. 2012 Jun;18(2):133–9.

[6] Wakhloo AK, Juengling FD, Van Velthoven V, Schumacher M, Hennig J, Schwechheimer K. Extended preoperative polyvinyl alcohol microembolization of intracranial meningiomas: assessment of two embolization techniques. AJNR Am J Neuroradiol. 1993 Jun;14(3):571–82.

[7] Gore P, Theodore N, Brasiliense L, Kim LJ, Garrett M, Nakaji P, et al. The utility of onyx for preoperative embolization of cranial and spinal tumors. Neurosurgery. 2008 Jun;62(6):1204–1211; discussion 1211–1212.
[8] Lanzino G. Embolization of meningiomas. J Neurosurg. 2013 Aug;119(2):362–3.
[9] Abdel Kerim A, Bonneville F, Jean B, Cornu P, LeJean L, Chiras J. Balloon-assisted embolization of skull base meningioma with liquid embolic agent. J Neurosurg. 2010 Jan;112(1):70–2.
[10] Koike T, Sasaki O, Tanaka R, Arai H. Long-term results in a case of meningioma treated by embolization alone--case report. Neurol Med Chir (Tokyo). 1990 Mar;30(3):173–7.
[11] Das D, Singh V. A sphenoid wing meningioma presenting with intraparenchymal and intraventricular hemorrhage treated with endovascular embolization alone: case report and radiologic follow-up. J Neurointerventional Surg. 2012 Nov;4(6):e36.
[12] Bendszus M, Martin-Schrader I, Schlake HP, Solymosi L. Embolisation of intracranial meningiomas without subsequent surgery. Neuroradiology. 2003 Jul;45(7):451–5.
[13] Morimura T, Takeuchi J, Maeda Y, Tani E. Preoperative embolization of meningiomas: its efficacy and histopathological findings. Nōshuyō Byōri Brain Tumor Pathol. 1994;11(2):123–9.
[14] Barresi V, Branca G, Granata F, Alafaci C, Caffo M, Tuccari G. Embolized meningiomas: risk of overgrading and neo-angiogenesis. J Neurooncol. 2013 Jun;113(2):207–19.
[15] Zilani G, Pereira EAC, Baig F, Uberoi R, Kuker W, Kerr RSC. Venoplasty and stenting of a jugular foramen meningioma. Br J Neurosurg. 2009;23(5):557–60.
[16] Ganesan D, Higgins JNP, Harrower T, Burnet NG, Sarkies NJC, Manford M, et al. Stent placement for management of a small parasagittal meningioma. Technical note. J Neurosurg. 2008 Feb;108(2):377–81.
[17] Chivoret N, Fontaine D, Lachaud S, Chau Y, Sedat J. Endovascular angioplasty before resection of a sphenoidal meningioma with vascular encasement. Interv Neuroradiol J Peritherapeutic Neuroradiol Surg Proced Relat Neurosci. 2011 Sep;17(3):391–4.
[18] Heye S, G. Maleux, Van Loon J, Wilms G. Symptomatic stenosis of the cavernous portion of the internal carotid artery due to an irresectable medial sphenoid wing meningioma: treatment by endovascular stent placement. AJNR Am J Neuroradiol. 2006 Aug;27(7):1532–4.
[19] Fernandez-Valverde F, Jimenez-Gomez E, Roldan-Romero E, Bravo-Rodriguez F. [Presurgical endovascular treatment of symptomatic carotid stenosis caused by a meningioma of the planum sphenoidale]. Rev Neurol. 2013 Feb 1;56(3):157–60.
[20] Ishikawa M, Nishi S, Aoki T, Takase T, Wada E, Oowaki H, et al. Predictability of internal carotid artery (ICA) dissectability in cases showing ICA involvement in parasellar meningioma. J Clin Neurosci Off J Neurosurg Soc Australas. 2001 May;8 Suppl 1:22–5.
[21] Shaffrey ME, Dolenc VV, Lanzino G, Wolcott WP, Shaffrey CI. Invasion of the internal carotid artery by cavernous sinus meningiomas. Surg Neurol. 1999 Aug;52(2):167–71.
[22] Zee C-S, Go JL, Hovanessian A, Creasy JL, Coombs BD, Runge V, et al. Imaging in Spinal Meningioma [Internet]. 2014 [cited 2014 Sep 18]. Available from: http://emedicine.medscape.com/article/341870-overview

[23] Charles YP, Barbe B, Beaujeux R, Boujan F, Steib J-P. Relevance of the anatomical location of the Adamkiewicz artery in spine surgery. 2011 Jan;3–9.

[24] Charles YP, Barbe B, Beaujeux R, Boujan F, Steib J-P. Relevance of the anatomical location of the Adamkiewicz artery in spine surgery. Surg Radiol Anat SRA. 2011 Jan;33(1):3–9.

[25] Shi Z-S, Feng L, Jiang X-B, Huang Q, Yang Z, Huang Z-S. Therapeutic embolization of meningiomas with Onyx for delayed surgical resection. Surg Neurol. 2008 Nov;70(5):478–81.

[26] Rosen CL. Meningiomas: the role of preoperative angiography and embolization. Neurosurg Focus. 2003 Oct 15;15(4):1 p following ECP4.

[27] Bendszus M, Monoranu CM, Schütz A, Nölte I, Vince GH, Solymosi L. Neurologic complications after particle embolization of intracranial meningiomas. AJNR Am J Neuroradiol. 2005 Jul;26(6):1413–9.

[28] Carli DFM, Sluzewski M, Beute GN, van Rooij WJ. Complications of particle embolization of meningiomas: frequency, risk factors, and outcome. AJNR Am J Neuroradiol. 2010 Jan;31(1):152–4.

[29] Kallmes DF, Evans AJ, Kaptain GJ, Mathis JM, Jensen ME, Jane JA, et al. Hemorrhagic complications in embolization of a meningioma: case report and review of the literature. Neuroradiology. 1997 Dec;39(12):877–80.

[30] Lefkowitz M, Giannotta SL, Hieshima G, Higashida R, Halbach V, Dowd C, et al. Embolization of neurosurgical lesions involving the ophthalmic artery. Neurosurgery. 1998 Dec;43(6):1298–303.

[31] Richter HP, Schachenmayr W. Preoperative embolization of intracranial meningiomas. Neurosurgery. 1983 Sep;13(3):261–8.

[32] Gruber A, Killer M, Mazal P, Bavinzski G, Richling B. Preoperative embolization of intracranial meningiomas: a 17-years single center experience. Minim Invasive Neurosurg MIN. 2000 Mar;43(1):18–29.

[33] Ng HK, Poon WS, Goh K, Chan MS. Histopathology of post-embolized meningiomas. Am J Surg Pathol. 1996 Oct;20(10):1224–30.

[34] Yu SCH, Boet R, Wong GKC, Lam WWM, Poon WS. Postembolization hemorrhage of a large and necrotic meningioma. AJNR Am J Neuroradiol. 2004 Mar;25(3):506–8.

[35] Hayashi T, Shojima K, Utsunomiya H, Moritaka K, Honda E. Subarachnoid hemorrhage after preoperative embolization of a cystic meningioma. Surg Neurol. 1987 Mar;27(3):295–300.

[36] Suyama T, Tamaki N, Fujiwara K, Hamano S, Kimura M, Matsumoto S. Peritumoral and intratumoral hemorrhage after gelatin sponge embolization of malignant meningioma: case report. Neurosurgery. 1987 Dec;21(6):944–6.

[37] Lasjaunias P. Craniofacial and Upper Cervical Arteries: Functional, Clinical and Angiographic Aspects. Baltimore: Williams & Wilkins; 1981.

[38] Barr JD, Mathis JM, Horton JA. Iatrogenic carotid-cavernous fistula occurring after embolization of a cavernous sinus meningioma. AJNR Am J Neuroradiol. 1995 Mar;16(3):483–5.

[39] Meguro T, Tomita Y, Tanabe T, Muraoka K, Terada K, Hirotsune N, et al. [Embolization of the feeding artery of a meningioma with dangerous vascular anastomosis between the middle meningeal artery and the ophthalmic artery]. No Shinkei Geka. 2013 Nov;41(11):995–9.

[40] Yasui K, Shoda Y, Suyama T, Numa Y, Amanouchi YY, Kawamoto K. Preoperative embolization for meningioma using lipiodol. Interv Neuroradiol J Peritherapeutic Neuroradiol Surg Proced Relat Neurosci. 1998 Nov 30;4 Suppl 1:63–6.
[41] Kirkman MA, Sethi H, Kitchen ND. Scalp necrosis following preoperative embolization for meningeal tumors: two cautionary tales. Acta Neurochir (Wien). 2013 Aug;155(8):1413–5.
[42] Adler JR, Upton J, Wallman J, Winston KR. Management and prevention of necrosis of the scalp after embolization and surgery for meningioma. Surg Neurol. 1986 Apr;25(4):357–60.
[43] Chan RC, Thompson GB. Ischemic necrosis of the scalp after preoperative embolization of meningeal tumors. Neurosurgery. 1984 Jul;15(1):76–81.
[44] Ng SH, Wan YL, Wong HF, Ko SF, Yen PS, See LC, et al. Preoperative embolization of meningiomas: comparison of superselective and subselective techniques. J Formos Med Assoc Taiwan Yi Zhi. 1998 Mar;97(3):153–8.
[45] Yen P-S, Lin C-C, Lee C-C, Harnod T, Loh T-W, Hsu Y-H. CNS Clostridium perfringens infection: a rare complication of preoperative embolization of meningioma. AJNR Am J Neuroradiol. 2006 Jul;27(6):1355–6.
[46] Terada T, Kinoshita Y, Yokote H, Tsuura M, Itakura T, Komai N, et al. Preoperative embolization of meningiomas fed by ophthalmic branch arteries. Surg Neurol. 1996 Feb;45(2):161–6.
[47] Terada T, Nakai E, Tsumoto T, Itakura T. Iatrogenic arteriovenous fistula of the middle meningeal artery caused during embolization for meningioma--case report. Neurol Med Chir (Tokyo). 1997 Sep;37(9):677–80.
[48] Kai Y, Hamada J-I, Morioka M, Yano S, Nakamura H, Makino K, et al. Preoperative cellulose porous beads for therapeutic embolization of meningioma: provocation test and technical considerations. Neuroradiology. 2007 May;49(5):437–43.
[49] Nania A, Granata F, Vinci S, Pitrone A, Barresi V, Morabito R, et al. Necrosis score, surgical time, and transfused blood volume in patients treated with preoperative embolization of intracranial meningiomas. Analysis of a single-centre experience and a review of literature. Clin Neuroradiol. 2014 Mar;24(1):29–36.
[50] Nakasu S, Nakajima M, Nakazawa T, Nakasu Y, Handa J. p53 accumulation and apoptosis in embolized meningiomas. Acta Neuropathol (Berl). 1997 Jun;93(6):599–605.
[51] Nakasu S, Nakajima M, Nakazawa T, Nakasu Y, Handa J. Alteration of bcl-2 and bax expression in embolized meningiomas. Brain Tumor Pathol. 1998;15(1):13–7.
[52] Tymianski M, Willinsky RA, Tator CH, Mikulis D, TerBrugge KG, Markson L. Embolization with temporary balloon occlusion of the internal carotid artery and in vivo proton spectroscopy improves radical removal of petrous-tentorial meningioma. Neurosurgery. 1994 Nov;35(5):974–977; discussion 977.
[53] Matsuda K, Takeuchi H, Arai Y, Kitai R, Hosoda T, Tsunetoshi K, et al. Atypical and ischemic features of embolized meningiomas. Brain Tumor Pathol. 2012 Jan;29(1):17–24.
[54] Jimenez O, Marcillo A, Levi AD. A histopathological analysis of the human cervical spinal cord in patients with acute traumatic central cord syndrome. Spinal Cord. 2000 Sep;38(9):532–7.

[55] Chun JY, McDermott MW, Lamborn KR, Wilson CB, Higashida R, Berger MS. Delayed surgical resection reduces intraoperative blood loss for embolized meningiomas. Neurosurgery. 2002 Jun;50(6):1231–1235; discussion 1235–1237.

[56] Waldron JS, Sughrue ME, Hetts SW, Wilson SP, Mills SA, McDermott MW, et al. Embolization of skull base meningiomas and feeding vessels arising from the internal carotid circulation. Neurosurgery. 2011 Jan;68(1):162–169; discussion 169.

[57] Macpherson P. The value of pre-operative embolisation of meningioma estimated subjectively and objectively. Neuroradiology. 1991;33(4):334–7.

[58] Raper DMS, Starke RM, Henderson F, Ding D, Simon S, Evans AJ, et al. Preoperative embolization of intracranial meningiomas: efficacy, technical considerations, and complications. AJNR Am J Neuroradiol. 2014 Sep;35(9):1798–804.

[59] Borg A, Ekanayake J, Mair R, Smedley T, Brew S, Kitchen N, et al. Preoperative particle and glue embolization of meningiomas: indications, results, and lessons learned from 117 consecutive patients. Neurosurgery. 2013 Dec;73(2 Suppl Operative):244–251; discussion 252.

[60] Bendszus M, Rao G, Burger R, Schaller C, Scheinemann K, Warmuth-Metz M, et al. Is there a benefit of preoperative meningioma embolization? Neurosurgery. 2000 Dec;47(6):1306–1311; discussion 1311–1312.

[61] Dean BL, Flom RA, Wallace RC, Khayata MH, Obuchowski NA, Hodak JA, et al. Efficacy of endovascular treatment of meningiomas: evaluation with matched samples. AJNR Am J Neuroradiol. 1994 Oct;15(9):1675–80.

[62] Quiñones-Hinojosa A, Kaprealian T, Chaichana KL, Sanai N, Parsa AT, Berger MS, et al. Pre-operative factors affecting resectability of giant intracranial meningiomas. Can J Neurol Sci J Can Sci Neurol. 2009 Sep;36(5):623–30.

[63] Manjila S, Cox EM, Smith GA, Corriveau M, Chhabra N, Johnson F, et al. Extracranial ligation of ethmoidal arteries before resection of giant olfactory groove or planum sphenoidale meningiomas: 3 illustrative cases with a review of the literature on surgical techniques. Neurosurg Focus. 2013 Dec;35(6):E13.

# INDEX

## #



## A

## B



## C

## D

## E



## F

## G



## H

## I



## J



## L



## M

## N

## O



## P

## Q



## R



## S

## T

## U



## V



## W



## X



## Z